Cataract Surgery in the Glaucoma Patient

Sandra Johnson

Editor

Cataract Surgery
in the Glaucoma Patient

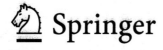 Springer

Editor
Sandra Johnson
University of Virginia School
    of Medicine
Charlottesville, VA 22908
USA

ISBN 978-0-387-09407-6   e-ISBN 978-0-387-09408-3
DOI 10.1007/978-0-387-09408-3
Springer Dordrecht Heidelberg London New York

Library of Congress Control Number: 2009931581

Cover illustration: Original cover photo courtesy of Pat Saine

Printed on acid-free paper

Springer is part of Springer Science+Business Media (www.springer.com)

Preface

Cataract surgery is one of the most frequently performed procedures in the United States, and cataracts are a leading cause of visual impairment in the world. Glaucoma is also a very common eye disease with an expected 3.3 million Americans afflicted with primary open angle glaucoma by 2020. It is also a leading cause of irreversible blindness worldwide. The coexistence of these two diseases is not uncommon, and how a cataract is approached can have an impact on the glaucoma status of a patient. After all, cataracts are rarely associated with permanent blindness as is glaucoma. Managing cataracts to the best advantage of the glaucoma should result in the best long-term visual outcomes for our patients with both diseases.

While detailed instruction on cataract surgery is reviewed in other texts, this book serves to focus on the management of cataract in the setting of glaucoma, using an evidence-based medicine approach. It is hoped to serve as a wonderful resource for ophthalmologists, residents, and glaucoma fellows.

Charlottesville, VA   Sandra M. Johnson, MD

Acknowledgments

I would like to acknowledge all the contributors of this book without whom it would not be published. The experience of our mentors and the contributors to our references, cited and uncited, helped provide us with our current insights. In addition, I thank the photographers who assisted the authors including those from Dartmouth Hitchcock Medical Center (Tom Monego and Pat Saine), Medical College of Georgia (Mike Stanley), and University of Virginia (Alan Lyon, Jared Watson, and Lloyd Situkali).

Sandra M. Johnson

Contents

Part I   Cataract Surgery   1

1   **Approach to Cataract Surgery in Glaucoma Patients**   3
Graham A. Lee and Ivan Goldberg

2   **Anesthesia**   17
Marlene R. Moster and Augusto Azuara-Blanco

3   **Management of the Small Pupil**   23
Cynthia Mattox

4   **Small Incision Cataract Surgery and Glaucoma**   35
Brooks J. Poley, Richard L. Lindstrom, Thomas W. Samuelson,
and Richard R. Schulze Jr.

5   **Elevated Intraocular Pressure After Cataract Surgery**   51
Parag A. Gokhale and Emory Patterson

Part II   Combined Surgery   57

6   **Combined Cataract and Trabeculectomy Surgery**   59
Sandra M. Johnson

7   **Managing Cataract and Glaucoma in the Developing
World – Manual Small Incision Cataract Surgery (MSICS)
Combined with Trabeculectomy**   73
Rengaraj Venkatesh, Rengappa Ramakrishnan, Ramasamy Krishnadas,
Parthasarathy Sathyan, and Alan L. Robin

8   **Antimetabolite-Augmented Trabeculectomy Combined with
Cataract Extraction for the Treatment of Cataract and Glaucoma**   83
Sumit Dhingra and Peng Tee Khaw

9   **Early Postoperative Bleb Maintenance**   91
Robert T. Chang and Donald L. Budenz

10   **Laser Suture Lysis and Releasable Sutures**   105
Anastasios Costarides and Prathima Neerukonda

11   **Cataract Surgery Combined with Glaucoma Drainage Devices**   109
Ramesh S. Ayyala and Brian J. Mikulla

12   **Choroidal Detachment Following Glaucoma Surgery**   119
Diego G. Espinosa-Heidmann

13 Cataract Extraction Combined with Endoscopic Cyclophotocoagulation **129**
Steven D. Vold

14 Approach to Cataract Extraction Combined with New Glaucoma Devices . . **135**
Diamond Y. Tam and Iqbal Ike K. Ahmed

Part III Glaucoma Conditions **159**

15 Cataract Surgery in Patients with Exfoliation Syndrome **161**
Anastasios G.P. Konstas, Nikolaos G. Ziakas, Miguel A. Teus,
Dimitrios G. Mikropoulos, and Vassilios P. Kozobolis

16 Cataract Surgery in the Presence of a Functioning Trabeculectomy Bleb . . **177**
Hylton R. Mayer and James C. Tsai

17 Cataract Extraction in Eyes with Prior GDD Implantation **187**
Ramesh Ayyala and Brian Mikulla

18 Cataract Surgery in the Primary Angle-Closure Patient **189**
Jimmy S.M. Lai

19 Nanophthalmos **197**
Carlos Gustavo Vasconcelos de Moraes and Remo Susanna Jr.

20 Cataract Induced Glaucoma: Phacolytic/Phacomorphic **207**
Sandra M. Johnson

21 Glaucoma Related to Pseudophakia **213**
Junping Li and Jason Much

22 Cataract and Glaucoma in Retinopathy of Prematurity **221**
Anthony J. Anfuso and M. Edward Wilson

23 Cataract Surgery in the Hypotonous Eye **227**
Devon Ghodasra and Sandra M. Johnson

Appendix: Index of Major Figures and Tables **233**

Index **239**

Contributors

Iqbal Ike K. Ahmed, MD, FRCSC Department of Ophthalmology, University of Toronto, Toronto, ONT, Canada, ikeahmed@mac.com

Anthony J. Anfuso, MD University of West Virginia, Morgantown, WV, USA, tony.anfuso@gmail.com

Ramesh S. Ayyala, MD, FRCS, FRCOphth Department of Ophthalmology, Tulane University School of Medicine, New Orleans, LA, USA, rayyala@tulane.edu

Augusto Azuara-Blanco, MD, PhD, FRCS(Ed) Department of Ophthalmology, The Eye Clinic, University of Aberdeen, Foresterhill, Aberdeen, Scotland, aazblanco@aol.com

Donald L. Budenz, MD, MPH Department of Ophthalmology, Bascom Palmer Eye Institute, Miller School of Medicine, University of Miami, Miami, FL, USA, dbudenz@med.miami.edu

Robert T. Chang, MD Department of Ophthalmology, Bascom Palmer Eye Institute, Miller School of Medicine, University of Miami, Miami, FL, USA, viroptic@yahoo.com

Anastasios Costarides, MD, PhD Emory University School of Medicine, Emory Eye Center, Atlanta, GA, USA, acostar@emory.edu

Carlos Gustavo Vasconcelos de Moraes, M.D. Department of Ophthalmology, Glaucoma Associates of New York, New York Eye and Ear Infirmary, New York, NY, USA, gustavousp@gmail.com

Sumit Dhingra, MBBCh, MA, MRCOphth Department of Ocular Repair and Regeneration BiologyNIHR Biomedical Research Centre, UCL Institute of Ophthalmology and Moorfields Eye Hospital, London, UK, drsumitdhingra@gmail.com

Diego G. Espinosa-Heidmann, MD Duke University Eye Center, Durham, NC, USA, diego.espinosa-heidmann@duke.edu

Devon Ghodasra, BS Medical College of Georgia, School of Medicine, Augusta, GA, USA, devonghodasra@gmail.com

Parag A. Gokhale, MD Department of Ophthalmology, Virginia Mason Medical Center, Seattle, WA, USA, ophpag@vmmc.org

Ivan Goldberg, MBBS, FRANZCO, FRACS Department of Ophthalmology, Sydney Eye Hospital, University of Sydney, Sydney, NSW, Australia, eyegoldberg@gmail.com

Sandra M. Johnson Department of Ophthalmology, Glaucoma Service, University of Virginia School of Medicine, Charlottesville, VA, USA, catglaubk@gmail.com

Peng Tee Khaw, PhD, FRCP, FRCS, FRCOphth, FIBiol, FRCPath, FmedSci Department of Ocular Repair and Regeneration BiologyNIHR Biomedical Research Centre, UCL Institute of Ophthalmology and Moorfields Eye Hospital, London, UK, p.khaw@ucl.ac.uk

Anastasios G.P. Konstas, MD, PhD 1st University Department of Ophthalmology, Head of the Glaucoma Unit, AHEPA Hospital, Thessaloniki, Greece, konstas@med.auth.gr

Vassilios P. Kozobolis, MD, PhD Department of Ophthalmology, University Hospital of Alexandroupolis, Medical School, Dragana, Alexandroupolis, Alexandroupoli, Greece, vkozobolis@yahoo.gr

Ramasamy Krishnadas, DO, DNB Aravind Eye Hospital and Postgraduate Institute of Ophthalmology, Madurai, TN, India, krishnadas@aravind.org

Jimmy S.M. Lai, FRCSOphth, FRCSEd, M.Med (Ophthalmology), M.D., L.L.B. Queen Mary Hospital, Eye Institute and Research Center for Heart Brain and Healthy Ageing, The University of Hong Kong, Cyberport, Hong Kong, China, laism@hku.hk

Graham A. Lee, MD, MBBS, FRANZCO Department of Ophthalmology, Royal Brisbane Hospital, Brisbane, QLD, Australia, eye@cityeye.com.au

Junping Li, MD, PhD Clinical Ophthalmology, University of Virginia, Chief of Ophthalmology, Salem Veterans Affairs Medical Center, Salem, VA, USA, junping.li2@va.gov

Richard L. Lindstrom, MD Department of Ophthalmology, University of Minnesota, Minnesota Eye Consultants, PA, Bloomington, MN, USA, rllindstrom@mneye.com

Cynthia Mattox, MD Department of Ophthalmology, New England Eye Center, Tufts University School of Medicine, Boston, MA, USA, cmattox@tuftsmedicalcenter.org

Hylton R. Mayer, MD Department of Ophthalmology, Yale University School of Medicine, New Haven, CT, USA, hylton.mayer@yale.edu

Dimitrios G. Mikropoulos, MD AHEPA Hospital, Thessaloniki, Greece, mikropou@med.auth.gr

Brian J. Mikulla, BS, MBA Department of Ophthalmology, Tulane University School of Medicine, New Orleans, LA, USA, bmikulla@tulane.edu

Marlene R. Moster, MD Department of Ophthalmology, Thomas Jefferson University Hospital, Philadelphia, PA, USA, marlenemoster@aol.com

Jason Much, MD Department of Ophthalmology, University of Virginia, Charlottesville, VA, USA, jwm7e@virginia.edu

Prathima Neerukonda, MD Department of Ophthalmology, Emory University, Atlanta, GA, USA, prathima77@gmail.com

Emory Patterson, MD Department of Ophthalmology, Medical College of Georgia, Augusta, GA, USA, epatterson@mcg.edu

Brooks J. Poley, MD Department of Ophthalmology, Volunteers in Medicine Clinic, Hilton Head Island, SC, USA, scbrooks@hargray.com

Rengappa Ramakrishnan, MD Department of Glaucoma, Aravind Eye Hospital, Tirunelveli, TN, India,drrk@tvl.aravind.org

Alan L. Robin, MD University of Maryland, Baltimore, MD, USA; Johns Hopkins University, Baltimore, MD, USA; Bloomberg School of Public Health, Johns Hopkins University, Baltimore, MD, USA, arobin@glaucomaexpert.com

Thomas W. Samuelson, MD Department of Ophthalmology, University of Minnesota, Phillips Eye Institute, Minneapolis, MN, USA, twsamuelson@mneye.com

Parthasarathy Sathyan, Dip.N.B. Department of Glaucoma, Aravind Eye Hospital, Peelamedu, Coimbatore, TN, India, dr.sathyan.p@gamil.com

Richard R. Schulze Jr., M. Phil. (Oxon), MD Schulze Eye Center, Savannah, GA, USA, richardschulze@comcast.net

Remo Susanna Jr., MD Department of Ophthalmology, University of São Paulo, São Paulo, Brazil, rsussana@terra.com.br

Diamond Y. Tam, MD Department of Ophthalmology, University of Toronto, Toronto, ONT, Canada, diamondtam@gmail.com

Miguel A. Teus, MD, PhD Department of Ophthalmology, Hospital Universitario "Principe de Asturias", Universidad de Alcalá, Madrid, Spain, mteus@teleline.es

James C. Tsai, MD, FACS Department of Ophthalmology & Visual Science, Department of Ophthalmology, Yale-New Haven Hospital, Yale University School of Medicine, New Haven, CT, USA, james.tsai@yale.edu

Rengaraj Venkatesh, MD Department of Glaucoma, Aravind Eye Hospital, Thavalakuppam, Pondicherry, India, venkatesh@pondy.aravind.org

Steven D. Vold, MD Boozman-Hof Regional Eye Clinic, P.A., Rogers, AR, USA, svold@cox.net

M. Edward Wilson Jr., MD Department of Ophthalmology, Storm Eye Institute, Medical University of South Carolina, Charleston, SC, USA, wilsonme@musc.edu

Nikolaos G. Ziakas, MD, PhD 1st University Department of Ophthalmology, AHEPA Hospital, Thessaloniki, Greece, nikolasziakas@yahoo.gr

Part I
Cataract Surgery

Chapter 1

Approach to Cataract Surgery in Glaucoma Patients

Graham A. Lee and Ivan Goldberg

Introduction

As both glaucoma and cataract are increasingly frequent with increasing age, glaucoma patients undergoing cataract surgery are common. These patients require a carefully planned approach to achieve not only a successful cataract extraction outcome but, more importantly, long-term control of their glaucoma.

Clinical History

Is cataract surgery necessary? Determine the degree of visual disability from the cataract versus that from the glaucoma; for the patient, it is the summed visual disability that affects him or her. To have realistic expectations of the potential visual benefits from surgery, patients need to understand the difference. Unless visual loss from glaucoma in the two eyes overlaps, the irreversible glaucoma damage may not be obvious to the patient. Cataract-induced visual loss presents as progressive reduction in visual acuity and in loss of fine detail and contrast (especially in low light), and glare; if allowed to progress, this may threaten a patient's ability to drive and his or her ambulatory vision. In patients with both glaucomatous and cataractous loss, this distinction may not be clear: Glaucoma can manifest as paracentral scotomas, while cortical cataract can present as peripheral loss.

Preoperative Assessment

Glaucoma patients require the same careful preoperative examination as all cataract patients. Secondary

glaucomas present specific challenges during cataract surgery; preoperative surgical planning minimizes risks of complications.

Cornea

In well-controlled glaucoma, the cornea in most patients is normal for their age. Epithelial and stromal edema (e.g., with high intraocular pressure [IOP], bullous keratopathy, and the iridocorneal endothelial [ICE] syndrome) interferes with visualization of intraocular structures (Figs. 1.1 and 1.2). Keratic precipitates may indicate previous uveitis (Fig. 1.3). Moderate endothelial loss of around 7% has been observed following trabeculectomy compared with a loss of 2.6% following deep sclerectomy.[1] More endothelial loss occurs with two-site phacotrabeculectomy compared with one-site.[2] This may influence choice of procedure in already

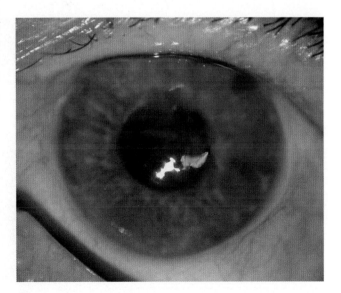

Fig. 1.1 Bullous keratopathy showing irregular ocular surface and stromal edema

G.A. Lee (✉)
Department of Ophthalmology, Royal Brisbane Hospital, Brisbane, QLD 4029, Australia
e-mail: eye@cityeye.com.au

S.M. Johnson (ed.), *Cataract Surgery in the Glaucoma Patient*, DOI 10.1007/978-0-387-09408-3_1,
© Springer Science+Business Media, LLC 2009

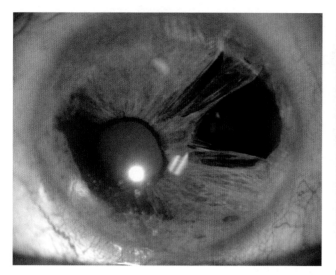

Fig. 1.2 Iridocorneal (ICE) Syndrome showing polycoria, corectopia, ectropian uveae, iris nodules, and iris stromal atrophy

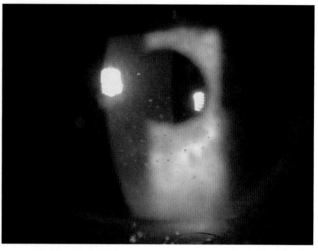

Fig. 1.3 Keratic precipitates in uveitic glaucoma

compromised corneas, but the degree of IOP lowering needed for a particular patient is more critical.

Gonioscopy

Vital in all patients, gonioscopic assessment of the angle is especially important in those with glaucoma. If less than 2.4 mm, anterior chamber depth is a significant risk factor for angle closure.[3] Occludable and partially closed angles often reopen following cataract removal (Fig. 1.4a, b); however, there may be persistent peripheral anterior synechial closure (Fig. 1.5). Intermittent iridotrabecular contact might explain

outflow damage despite an apparently open angle.[4] Trabecular meshwork pigment with radial transillumination defects indicates pigment dispersion (Fig. 1.6a, b). Pseudoexfoliative (PXF) material on the anterior lens capsule, iris, and meshwork indicates an increased risk of zonular and capsular weakness, and of lens dislocation (Fig. 1.7; see also Chapter 15).

Optic Nerve

The neuroretinal rim is the key to diagnose glaucoma and to stage damage. Visual field loss should correspond to optic

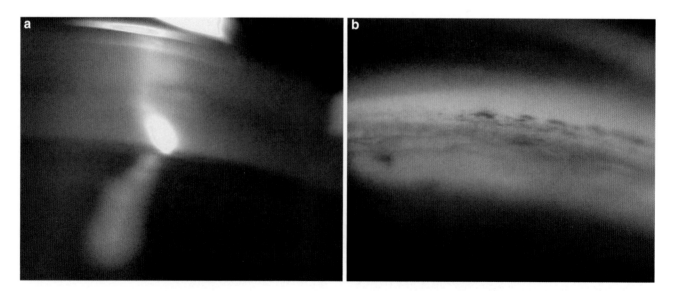

Fig. 1.4 (a) Gonioscopic view of superior angle pre-cataract extraction in angle-closure glaucoma. (b) Gonioscopic view of superior angle post-cataract extraction in angle-closure glaucoma

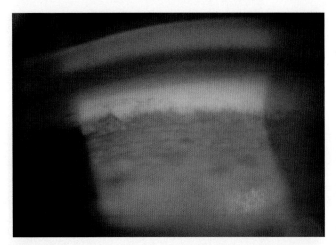

Fig. 1.5 Gonioscopic view showing peripheral anterior synechiae following cataract extraction

nerve rim thinning and nerve fiber layer defects. Without such correlation, suspect non-glaucomatous causes. Dense cataract can make disc assessment difficult or impossible. While advanced damage suggests a poorer visual prognosis following cataract surgery, removal of a dense cataract might improve both vision and IOP control (see Chapter 3). Look for shunt vessels (previous branch or central retinal vein occlusions) (Fig. 1.8), disc hemorrhages (increased risk of glaucoma progression) (Fig. 1.9), neovascularization, and disc drusen.

Silicone Oil

Silicone oil retinal tamponade following complicated vitreoretinal surgery may precipitate posterior subcapsular lens

opacities and/or secondary glaucoma. Biometry in the presence of silicone oil is altered; Murray et al.[5] reported a mean ratio of true axial length to measured axial length of 0.71 (Fig. 1.10). Calculated intraocular lens (IOL) power depends on whether the oil is to be retained or removed at the time of cataract surgery. Preserving the integrity of the posterior capsule is important to keep oil from entering the anterior segment; this reduces the probability of silicone oil-induced IOP increases and potential silicone oil keratopathy (Fig. 1.11).

Investigations

Field Analysis

Mean deviation (MD) levels in standard automated perimetry indicate severity of visual loss from both glaucoma and cataract. Pattern standard deviation (PSD) or its equivalent reduces the effect of overall field depression from a uniform cataract (Fig. 1.12a, b). Visual field changes after cataract extraction in patients with advanced field loss[6] showed mean values for MD and PSD of –13.2 and 6.4 dB before and –11.9 and 6.8 dB after cataract surgery ($P \leq 0.001$ for all comparisons). Mean ($\pm$ SD) number of abnormal points on pattern deviation plot was 26.7 ± 9.4 and 27.5 ± 9.0 before and after cataract surgery, respectively ($P = 0.02$). Scotoma depth index did not change after cataract extraction (–19.3 versus –19.2 dB, $P = 0.90$). Cataract extraction generally improved the visual field; this was most marked in eyes with less advanced glaucomatous damage. Enlargement of scotomas was statistically significant, but was not clinically

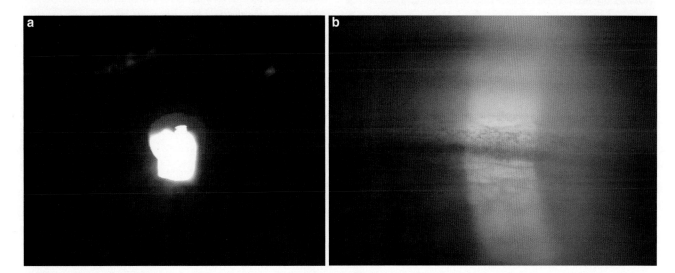

Fig. 1.6 (a) Retroillumination of the iris demonstrating transillumination defects in pigment dispersion syndrome. (b) Gonioscopic view of increased pigmentation of the posterior trabecular meshwork in pigment dispersion syndrome

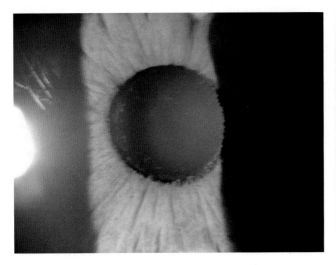

Fig. 1.7 Pseudoexfoliation (PXF) syndrome with material deposited on anterior lens capsule and pupil margin

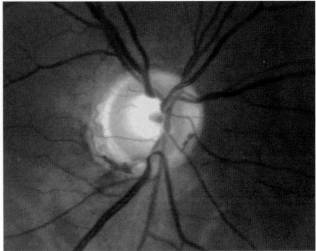

Fig. 1.9 Disc hemorrhage at 7 o'clock at the disc rim

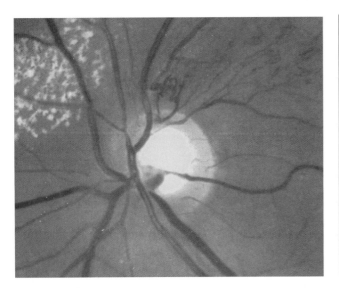

Fig. 1.8 Shunt vessels at the disc following branch retinal vein occlusion

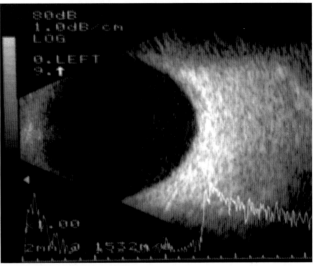

Fig. 1.10 Ultrasound of eye filled with silicone oil. The silicone oil artifactually "elongates" the axial length of the globe

meaningful. No improvement of sensitivity was observed in the deepest part of the scotomas. In a subset of the Collaborative Initial Glaucoma Treatment Trial, visual field testing before and after cataract extraction showed an improved MD but a worse PSD.[7] Other studies have found improvement of the MD with no change in mean PSD on SITA perimetry.[8] Cai et al. showed the amplitude of the AccuMap (objective multifocal visual evoked potential perimetry) was increased after cataract surgery (382.6 nV ± 146.7 nV versus 308.0 nV ± 96.6 nV; $P < 0.01$). The AccuMap severity index (ASI) was decreased following lens removal (48.6 ± 42.4 versus 90.0 ± 54.8, $P < 0.001$; $P < 0.001$).[9]

Focal lens opacities or cortical changes may simulate glaucomatous patterns of field loss, making it more difficult to separate the effects of the two pathologies. Advanced age-related cataracts may cause apparent false-positive responses with screening frequency doubling perimetry; even mild posterior subcapsular opacities may yield false-positive errors.[10]

Ultrasonic Biometry

A-scan biometry measures anterior chamber depth and axial lengths. In angle closure, by removing a cataractous lens with a thickness of more than 4.5 mm and replacing it with a 1-mm-thick intraocular lens (IOL), cataract surgery

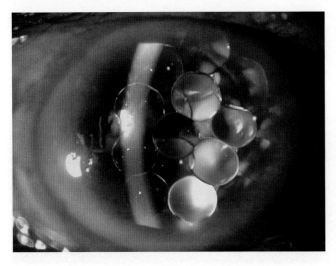

Fig. 1.11 Silicone oil droplets in anterior chamber of aphakic eye

cally shifted prediction of refractive error is significantly more frequent following posterior chamber intraocular lens implantation with phacotrabeculectomy compared with phacoemulsification, even when surgery was uncomplicated and performed by the same surgeon.[11] Another study comparing refractive outcome from cataract surgery after successful trabeculectomy to cataract surgery only found no significant difference from the predicted refraction.[12] Combined cataract surgery and trabeculectomy with mitomycin C tends to shorten the axial length and induces a corneal astigmatism and increased mean keratometry.[13] Despite this alteration of the axial length and corneal curvature, the refractive outcome after a combined operation did not differ significantly from the predicted refraction. At present there is insufficient evidence to make firm recommendations as to the use of multifocal lenses in patients with glaucoma.[14]

deepens the anterior chamber and opens the angle (Fig. 1.13a, b). In eyes with shallow anterior chambers, the IOL position is usually more posterior than was the crystalline lens; an increase of 0.5 diopters to the calculated IOL power will be closer to emmetropia. A shallow anterior chamber presents an intraoperative challenge by increasing the risk of trauma to the corneal endothelium and iris. Myopi-

Specular Microscopy/Pachymetry

Look for corneal endothelial compromise; expect it in the ICE syndrome or after penetrating keratoplasty. If the cell count is less than 500 viable cells/square millimeter and/or

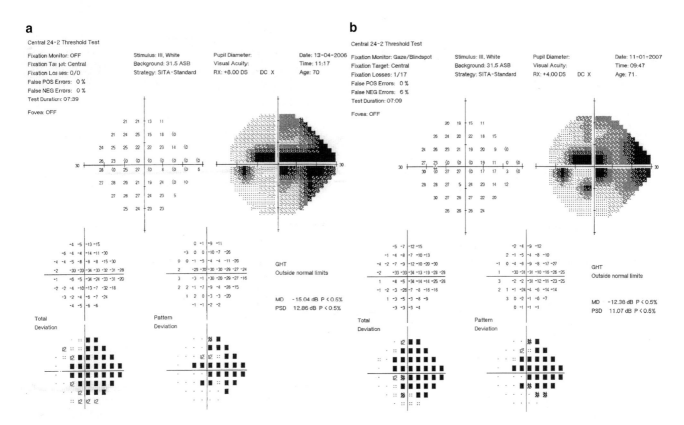

Fig. 1.12 (**a**) Humphrey field analysis (Central 24-2) demonstrating glaucomatous field loss in the presence of dense nuclear sclerosis. (**b**) Humphrey field analysis (Central 24-2) demonstrating improvement in MD and to a lesser extent the PSD following cataract surgery

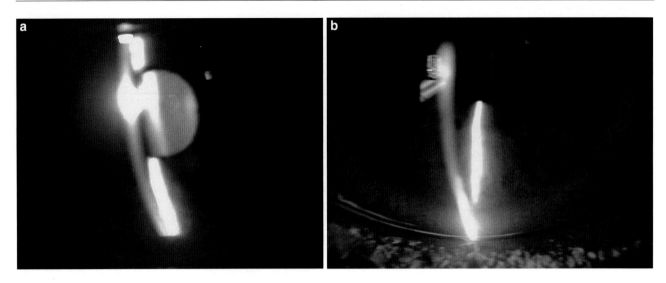

Fig. 1.13 (**a**) Narrowing of the anterior chamber pre-cataract surgery. (**b**) Widening of the anterior chamber post-cataract surgery

the central corneal thickness is greater than 640 μm, there is a significant risk of corneal decompensation post cataract surgery.[15] Combined corneal grafting and cataract removal is an option.

Imaging of the Nerve Fiber Layer

The thickness of the nerve fiber layer is a measure of optic nerve structural integrity. While it complements the clinical assessment of the neuroretinal rim, it may be useful in anomalous discs and when cup:disc ratio is not assessable (Fig. 1.14a, b). If imaging demonstrates good preservation of the nerve fiber layer, then visual improvement following cataract surgery is more likely. Dense media opacities interfere with scan quality and thus measurement reliability. Savini et al. reported that cataract density influenced retinal nerve fiber layer (RNFL) thickness, as measured by optical coherence tomography (OCT) (Carl Zeiss Meditec, Dublin, CA). Postoperative measurements were higher than preoperative measurements in all quadrants (temporal $P = 0.011$; superior $P = 0.0098$; nasal $P< 0.0001$; inferior $P = 0.0081$) and in 360° averages ($P < 0.0001$). More advanced lens opacities correlated with a higher apparent decrease in RNFL thickness ($r = 0.4071$, $P = 0.0434$). While pupil size only marginally affected RNFL measurements performed by Stratus OCT, the presence and degree of cataract seemed to be significant. Consider this when using OCT to help diagnose glaucoma and other neuro-ophthalmologic disorders affecting the RNFL in the presence of a cataract.[16]

Visante/Pentacam/Orb Scan

Various technologies image the anterior segment in detail. These are particularly useful in patients with crowded anterior segments (Figs. 1.15a, b and 1.16a, b). When planning anterior segment surgery in complex eyes, such technology can provide guidance. Dawczynski et al. studied the effect of phacoemulsification on the anterior chamber depth (ACD) and angle (ACA) in primary open angle glaucoma (POAG) and angle-closure glaucoma (ACG) compared with normals.[17] After cataract extraction, ACD and ACA increased significantly in the ACG group (3.1 ± 0.4 mm versus 1.8 ± 0.2 mm, $P < 0.005$; and $32.3° \pm 7.7°$ versus $16.0°$ $\pm 4.7°$, $P < 0.005$). In the POAG and control groups, ACD and ACA also increased postoperatively, but not as much as in the ACG group

Consent

Patients undergoing cataract surgery expect a good visual outcome. Glaucoma patients with vision compromised by optic nerve damage that will not be improved by cataract removal need to be realistic in their expectations: their surgery is NOT necessarily the same as that performed for their friends and relatives. The consent process needs to address this carefully and unambiguously so that the doctor and the patient have aligned hopes and expectations.

"Snuff-out" syndrome is the loss of the remaining central visual field during or following any intraocular surgery. It is usually irreversible. Retro- or peribulbar anesthetic injection

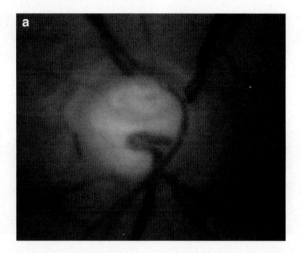

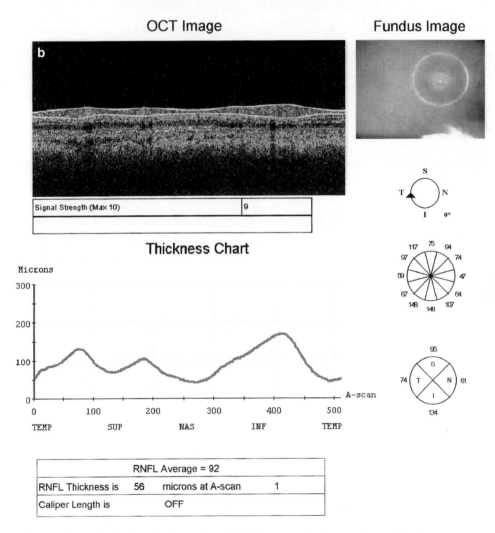

Fig. 1.14 (**a**) Anomalous cupping at the disc in a healthy patient. (**b**) OCT scan confirming normal nerve fiber layer

with a Honan's balloon or a similar device can raise IOP to over 50 mmHg.[18] Topical anesthesia may be the preferred technique to try to avoid excess pressure on the globe (see Chapter 2). Eyes with absolute splitting of fixation (<0 sensitivity, 1° from fixation on perimetric testing) are more at risk.[19]

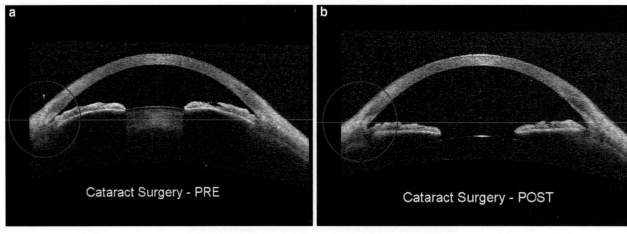

Fig. 1.15 (a) Visante anterior segment image of angle-closure glaucoma demonstrating closing of angle and shallow anterior chamber. (b) Visante anterior segment image of angle-closure glaucoma demonstrating angle opening following cataract removal (Horizontal line in Fig. 1.15 represents the interscleral spur line) (Figures courtesy of Dr. Lance Liu)

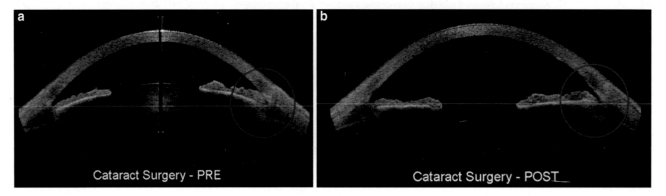

Fig. 1.16 (a) Visante anterior segment image of plateau iris syndrome demonstrating crowding of the angle. (b) Visante anterior segment image of plateau iris syndrome demonstrating limited angle opening following cataract removal (Horizontal line in Fig. 1.16 represents the interscleral spur line) (Figures courtesy of Dr. Lance Liu)

The aims of surgery need to be clearly stated. In angle-closure patients where cataract removal aims to reopen the angle, the corrected vision may still be good, with minimal lens opacities. Vision is less likely to be improved but the aim is to improve IOP control, and to protect the angle structures from further damage (see Chapter 18). Often these patients are hyperopic, with the surgery able to correct the refractive error. Cataract removal and IOL insertion in the other eye might be needed to correct anisometropia.

Preoperative Preparation for Cataract Surgery in the Glaucoma Patient

Most glaucoma patients instill one or more medications prior to cataract surgery. Commonest are the prostaglandin analogues (latanoprost, travoprost, or bimatoprost). This medication class, prior to and in the early postoperative phase, has been associated with cystoid macular edema.[20-22] The literature offers conflicting advice whether to withdraw a drug of this type. In advanced glaucomatous optic nerve atrophy where IOP fluctuation could result in visually significant compromise, glaucoma medications should be continued. In earlier stages of glaucoma when the IOP control is less critical, ceasing the glaucoma medications postoperatively provides an opportunity to assess the degree of IOP lowering from the cataract surgery alone, with the potential to reduce the number of medications and to avoid the increased risk of cystoid macula edema (see Chapter 4). A reverse therapeutic trial postoperatively may permit controlled cessation of one medication at a time. Chronic use of pilocarpine results in a small pupil that poorly dilates; previous cessation may make no difference. Pupil stretching or expanders are often required and should be anticipated (see Chapter 3).

Especially in advanced glaucoma, IOP fluctuations might critically destroy surviving nerve fibers. Anticipate and manage them: a history of high IOP is a strong risk factor.[23] For example, it has been shown that IOP spikes greater than 30 mmHg in the first 24 h might be prevented by timolol maleate 0.5% at the end of the cataract procedure.[24]

Preoperative Peripheral Iridotomy

Angle-closure patients are at risk of pupil block if dilated. Peripheral iridotomy might be indicated to allow safe fundal examination preoperatively and if there is a delay in performing the surgery.

Anticoagulants

Patients on anticoagulants (including aspirin, non-steroidal anti-inflammatory drugs, warfarin, and clopidogrel) are at increased risk of hemorrhage. In some patients these medications can be ceased safely 10 days pre-surgery (4 days for warfarin) and restarted afterward. When it is critical for the patient to remain on the anticoagulant, consult with other doctors caring for the patient, and consider switching to heparin (e.g., subcutaneous enoxaparin) until the day of surgery. If anticoagulants cannot be ceased, a topical approach is preferable to avoid the bleeding risks of injection. Patients who are unsuitable for topical surgery may need a general anesthetic. Systemic anticoagulation has also been associated with the risk of suprachoroidal hemorrhage.[25]

Steroids

Topical and even oral steroids used preoperatively might help patients at risk of heightened inflammation. In uveitic glaucoma patients, quiet the eye as much and for as long as possible prior to surgery. With adequate inflammation suppression, phacotrabeculectomy with mitomycin C can be an effective and safe therapeutic option for secondary cataract and glaucoma in uveitic eyes. Lower surgical success rates might follow later resurgence of inflammation.[26] A combined cataract surgery with glaucoma drainage device is an alternative to phacotrabeculectomy. See Chapter 11.

Approach to Surgery

Glaucoma patients can present with visual loss from cataract and cataract patients can present with glaucoma.[27] The aims of surgery in each situation need to be defined clearly,

with the doctor and patient reaching a common understanding. For most patients the perceived goal is often improved vision. This may not be achievable. It is for the doctor to communicate realistic aims, which include the following:

1. Improvement of vision if cataract is a significant cause of loss—the greater the loss from glaucoma, the less certain is such improvement.
2. Maintenance of vision if further loss from glaucoma is threatened.
3. Control of IOP if the cataract is involved in the mechanisms raising IOP or if a filtration operation is being performed to improve IOP control, or to allow cessation of medications with the concurrent existence of cataract to be managed.

Cataract Only

If visual field loss has been stabilized by adequate IOP control, perform cataract surgery when reduction in visual function interferes with daily living. Consider cataract surgery alone if glaucoma damage is relatively mild, when there are no other relevant ocular pathologies and visual improvement is likely. Provided IOP control is maintained postoperatively, no further procedure should be necessary.

In other patients with mild-to-moderate elevation of IOP, cataract extraction alone may lower IOP adequately. Mathalone et al. evaluated long-term IOP control after sutureless clear corneal phacoemulsification in eyes with medically controlled glaucoma. At 12 months, mean IOP decrease was 1.5 mmHg $\pm$ 4.4 (SD), and 1.9 $\pm$ 4.9 mmHg at 24 months. The mean decrease in the number of medications was 0.53 $\pm$ 0.86 ($P = 0.4$) at 12 months and 0.38 $\pm$ 0.9 ($P = 0.4$) at 24 months.[28] Phacoemulsification in non-glaucomatous pseudoexfoliation syndrome patients significantly reduced IOP by about 3.5 mmHg at 1 year.[29] Pseudoexfoliative glaucoma patients demonstrated more IOP reduction than did normals and primary open angle glaucoma patients undergoing phacoemulsification.[30] In patients with primary angle-closure, both IOP and the need for glaucoma drugs could be reduced by phacoemulsification alone.[31] IOP fell from a mean preoperative level of 19.7 $\pm$ 6.1 mmHg (range 11–40 mmHg) to 15.5 $\pm$ 3.9 mmHg (range 9–26 mmHg) at final follow-up ($P = 0.022$) (paired t-test), while the number of glaucoma agents fell from a mean 1.91 $\pm$ 0.77 (range 1–3) to 0.52 $\pm$ 0.87 (range 0–3) at final follow-up ($P <$ 0.001; paired t-test). Early phacoemulsification appeared to be more effective to prevent an IOP rise than laser peripheral iridoplasty in patients who had had an aborted episode of acute primary angle closure.[32] Phacoemulsification reduced the mean number of medications and consistently increased Shaffer gonioscopy grading. The effect of peripheral laser iridotomy compared with cataract surgery on the angle showed residual angle closure after iridotomy in 27 (38.6%) of 70 eyes; this was confirmed functionally by the dark room prone test and morphologically by ultrasound biomicroscopy (UBM). Eyes with IOP of ≥ 20 mmHg or with a glaucomatous visual field defect before iridotomy had a significantly higher prevalence of residual angle closure after iridotomy than did eyes without these findings ($P<0.05$). In all the eyes with residual angle closure after iridotomy, the response to the prone test became negative after cataract surgery, with significant lowering of IOP ($P < 0.01$).[33] Residual angle closure after iridotomy was common, especially in eyes with primary angle closure and poorly controlled IOP or glaucomatous optic neuropathy. Cataract surgery effectively resolved residual angle closure after iridotomy and lowered IOP. Using UBM, Nonaka et al. measured anterior chamber depth (ACD), angle opening distance at points 500 μm from the scleral spur (AOD500), and trabecular-ciliary process distance (TCPD).[34] Correlated with one another, all parameters increased significantly after cataract surgery ($P < 0.001$). Cataract surgery not only eliminated pupillary block but also attenuated any anterior positioning of the ciliary processes.

In 12 consecutive patients with end-stage glaucoma who underwent cataract surgery, 6 months postoperatively, Altmeyer et al. reported[35] improved mean visual acuity (from 0.3 to 0.5; $P = 0.007$) and decreased IOP (by 4.4 mmHg; $P = 0.007$); anti-glaucomatous drugs decreased in number from 1.5 preoperatively to 0.8, and mean deviation (MD) improved from -27.5 to -26.4 dB ($P = 0.036$). Thus patients with progressive cataract and end-stage glaucoma can benefit from cataract surgery.

Cataract and Glaucoma Surgery

Glaucoma patients with progressive visual loss and higher than desirable IOP, despite medical and laser strategies, require drainage surgery. In the presence of a visually significant cataract, determine whether cataract or glaucoma surgery or both are needed.

If the cataract is extracted first, IOP might fall. This is particularly likely if an angle-closure mechanism is eliminated before trabecular function has been damaged.[36] In open angle glaucoma patients, the reasons for reduced IOP after cataract surgery are less obvious.

Routine cataract surgery provokes subclinical inflammation. Increased flare after routine cataract surgery has been measured for up to 30 days postoperatively.[37] As this implies exaggerated wound healing, to optimize trabeculectomy

function, it could be better to delay drainage at least until after this period. If IOP control is poor following cataract surgery, despite maximal tolerable medication, then drainage will be needed under suboptimal conditions, increasing likely benefit from anti-metabolite augmentation and/or pre- as well as postoperative topical and even oral steroids. Luo et al. measured mean aqueous flare values of 15.12 ± 2.87, 40.24 ± 3.75, 24.33 ± 3.38, 21.18 ± 1.77, and 16.51 ± 1.70 (photon counts/ms) preoperatively and on days 1, 7, 30, and 90, respectively, after trabeculectomy ($P < 0.05$) compared with 6.94 ± 2.34, 26.27 ± 10.21, 13.96 ± 6.44, 9.07 ± 2.67, and 7.16 ± 1.89, respectively, after phacoemulsification ($P < 0.05$). Trabeculectomy disrupted the blood-aqueous barrier permanently whilst phacoemulsification affected it transiently.[37]

Drainage Surgery Followed by Cataract Surgery

In patients with uncontrolled IOP it might be urgent to perform drainage prior to cataract surgery. When IOP is high and/or there is advanced glaucoma damage threatening fixation, there is potential for visual "snuff-out," especially with IOP spikes. Trabeculectomy was associated with progressive cataract—predominantly the posterior subcapsular variety.[38]

Previously functioning drainage procedures can fail after cataract surgery, most likely by bleb exposure to induced inflammatory mediators. Approximately 50% of patients undergoing clear cornea phacoemulsification after trabeculectomy will require either further medication or further surgery to maintain target IOP.[39,40] Identified risk factors for bleb failure include cataract extraction, age greater than 60 years, interval of 5 months or less between trabeculectomy and cataract extraction, use of pre-cataract extraction glaucoma medications, and postoperative IOP >19 mmHg within 2 weeks.[41] Cataract surgery after previously successful bleb needling revision significantly compromised bleb function.[42]

To reduce the potential for fibrosis, subconjunctival 5-fluorouracil (5-FU) with or without needling can be useful. Sharma et al. retrospectively evaluated the protective role of subconjunctival 5-FU on a preexisting bleb in patients with primary open angle glaucoma undergoing phacoemulsification more than 12 months post-trabeculectomy. Data were collected for two groups of patients: Group 1 (22 patients) received 5-FU at the end of successful phacoemulsification, whereas group 2 (25 patients) did not. Reduced IOP control was seen in 13.6% of the patients in group 1 and in 36.4% in group 2 ($P = 0.03$). 5-FU seemed to protect bleb function.[43] Consider it at the end of phacoemulsification in such cases. See also Chapter 16.

Table 1.1 Filtration surgeries reported combined with cataract surgery

- Trabeculectomy
- Glaucoma drainage device
- EX-PRESS mini shunt
- Viscocanulostomy
- Canaloplasty
- Non-penetrating deep sclerectomy
- Goniotomy/trabeculotomy
- Eyepass shunt

Combined Surgery

Many studies address outcomes of combined versus separate glaucoma and cataract surgery (Table 1.1). Jin et al. reviewed two-site phacotrabeculectomy in 60 eyes of 43 patients. An IOP 21 mmHg or less was achieved in 95% with or without medications; however, only 50% had an IOP of 15 mmHg or lower.[44] This suggests less effective overall IOP reduction compared with trabeculectomy with mitomycin-C alone. Murthy et al. compared the 2-year outcomes of trabeculectomy with mitomycin-C (trabMMC) versus phacotrabeculectomy with mitomycin-C (phacotrabMMC).[45] Mean IOP drop from baseline was significantly greater with trabMMC throughout the study (-10.87 ± 8.33 mmHg in trabMMC versus -6.15 ± 7.01 mmHg in phacotrabMMC at 2 years, $P = 0.003$); however, baseline IOP was also higher in the trabMMC group (26.1 mmHg versus 20.3 mmHg, $P < 0.0001$). TrabMMC and phacotrabMMC may be equally safe and effective in bringing IOP to within an acceptable target range over 2 years in advanced glaucoma patients at increased risk for filtering surgery failure, although trabMMC appears to be associated with greater IOP reduction.

Same-site or two-site combined surgery has been assessed with no clear superiority of either.[2,45–47] The role of combined surgery is advantageous in elderly patients who are unsuitable for multiple procedures. Cotran et al. studied one-site versus two-site phacotrabeculectomy over a 3-year period.[48] The mean preoperative IOP was 20.1 ± 3.8 mmHg in the one-site group and 19.5 ± 5.3 mmHg in the two-site group ($P = 0.56$) using 2.3 ± 0.9 and 2.5 ± 0.9 anti-glaucoma medications, respectively ($P = 0.27$). After 3 years, mean IOP was 12.6 ± 4.8 mmHg in the one-site group and 11.7 ± 4.0 mmHg in the two-site group ($P = 0.40$), instilling 0.3 ± 0.7 and 0.4 ± 0.9 medications, respectively ($P = 0.59$). At the end of the study, 73% of one-site eyes and 78.4% of two-site eyes had IOPs less than 18 mmHg on no anti-glaucoma medications ($P = 0.59$). Operating time was less in the one-site group ($P < 0.0001$). One-site fornix-based and two-site limbus-based phacotrabeculectomy were similarly effective in lowering IOP and in reducing the need for anti-glaucoma medications over a 3-year follow-up period. See Chapter 6.

Phacoemulsification can also be combined with a glaucoma drainage device, such as an Ahmed valve. Nassiri et al. reviewed 41 eyes in 31 patients who underwent combined phacoemulsification and Ahmed valve implantation. The mean IOP lowered from 28.2 ± 3.1 to 16.8 ± 2.1, while the number of anti-glaucoma medications fell from 2.6 ± 0.66 to 1.2 ± 1.4. An IOP of <21 mmHg on no medications or on one or more medications was achieved in 56.1 and 31.7%, respectively. Five eyes (12.2%) were considered failures (IOP < 6 mmHg or > 21 mmHg).[49] Other devices, such as the Eyepass glaucoma implant are under trial, but may not achieve consistent low target IOPs.[50] Traverso et al. and Rivier et al. have studied a stainless steel glaucoma drainage implant (Ex-PRESS). With a subconjunctival position, conjunctival erosion and extrusion were significant problems.[51,52] Positioned under a scleral trapdoor, these problems have been addressed.[53] Combined phacoemulsification and ab interno trabeculectomy and endoscopic-controlled erbium:YAG-laser goniotomy require more extensive study.[54,55]

Deep sclerectomy with phacoemulsification may be viable if augmented with intraoperative mitomycin C. There is reduced hypotensive efficacy compared with trabeculectomy but with less chance of cystic blebs, delayed bleb leaks, and infection.[56] Viscocanalostomy has also been combined with phacoemulsification.[57–61] Non-penetrating glaucoma surgery may not achieve low enough IOPs, especially for more advanced glaucoma patients.[62,63] Larger long-term IOP fluctuations after this type of triple procedure were associated with progressive visual field deterioration even though patients with glaucoma maintained their IOPs.[64] Combined phacoemulsification and cyclophotocoagulation, either transscleral or endoscopic, is an option, particularly in patients unsuitable for drainage surgery. Problems are the narrow margins for success, with significant risks of uncontrolled IOP needing additional photocoagulation on the one hand, and of induced phthisis on the other.[65,66] See Chapter 13.

Phacotrabeculectomy can be supplemented with early and repeated needle revisions with 5-FU to improve outcomes.[67] In "normal pressure glaucoma," phacoviscocanalostomy achieved 20% and 30% IOP reductions with (or without) medications in 78.5% (67.4%) and 35.5% (37.4%) of patients at 24 months, and 58.0% (44.2%) and 28.0% (26.6%) of patients at 48 months; these were better than in the cataract-extraction-only group, with only 16.0% (9.5%) and 5.7% (2.9%) at 24 months ($P < 0.001$ for each comparison, Kaplan-Meier life-table analysis with log-rank test).[61] Microincision bimanual phacotrabeculectomy may be an option as incision sizes reduce in future.[68]

In aqueous misdirection glaucoma, a sequential three-step surgical approach has been suggested[69]: initial vitrectomy, phacoemulsification, and definitive vitrectomy. Step 1: preliminary limited core vitrectomy to "debulk" the vitreous and soften the eye. Step 2: phacoemulsification performed in a standard manner. Step 3: residual vitrectomy, zonulo-hyaloidectomy, and peripheral iridectomy (if not already present) to create free communication between the posterior and anterior segments.[69]

A novel combined approach is circumferential viscodilation and tensioning of the inner wall of Schlemm's canal (canaloplasty) to treat open angle glaucoma (OAG), combined with clear corneal phacoemulsification and posterior chamber IOL implantation.[70] The mean preoperative baseline IOP was 24.4 ± 6.1 mmHg (SD) with a mean of 1.5 ± 1.0 medications per eye. In all eyes, the mean postoperative IOP was 13.6 ± 3.8 mmHg at 1 month, 14.2 ± 3.6 mmHg at 3 months, 13.0 ± 2.9 mmHg at 6 months, and 13.7 ± 4.4 mmHg at 12 months. Medication use dropped to a mean of 0.2 ± 0.4 per patient at 12 months. Surgical complications were reported in five eyes (9.3%): hyphema ($n = 3$, 5.6%), Descemet's tear ($n = 1$, 1.9%), and iris prolapse ($n = 1$, 1.9%). Transient IOP elevation of >30 mmHg was observed in four eyes (7.3%) 1 day postoperatively. Canaloplasty is a complex procedure requiring expensive equipment; its long-term value remains to be demonstrated.

Summary

A careful history, thoughtful and thorough clinical assessment with the aid of emerging technologies, planned surgical steps, and a fully informed consent process will increase the chances of a satisfactory outcome for the majority of patients. The approach to surgery and the postoperative care is just as important as the surgery itself.

References

1. Arnavielle S, Lafontaine PO, Bidot S, et al. Corneal endothelial cell changes after trabeculectomy and deep sclerectomy. *J Glaucoma*. 2007;16(3):324–8.
2. Buys YM, Chipman ML, Zack B, et al. Prospective randomized comparison of one- versus two-site Phacotrabeculectomy two-year results. *Ophthalmology*. 2008;115(7):1130–3 e1.
3. Aung T, Nolan WP, Machin D, et al. Anterior chamber depth and the risk of primary angle closure in 2 East Asian populations. *Arch Ophthalmol*. 2005;123(4):527–32.
4. Mapstone R. One gonioscopic fallacy. *Br J Ophthalmol*. 1979;63(4):221–4.
5. Murray DC, Potamitis T, Good P, et al. Biometry of the silicone oil-filled eye. *Eye*. 1999;13(Pt 3a):319–24.
6. Koucheki B, Nouri-Mahdavi K, Patel G, et al. Visual field changes after cataract extraction: the AGIS experience. *Am J Ophthalmol*. 2004;138(6):1022–8.
7. Musch DC, Gillespie BW, Niziol LM, et al. Cataract extraction in the collaborative initial glaucoma treatment study: incidence, risk factors, and the effect of cataract progression and extraction on clinical and quality-of-life outcomes. *Arch Ophthalmol*. 2006;124(12):1694–700.
8. Rehman Siddiqui MA, Khairy HA, Azuara-Blanco A. Effect of cataract extraction on SITA perimetry in patients with glaucoma. *J Glaucoma*. 2007;16(2):205–8.
9. Cai Y, Lim BA, Chi L, et al. Effects of lens opacity on AccuMap multifocal objective perimetry in glaucoma. *Zhonghua Yan Ke Za Zhi*. 2006;42(11):972–6.
10. Casson RJ, James B. Effect of cataract on frequency doubling perimetry in the screening mode. *J Glaucoma*. 2006;15(1):23–5.
11. Chan JC, Lai JS, Tham CC. Comparison of postoperative refractive outcome in phacotrabeculectomy and phacoemulsification with posterior chamber intraocular lens implantation. *J Glaucoma*. 2006;15(1):26–9.
12. Tan HY, Wu SC. Refractive error with optimum intraocular lens power calculation after glaucoma filtering surgery. *J Cataract Refract Surg*. 2004;30(12):2595–7.
13. Law SK, Mansury AM, Vasudev D, Caprioli J. Effects of combined cataract surgery and trabeculectomy with mitomycin C on ocular dimensions. *Br J Ophthalmol*. 2005;89(8):1021–5.
14. Kumar BV, Phillips RP, Prasad S. Multifocal intraocular lenses in the setting of glaucoma. *Curr Opin Ophthalmol*. 2007;18(1):62–6.
15. Seitzman G. Cataract surgery in Fuchs' dystrophy. *Curr Opin Ophthalmol*. 2005;16(4):241–5.
16. Savini G, Zanini M, Barboni P. Influence of pupil size and cataract on retinal nerve fiber layer thickness measurements by Stratus OCT. *J Glaucoma*. 2006;15(4):336–40.
17. Dawczynski J, Koenigsdoerffer E, Augsten R, et al. Anterior segment optical coherence tomography for evaluation of changes in anterior chamber angle and depth after intraocular lens implantation in eyes with glaucoma. *Eur J Ophthalmol*. 2007;17(3):363–7.
18. Morgan JE, Chandna A. Intraocular pressure after peribulbar anaesthesia: is the Honan balloon necessary? *Br J Ophthalmol*. 1995;79(1):46–9.
19. Kolker AE. Visual prognosis in advanced glaucoma: a comparison of medical and surgical therapy for retention of vision in 101 eyes with advanced glaucoma. *Trans Am Ophthalmol Soc*. 1977;75:539–55.
20. Miyake K, Ibaraki N. Prostaglandins and cystoid macular edema. *Surv Ophthalmol*. 2002;47(Suppl 1):S203–18.
21. Altintas O, Yuksel N, Karabas VL, Demirci G. Cystoid macular edema associated with latanoprost after uncomplicated cataract surgery. *Eur J Ophthalmol*. 2005;15(1):158–61.
22. Henderson BA, Kim JY, Ament CS, et al. Clinical pseudophakic cystoid macular edema. Risk factors for development and duration after treatment. *J Cataract Refract Surg*. 2007;33(9):1550–8.
23. Dietlein TS, Jordan J, Dinslage S, et al. Early postoperative spikes of the intraocular pressure (IOP) following phacoemulsification in late-stage glaucoma. *Klin Monatsbl Augenheilkd*. 2006;223(3):225–9.
24. Levkovitch-Verbin H, Habot-Wilner Z, Burla N, et al. Intraocular pressure elevation within the first 24 hours after cataract surgery in patients with glaucoma or exfoliation syndrome. *Ophthalmology*. 2008;115(1):104–8.
25. Jeganathan VSE, Ghosh S, Ruddle JB, et al. Risk factors for delayed suprachoroidal haemorrhage following glaucoma surgery. *Br J Ophthalmol*. 2008;92:1393–6.
26. Park UC, Ahn JK, Park KH, Yu HG. Phacotrabeculectomy with mitomycin C in patients with uveitis. *Am J Ophthalmol*. 2006;142(6):1005–12.

27. Chandrasekaran S, Cumming RG, Rochtchina E, Mitchell P. Associations between elevated intraocular pressure and glaucoma, use of glaucoma medications, and 5-year incident cataract: the Blue Mountains Eye Study. *Ophthalmology*. 2006;113(3): 417–24.

28. Mathalone N, Hyams M, Neiman S. Long-term intraocular pressure control after clear corneal phacoemulsification in glaucoma patients. *J Cataract Refract Surg*. 2005;31(3):479–83.

29. Cimetta DJ, Cimetta AC. Intraocular pressure changes after clear corneal phacoemulsification in nonglaucomatous pseudoexfoliation syndrome. *Eur J Ophthalmol*. 2008;18(1):77–81.

30. Damji KF, Konstas AG, Liebmann JM, et al. Intraocular pressure following phacoemulsification in patients with and without exfoliation syndrome: a 2 year prospective study. *Br J Ophthalmol*. 2006;90(8):1014–8.

31. Lai JS, Tham CC, Chan JC. The clinical outcomes of cataract extraction by phacoemulsification in eyes with primary angle-closure glaucoma (PACG) and co-existing cataract: a prospective case series. *J Glaucoma*. 2006;15(1):47–52.

32. Lam DS, Leung DY, Tham CC, et al. Randomized trial of early phacoemulsification versus peripheral iridotomy to prevent intraocular pressure rise after acute primary angle closure. *Ophthalmology*. 2007;115(7):1134–40.

33. Nonaka A, Kondo T, Kikuchi M, et al. Cataract surgery for residual angle closure after peripheral laser iridotomy. *Ophthalmology*. 2005;112(6):974–9.

34. Nonaka A, Kondo T, Kikuchi M, et al. Angle widening and alteration of ciliary process configuration after cataract surgery for primary angle closure. *Ophthalmology*. 2006;113(3):437–41.

35. Altmeyer M, Wirbelauer C, Häberle H, Pham DT. Cataract surgery in patients with end-stage glaucoma. *Klin Monatsbl Augenheilkd*. 2006;223(4):297–302.

36. Bleckmann H, Keuch R. Cataract extraction including posterior chamber lens implantation in the treatment of acute glaucoma. *Ophthalmologe*. 2006;103(3):199–203.

37. Luo LX, Liu YZ, Ge J, Zhang XY, Liu YH, Wu MX. Changes of blood-aqueous barrier after phacoemulsification in patients with previous glaucoma filtering surgery. *Zhonghua Yan Ke Za Zhi*. 2005;41(2):132–5.

38. Husain R, Aung T, Gazzard G, et al. Effect of trabeculectomy on lens opacities in an East Asian population. *Arch Ophthalmol*. 2006;124(6):787–92.

39. Ehrnrooth P, Lehto I, Puska P, Laatikainen L. Phacoemulsification in trabeculectomized eyes. *Acta Ophthalmol Scand*. 2005;83(5):561–6.

40. Klink J, Schmitz B, Lieb WE, et al. Filtering bleb function after clear cornea phacoemulsification: a prospective study. *Br J Ophthalmol*. 2005;89(5):597–601.

41. Mandal AK, Chelerkar V, Jain SS, et al. Outcome of cataract extraction and posterior chamber intraocular lens implantation following glaucoma filtration surgery. *Eye*. 2005;19(9): 1000–8.

42. Rotchford AP, King AJ. Cataract surgery after needling revision of trabeculectomy blebs. *J Glaucoma*. 2007;16(6):562–6.

43. Sharma TK, Arora S, Corridan PG. Phacoemulsification in patients with previous trabeculectomy: role of 5-fluorouracil. *Eye*. 2007;21(6):780–3.

44. Jin GJ, Crandall AS, Jones JJ. Phacotrabeculectomy: assessment of outcomes and surgical improvements. *J Cataract Refract Surg*. 2007;33(7):1201–8.

45. Murthy SK, Damji KF, Pan Y, Hodge WG. Trabeculectomy and phacotrabeculectomy, with mitomycin-C, show similar two-year target IOP outcomes. *Can J Ophthalmol*. 2006;41(1):51–9.

46. Tous HM, Nevarez J. Comparison between the outcomes of combined phaco/trabeculectomy by cataract incision site. *P R Health Sci J*. 2007;26(1):29–33.

47. Shingleton BJ, Price RS, O'Donoghue MW, Goyal S. Comparison of 1-site versus 2-site phacotrabeculectomy. J Cataract Refract Surg. 2006;32(5):799–802.

48. Cotran PR, Roh S, McGwin G. Randomized comparison of 1-Site and 2-Site phacotrabeculectomy with 3-year follow-up. *Ophthalmology*. 2008;115(3):447–54 e1.

49. Nassiri N, Nassiri N, Sadeghi Yarandi S, Mohammadi B, Rahmani L. Combined phacoemulsification and Ahmed valve glaucoma drainage implant: a retrospective case series. *Eur J Ophthalmol*. 2008;18(2):191–8.

50. Dietlein TS, Jordan JF, Schild A, et al. Combined cataract-glaucoma surgery using the intracanalicular Eyepass glaucoma implant: first clinical results of a prospective pilot study. *J Cataract Refract Surg*. 2008;34(2):247–52.

51. Traverso CE, De Feo F, Messas-Kaplan A, et al. Long term effect on IOP of a stainless steel glaucoma drainage implant (Ex-PRESS) in combined surgery with phacoemulsification. *Br J Ophthalmol*. 2005;89(4):425–9.

52. Rivier D, Roy S, Mermoud A. Ex-PRESS R-50 miniature glaucoma implant insertion under the conjunctiva combined with cataract extraction. *J Cataract Refract Surg*. 2007;33(11): 1946–52.

53. Dahan E, Carmichael TR. Implantation of a miniature glaucoma device under a scleral flap. *J Glaucoma*. 2005;14(2):98–102.

54. Ferrari E, Bandello F, Roman-Pognuz D, Menchini F. Combined clear corneal phacoemulsification and ab interno trabeculectomy: three-year case series. *J Cataract Refract Surg*. 2005;31(9): 1783–8.

55. Philippin H, Wilmsmeyer S, Feltgen N, Ness T, Funk J. Combined cataract and glaucoma surgery: endoscope-controlled erbium:YAG-laser goniotomy versus trabeculectomy. *Graefes Arch Clin Exp Ophthalmol*. 2005;243(7):684–8.

56. Funnell CL, Clowes M, Anand N. Combined cataract and glaucoma surgery with mitomycin C: phacoemulsification-trabeculectomy compared to phacoemulsification-deep sclerectomy. *Br J Ophthalmol*. 2005;89(6):694–8.

57. Hassan KM, Awadalla MA. Results of combined phacoemulsification and viscocanalostomy in patients with cataract and pseudoexfoliative glaucoma. *Eur J Ophthalmol*. 2008;18(2):212–9.

58. Wishart MS, Dagres E. Seven-year follow-up of combined cataract extraction and viscocanalostomy. *J Cataract Refract Surg*. 2006;32(12):2043–9.

59. Kobayashi H, Kobayashi K. Randomized comparison of the intraocular pressure-lowering effect of phacoviscocanalostomy and phacotrabeculectomy. *Ophthalmology*. 2007;114(5): 909–14.

60. Park M, Hayashi K, Takahashi H, Tanito M, Chihara E. Phacoviscocanalostomy versus phaco-trabeculotomy: a middle-term study. *J Glaucoma*. 2006;15(5):456–61.

61. Shoji T, Tanito M, Takahashi H. Phacoviscocanalostomy versus cataract surgery only in patients with coexisting normal-tension glaucoma: midterm outcomes. *J Cataract Refract Surg*. 2007;33(7):1209–16.

62. Hondur A, Onol M, Hasanreisoglu B. Nonpenetrating glaucoma surgery: meta-analysis of recent results. *J Glaucoma*. 2008;17(2):139–46.

63. Lüke C, Dietlein TS, Lüke M, Konen W, Krieglstein GK. Phacotrabeculotomy combined with deep sclerectomy, a new technique in combined cataract and glaucoma surgery: complication profile. *Acta Ophthalmol Scand*. 2007;85(2):143–8.

64. Hong S, Seong GJ, Hong YJ. Long-term intraocular pressure fluctuation and progressive visual field deterioration in patients with glaucoma and low intraocular pressures after a triple procedure. *Arch Ophthalmol*. 2007;125(8):1010–3.

65. Janknecht P. Phacoemulsification combined with cyclophotocoagulation. *Klin Monatsbl Augenheilkd*. 2005;222(9):717–20.

66. Lin SC. Endoscopic and transscleral cyclophotocoagulation for the treatment of refractory glaucoma. *J Glaucoma*. 2008;17(3): 238–47.

67. Li G, Kasner O. Review of consecutive phacotrabeculectomies supplemented with early needle revision and antimetabolites. *Can J Ophthalmol*. 2006;41(4):457–63.

68. Tham CC, Li FC, Leung DY, Kwong YY, Yick DW, Lam DS. Microincision bimanual phacotrabeculectomy in eyes with coexisting glaucoma and cataract. *J Cataract Refract Surg*. 2006;32(11):1917–20.

69. Sharma A, Sii F, Shah P, Kirkby GR. Vitrectomy-phacoemulsification-vitrectomy for the management of aqueous misdirection syndromes in phakic eyes. *Ophthalmology*. 2006;113(11):1968–73.

70. Shingleton B, Tetz M, Korber N. Circumferential viscodilation and tensioning of Schlemm canal (canaloplasty) with temporal clear corneal phacoemulsification cataract surgery for open-angle glaucoma and visually significant cataract: one-year results. *J Cataract Refract Surg*. 2008;34(3): 433–40.

Chapter 2

Anesthesia

Marlene R. Moster and Augusto Azuara-Blanco

Introduction

There are numerous modes of anesthesia from which an eye surgeon can choose. Overall, there is not one type of anesthesia that is right for all cases. The best choice varies from surgeon to surgeon and from patient to patient. As cataract removal has become faster, safer, and less traumatic, the need for akinesia and anesthesia has declined significantly and the use of general anesthesia or regional (i.e., retrobulbar or peribulbar) block has largely been replaced with other safer and equally effective means of local anesthesia including sub-Tenon's, subconjunctival, intracameral, and topical. These newer and less invasive methods have not only reduced the potential for catastrophic surgical complications, but also increased the efficiency of cataract surgery and hastened the process of visual rehabilitation.

The goal of this chapter is to review the current choices for local ocular anesthesia in patients with glaucoma undergoing cataract surgery, helping to select the most appropriate type of anesthesia for each patient.

Preoperative Assessment of Patients

The preoperative assessment and preparation of patients undergoing ophthalmic surgery under local anesthesia varies worldwide. Routine investigation of patients undergoing cataract surgery is not essential.

The standard preoperative assessment includes specific enquiries about bleeding disorders and drugs. There is an increased risk of hemorrhage in patients receiving anticoagulants, and a clotting profile assessment is required prior to injection techniques.[1] Patients receiving anticoagulants are advised to continue medication. Clotting results should be within the recommended therapeutic range. Currently there is no recommendation (lack of data) for patients receiving antiplatelet agents. Sub-Tenon's block and topical anesthetic are the favored techniques in these patients.

Topical Anesthesia

Topical ocular anesthesia has been demonstrated to be a safe and effective alternative to retrobulbar or peribulbar anesthesia for cataract surgery.[2-4] However, topical anesthesia does not provide ocular akinesia and may provide inadequate sensory blockade for the iris and ciliary body. This is relevant for patients with glaucoma and shallow anterior chamber, small pupil, or posterior synechiae. Overall, in the majority of glaucoma patients undergoing cataract surgery, topical anesthesia is a suitable option.

The first approach simply involves administering local anesthetic eye drops—most commonly proparacaine, tetracaine, lidocaine, or bupivacaine—to the operative eye three or four times, usually separated by a few minutes just prior to surgery (Fig. 2.1).[4] The choice of which of these

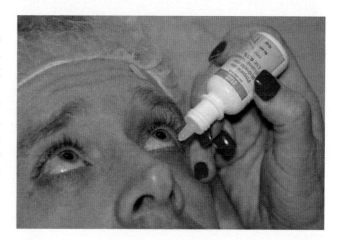

Fig. 2.1 A drop of topical anesthetic (proparacaine) is instilled in the eye

M.R. Moster (✉)
Department of Ophthalmology, Thomas Jefferson University Hospital, Philadelphia, PA 19107, USA
e-mail: marlenemoster@aol.com

S.M. Johnson (ed.), *Cataract Surgery in the Glaucoma Patient*, DOI 10.1007/978-0-387-09408-3_2,
© Springer Science+Business Media, LLC 2009

local anesthetics to use can be based on concerns regarding corneal epithelial toxicity, patient comfort, and patient's history of local anesthetic allergies. Overall, all of these local anesthetics are safe and effective in brief perioperative exposure. Tetracaineis the most irritating of the anesthetic eye drops mentioned and is an ester anesthetic and should be avoided in patients allergic to that family of local anesthetics.

Another popular practice is the administration of topical anesthesia using viscous lidocaine gel instead of or in addition to drops (Fig. 2.2). A common adjunct to topical anesthetic eye drops is intracameral injection of local anesthetics, mainly preservative-free 1% lidocaine injected in doses of 0.1–0.5 ml instilled into the anterior chamber (Figs. 2.3a, b).[3] Intracameral injection may provide sensory blockade for the iris and ciliary body, relieving discomfort that patients may have when iris manipulation is required in patients with poor pupil dilation and/or posterior synechiae.[4]

Regarding the safety of intracameral anesthesia, short-term studies seem to indicate that preservative-free 1% lidocaine in doses of 0.1–0.5 ml is well tolerated by the corneal endothelium, whereas higher concentrations are toxic.[5] Intracameral lidocaine alone has been shown to be a good pupillary dilator. This may be due to its direct action on the iris, causing muscle relaxation.

Intracameral preservative-free 1:10,000 epinephrine may be used when the pupil does not dilate fully or in patients using alpha-blockers such as tamsulosin with floppy iris.[6]

Sub-Tenon's Anesthesia

The sub-Tenon's anesthesia/block is a simple, safe, effective, and versatile alternative to a sharp needle block for orbital anesthesia. The exact frequency of the use of this technique is not known, but its use appears to have increased among glaucoma surgeons.[7,8]

Regarding the technique, access to the space by the inferonasal quadrant is the most commonly described approach because the placement of the cannula in this quadrant allows good fluid distribution superiorly while avoiding the area of surgery and reducing the risk of damage to the vortex veins.[8] After instillation of local anesthetic eye drops (e.g., proxymetacaine 0.5% or tetracaine 1%), the eye is cleaned with specially formulated 5% aqueous povidone iodine solution. An eyelid speculum is used to keep the eyelids apart. The patient is asked to look upward and outward, to expose the inferonasal quadrant. The conjunctiva and Tenon capsule are

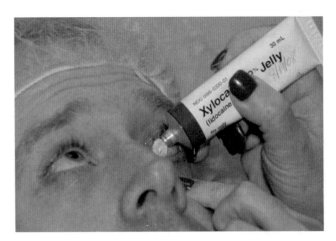

Fig. 2.2 Xylocaine (lidocaine) 2% Jelly (AstraZeneca) is placed in the eye in the preoperative area and allowed to remain in place for about 5 min before the patient is prepped and draped in the operating room

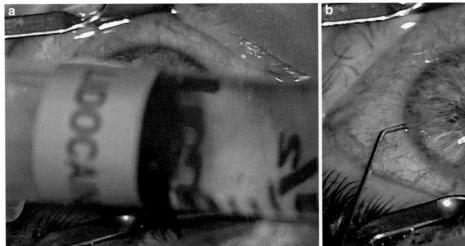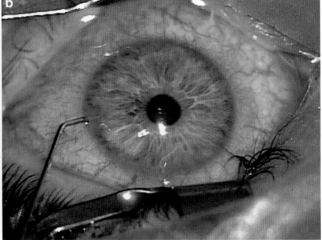

Fig. 2.3 (**a**) One percent non-preserved lidocaine (Xylocaine) is (**b**) introduced into the anterior chamber via a paracentesis with a 27-gauge cannula

gripped with non-toothed forceps 5–10 mm away from the limbus. A small incision is made through these layers with scissors and the sclera is exposed.[7]

A blunt curved metal sub-Tenon cannula (19G, 25 mm long, curved, with a flat profile with end hole), such as the Steven's cannula (Figs 2.4a, b), or others, such as the Connor cannula (Fig. 2.5), securely mounted onto a 5-ml syringe containing the local anesthetic solution, is inserted through the hole along the curvature of the sclera. If resistance is encountered, a gentle pressure is applied and hydrodissection usually helps in advancing the cannula. The resistance felt during insertion of the cannula is due to the intermuscular septum, but usually the cannula passes into the posterior sub-Tenon's space. If the hydrodissection does not help or the resistance encountered is too great, it is advisable to reposition or reintroduce the cannula because the muscle insertions vary and the cannula may be transversing the muscle's Tenon's sheath rather than following the globe surface. The local anesthetic agent of choice is injected slowly and the cannula is removed. A gentle pressure is applied over the globe to favor the spread of the local anesthetic agent.[7]

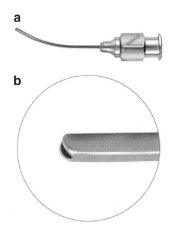

a

b

Fig. 2.4 (**a**) Steven's sub-Tenon cannula. (**b**) A close-up of the tip. *Images courtesy of the manufacturer—Katena Products Inc, Denville, NJ*

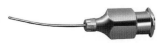

Fig. 2.5 E4999 Connor Anesthesia Cannula. *Image courtesy of the manufacturer—Storz Instruments, a division of Bausch & Lomb, Rochester, NY*

With the above technique, adequate anesthesia is achieved for the majority of ocular surgeries. Akinesia is volume dependent and if 4–5 ml of local anesthetic agent is injected, most patients develop akinesia.[9] However, superior oblique

muscle and lid movements may remain active in a small but significant number of patients.

There are other variations of the sub-Tenon's technique that relate to route of access, cannula, local anesthetic agent, volume, and the adjuvant used.

There are several advantages of sub-Tenon's block: it eliminates the risks of sharp needle techniques, provides reliable anesthesia, has the potential for further supplementation for prolonged anesthesia and postoperative pain relief, and can be safely used in patients with a long globe.[7,8] There are numerous studies demonstrating its effectiveness compared to retrobulbar, peribulbar, and topical anesthesia alone.[7,8] Sub-Tenon's block has been used for a large number of ophthalmic surgical procedures, including cataract and glaucoma surgeries. Recent reviews suggest that sub-Tenon's block may be used safely in patients receiving anticoagulants and antiplatelet agents, provided clotting results are in the normal therapeutic range.[10] Despite the reporting of a few major complications, it has one of the highest safety profiles of any regional anesthetic technique.

Patients may experience pain during the block. The origin of pain is multifactorial. The incidence of pain during sub-Tenon's injection with a posterior metal cannula is reported in up to 44% of patients.[7] Preoperative explanation of the procedure, good surface anesthesia, gentle technique, slow injection of warm local anesthetic agent, and reassurance are considered good practice and may reduce the discomfort and anxiety during the injection.

Fine vessels are inevitably severed on making the conjunctival dissection, causing some degree of subconjunctival hemorrhage, which typically does not have clinical relevance. Patients should receive adequate warning of this possibility.

Sight- and life-threatening complications have been reported but are very rare.[7] These include short-lived muscle paresis and orbital and retrobulbar hemorrhage. Trauma to inferior and medial rectus muscles leading to restrictive functions resulting in diplopia has been reported following damage to the muscles by a metal cannula.[7] Other complications relate to optic neuropathy and afferent pupillary and accommodation defects.[7] Retinal and choroidal vascular occlusion and a case of central spread of the local anesthetic agent leading to cardiorespiratory collapse have been reported.[7]

The rise in intraocular pressure (IOP) after administration of sub-Tenon's block is small or even non-significant.[11,12] This is a relevant finding for patients with glaucoma. However, pulsatile ocular blood flow may be affected by sub-Tenon's block in a similar way as retrobulbar and peribulbar injections.[12] Therefore, caution is required in the management of glaucoma patients with advanced optic nerve damage who may be at risk of wipe-out (see *Wipe-Out in Glaucoma Patients* section).

Retrobulbar and Peribulbar Techniques

The current retrobulbar technique used by most ophthalmologists today was described by Atkinson in 1934, and until recently served as the most commonly used technique for intraocular surgery.[13] Davis and Mandel are credited with introducing the peribulbar block in 1986 as a less dangerous alternative to retrobulbar anesthesia.[14] The decision between retrobulbar anesthesia and peribulbar anesthesia presents the surgeon with a choice between speed and safety. With a retrobulbar block, a surgeon can ensure that adequate akinesia and anesthesia will result for cataract surgery; however, a blind injection into the orbit poses several potential complications, including, but not limited to, retrobulbar hemorrhage, globe perforation, optic nerve damage, and brainstem anesthesia. Peribulbar anesthesia, involving the injection of local anesthetic external to the muscle cone, is thought to decrease the likelihood of optic nerve and globe perforation while maintaining the desirable qualities of excellent akinesia and anesthesia. However, the potential need for reinjection, the higher volume of injectate required, and the longer duration of onset associated with peribulbar blocks may make it a less attractive alternative.

Patient Monitoring

Presence of Anesthesiologists

The presence of the anesthesiologists during sub-Tenon's, retrobulbar, or peribulbar block may not be required, but their skills in managing life-threatening cardiorespiratory events must be available from the other staff in the operating room or ambulatory surgical center. It is also recommended that monitoring should be by a member of the staff who remains with the patient at all times throughout the monitoring period and whose sole responsibility is to the patient. This person must be trained to detect and act on any adverse events, and this person may be an anesthesiologist, a nurse, or an operating department practitioner as long as he or she is trained in life support.[7,15]

Monitoring During Block Procedure

Blood pressure, oxygen saturation, and electrocardiogram (ECG) leads are connected and baseline recordings are routinely obtained. Although the insertion of an intravenous line has been questioned for topical and sub-Tenon's techniques, it is considered good practice, in general, and necessary in retrobulbar and peribulbar block.[7,15]

Intraoperative Monitoring

The patient should be comfortable and soft pads are placed under the pressure areas. All patients undergoing eye surgery under local anesthesia should be monitored with pulse oximetry, ECG, non-invasive blood pressure measurement, and maintenance of verbal contact. Patients should receive an oxygen-enriched breathing atmosphere to prevent hypoxia and with a flow rate high enough to prevent hypercarbia if enclosed in surgical drapes. ECG and pulse oximetry should be continued. Once the patient is under the drapes, verbal and tactile contacts are maintained.[7,15]

Sedation During Regional or Local Anesthesia

The patient undergoing ophthalmic surgical procedures, irrespective of type of regional anesthesia employed, should be fully conscious, responsive, and free of anxiety, discomfort, and pain.[7] The aim of sedation is to minimize anxiety while providing the maximum degree of safety. Sedation is commonly used during cataract surgery under topical anesthesia but only selected patients receiving sub-Tenon's or other orbital regional block, in which explanation and reassurance have proved inadequate, may benefit from sedation. Short-acting benzodiazepines, opioids, or intravenous anesthetic agents in minimum dosages are used. However, there is an increased risk of an intraoperative event when sedation is used. A means of providing supplementation oxygen must be available when sedation is administered.[7,15]

General Anesthesia

General anesthesia provides excellent anesthesia, analgesia, and akinesia. This provides the most controlled environment for surgery. However, general anesthesia is associated with an increased risk of systemic complications (e.g., malignant hyperthermia, hemodynamic fluctuation, myocardial infarction, postoperative nausea, and vomiting) and requires more medication, equipment, and personnel. As a result, it is the most costly form of anesthesia. General anesthesia remains the technique of choice for children and mentally retarded, demented, or psychologically unstable patients. Patients may ultimately feel that they will not be able to cooperate during surgery and request general anesthesia.[16]

There are patients in which general anesthesia is contraindicated or should be undertaken with caution. Myotonic dystrophy patients develop cataracts at a younger age; these patients are at risk of cardiac and respiratory complications under general anesthesia.[17] Marfan's patients are subject to lens subluxation and dislocation; they are also at increased risk of cardiac and pulmonary complications under general anesthesia.[18] Thorough review of medications is necessary, since some ocular medications may interfere with general anesthesia. Topical epinephrine used to treat glaucoma may interact with halogenated hydrocarbon anesthetics, leading to ventricular fibrillation.[4] Echothiophate, which in the past was used to treat glaucoma, inhibits plasma pseudocholinesterase, which also metabolizes anesthetics including succinylcholine, leading to overdosing and a prolonged dependency on mechanical ventilation.[4]

Current Trends

In the most recent published study of the practice styles and preferences of American Society of Cataract and Refractive Surgery (ASCRS) members,[19] it was found that retrobulbar block without facial block was used by 11% of surgeons and retrobulbar injection with facial block by 9% (down from 76% in 1985, 32% in 1995, and 14% in 2000). The peribulbar block was used by 17% of surgeons (down from 38% in 1995). Topical anesthesia was used by 61% (up from 8% in 1995 and 51% in 2000). Of those surgeons electing to use topical, 73% of surgeons also used concomitant intracameral lidocaine. The use of topical also varied with surgical volume. Those performing one to five cataract procedures per month employed topical 38% of the time and those doing more than 75 procedures used it in 76% of cases. Clearly the trend has been to transition from retrobulbar anesthesia to topical, and this pattern parallels the increase in the use of temporal clear corneal incisions. To our knowledge there is no data regarding patients with glaucoma undergoing cataract surgery.

Wipe-Out in Glaucoma Patients

The phenomenon of severe visual loss after surgery, with no obvious cause, is known as "wipe-out" or "snuff syndrome." Wipe-out may affect patients who have very severe glaucomatous damage and, overall is a very uncommon complication but remains an important concern among glaucoma surgeons.

With modern cataract and glaucoma surgical techniques it is becoming increasingly rare.[20,21] Among the possible mechanisms, direct damage to the optic nerve from anesthetic technique has been proposed. Because glaucoma is a chronic condition characterized by progressive pressure/ischemic damage to the optic nerve head, glaucoma patients may be at risk of further optic nerve damage (and possibly wipe-out) in severe disease from orbital retrobulbar and peribulbar anesthesia, as there is potential for direct trauma, pressure on the nerve, and/or ischemia. Local pressure to the optic nerve may result from a hematoma in the optic nerve sheath, a retrobulbar hematoma, or simply from the volume of anesthetic injected.[22] Even with a low volume of local anesthetic (LA), if the LA were to become trapped between fascial layers, this could lead to a "compartment syndrome." Localized pressure may also induce ischemia of the nerve, as may epinephrine (adrenaline) if used in the LA mixture. For patients whose optic nerve is already damaged by glaucoma, this could result in wipe-out.[22]

Doppler imaging studies have shown that retrobulbar, peribulbar, and sub-Tenon's injections can cause a marked reduction in blood flow in the arteries supplying the anterior optic nerve, particularly if epinephrine is included in the LA mixture.[22] Current high index of suspicion means that many glaucoma specialists now try to avoid using these LA techniques for any surgery on glaucoma patients, including cataract surgery. Currently preferred techniques are anterior sub-Tenon's, subconjunctival, topical, and intracameral anesthesia. These "newer" techniques appear to be successful in terms of safety and patient acceptability.[4,19,22]

Summary

Given the choices for ocular anesthesia today, one thing remains clear: No single mode of anesthesia can serve as a universal choice for all patients and all surgeons. The decision to choose one of these methods ultimately falls upon the surgeon, and the surgeon should carefully tailor his approach to each individual patient. The decision of which type of anesthesia to use is not only dependent on a number of patient factors but also dependent on the surgeon and the surgeon's level of expertise and facility with the surgery to be performed.

It is essential that the surgeon, the patient, and the anesthesia staff work together and be involved in the selection and execution of anesthesia during the surgery. Involving the patient in this decision by describing the patient experience prior to and during surgery is critical. Fear and anxiety result when things are unknown or unexpected. If patients are prepared, they are better equipped to cope with the sensations they may feel during and after surgery.

References

1. Sweitzer BJ. Preoperative medical testing and preparation for ophthalmic surgery. *Ophthalmol Clin North Am.* 2006;19: 163–77

2. Patel BC, Burns TA, Crandall A, et al. A comparison of topical and retrobulbar anesthesia for cataract surgery. *Ophthalmology.* 1996;103:1196–203.

3. Crandall AS, Zabriskie NA, Patel BC, et al. A comparison of patient comfort during cataract surgery with topical anesthesia versus topical anesthesia and intracameral lidocaine. *Ophthalmology.* 1999;106:60–6.

4. Navaleza JS, Pendse SJ, Blecher MH. Choosing anesthesia for cataract surgery. *Ophthalmol Clin North Am.* 2006;19:233–7.

5. Karp CL, Cox TA, Wagoner MD, Ariyasu RG, Jacobs DS. Intracameral anesthesia: a report by the American Academy of Ophthalmology. *Ophthalmology.* 2001;108:1704–10.

6. Lee JJ, Moster MR, Henderer JD, Membreno JH. Pupil dilation with intracameral 1% lidocaine during glaucoma filtering surgery. *Am J Ophthalmol.* 2003;136:201–3.

7. Kumar CM, Dodds C. Sub-Tenon's anesthesia. *Ophthalmol Clin North Am.* 2006;19:209–19.

8. Kumar CM, Williamson S, Manickam B. A review of sub-Tenon's block: current practice and recent development. *Eur J Anaesthesiol.* 2005;22:567–77.

9. Kumar CM, Dodds C. Evaluation of the Greenbaum sub-Tenon's block. *Br J Anaesth.* 2001;87:631–3.

10. Katz J, Feldman MA, Bass EB, et al. Study of medical testing for cataract surgery team. Risks and benefits of anticoagulant and antiplatelet medication use before cataract surgery. *Ophthalmology.* 2003;110:1784–8.

11. Alwitry A, Koshy Z, Browning AC, Kiel W, Holden R. The effect of sub-Tenon's anaesthesia on intraocular pressure. *Eye.* 2001;15:733–5.

12. Pianka P, Weintraub-Padova H, Lazar M, Geyer O. Effect of sub-Tenon's and peribulbar anesthesia on intraocular pressure and ocular pulse amplitude. *J Cataract Refract Surg.* 2001;27:1221–6.

13. Atkinson WS. Retrobulbar injection of anesthetic within the muscular cone. *Arch Ophthalmol.* 1936;16:494–503.

14. Davis DB 2nd, Mandel MR. Posterior peribulbar anesthesia: an alternative to retrobulbar anesthesia. *J Cataract Refract Surg.* 1986;12:182–4.

15. Astbury N, Bagshaw H, Desai P, et al. Local anesthesia for intraocular surgery. London: The Royal College of Anaesthetists and the Royal College of Ophthalmologists; 2001.

16. McGoldrick KE, Foldes PJ. General anesthesia for ophthalmic surgery. *Ophthalmol Clin North Am.* 2006;19:179–91.

17. Aldridge LM. Anaesthetic problems in myotonic dystrophy. A case report and review of the Aberdeen experience comprising 48 general anaesthetics in a further 16 patients. *Br J Anaesth.* 1985;57:1119–30.

18. Wells DG, Podolakin W. Anaesthesia and Marfan's syndrome: case report. *Can J Anaesth.* 1987;34:311–4.

19. Leaming DV. Practice styles and preferences of ASCRS members–2003 survey. *J Cataract Refract Surg.* 2004;30:892–900.

20. Law SK, Nguyen AM, Coleman AL, Caprioli J. Severe loss of central vision in patients with advanced glaucoma undergoing trabeculectomy. *Arch Ophthalmol.* 2007;125:1044–50.

21. Topouzis F, Tranos P, Koskosas A, et al. Risk of sudden visual loss following filtration surgery in end-stage glaucoma. *Am J Ophthalmol.* 2005;140:661–6.

22. Eke T. Anesthesia for glaucoma surgery. *Ophthalmol Clin North Am.* 2006;19:245–55.

Chapter 3

Management of the Small Pupil

Cynthia Mattox

Introduction

A small pupil, defined as a pupil that enlarges poorly after dilation, is likely the most common condition surgeons encounter when approaching glaucoma patients with cataract. Poor pupil dilation increases the risk of having complications during cataract surgery. Small pupils have numerous causes. Recognition of the cause of the small pupil and careful preoperative planning will ensure successful operative management (Fig. 3.1).

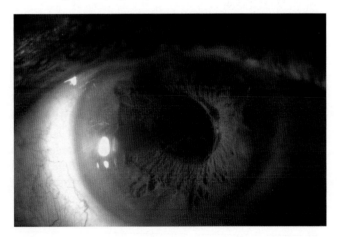

Fig. 3.1 Eye with small pupil, chronic angle closure, and posterior synechiae

Small Pupils and Their Etiology

A variety of conditions can lead to small pupils, many of them associated with glaucomas. By taking a careful history and performing a focused examination the surgeon will

C. Mattox (✉)
Department of Ophthalmology, New England Eye Center, Tufts University School of Medicine, Boston, MA 02493, USA
e-mail: cmattox@tuftsmedicalcenter.org

usually be able to determine the etiology of the small pupil. Many times the underlying or associated condition will guide the surgeon to a specific surgical plan.

Small Pupils Caused by Medication

Parasympathomimetics

In the second half of the twentieth century, the most common medication-induced cause of small pupils was undoubtedly the use of miotic glaucoma medications. Pilocarpine and the other parasympathomimetics were commonly used chronically to treat glaucoma before the advent of more modern medications with fewer side effects. The drugs themselves are cataractogenic and aggravate vision loss in patients with central lens opacification. The continuous constriction of the pupil from contraction of the pupillary sphincter usually leads to atrophy of the pupil dilator muscle, so these eyes rarely dilate well even with the use of multiple mydriatic and cycloplegic eye drops. The miosis may cause posterior synechiae to the anterior lens capsule to develop in phakic patients. In some patients, a low-grade inflammation can be present as well as a disruption of the blood-aqueous barrier. Fortunately, because of the newer medications available to treat glaucoma, it is relatively rare to find a cataract patient with recently diagnosed open angle glaucoma on a miotic medication. However, some glaucomas, such as pigmentary and plateau iris syndrome, will benefit from the use of miotics. Many times these glaucoma patients are younger and may be treated for many years with miotics before having to deal with a cataract. Fortunately, for most typical glaucoma patients these days, miotics are reserved for patients who are pseudophakic and unresponsive to other medications or unable to undergo surgical treatment for their glaucoma.

Diagnostic Keys

Usually the patient's history is sufficient, but keep in mind that patients treated with miotics for long periods in the past may have been switched to newer medications in recent years. These patients may still fail to dilate adequately. Examination should evaluate the size of the pupil as well as the location of posterior synechiae.

Surgical Planning Tips

It is best to discontinue miotics for at least 1 week prior to cataract surgery. Although this is not likely to enhance pupil dilation at the time of surgery, it often will reduce the postoperative inflammation that may occur in eyes with chronic breakdown of the blood-aqueous barrier. The surgeon may also consider prescribing preoperative and postoperative non-steroidal anti-inflammatory drops (NSAIDs) in addition to the usual postoperative corticosteroids in these eyes.

Surgical Techniques (See Specific Surgical Techniques Section Below)

Usually manual pupil stretching techniques are useful in these eyes, but a more gentle, slow stretch is employed to avoid tearing the iris stroma in these atrophic irides. The surgeon should watch for small microtears developing in the sphincter as the stretch is performed and stop manipulation when adequate relaxation of the sphincter ring is achieved. Alternatively, pupil expansion rings can be employed with care. It may be best to choose a pupil expansion ring that provides only moderate dilation to avoid iris stromal tearing. Vigorous stretching with iris retractors is more likely to cause trauma in these eyes.

Systemic Alpha-1 Antagonists

There are several popular systemic alpha-1 blockers used to treat urinary symptoms associated with benign prostatic hypertrophy in men and occasionally in women with urinary retention. In 2005, Chang and Campbell[1] reported on intraoperative floppy iris syndrome (IFIS) where abrupt billowing, constriction, and prolapse of the iris occur during routine cataract surgery. They associated IFIS with patients taking the alpha-1 blocker Flomax. IFIS is less likely to be caused by other alpha-1 blockers listed in Table 3.1.

The difference is that Flomax has an extremely high affinity for the alpha-1A receptor subtype, while the others are less subtype specific. The prostate and the iris dilator muscle are rich in alpha-1A receptors, and the use of these medications, even months or years in the past, can produce a permanent severe loss of tone or even atrophy in the iris dilator muscle.

Table 3.1 Alpha-1 blockers[3,30–32]

Alpha-1 blockers	Manufacturer
Flomax (tamsulosin)	Boehringer-Ingleheim pharmaceuticals, Ridgefield, CT
Hytrin (terazosin)	Abbott laboratories, Abbott Park, IL
Cardura (doxazosin mesylate)	Pfizer, New York, NY
Uroxatral (alfuzosin)	Sanofi-Aventis, Paris, France

Diagnostic Tips

A careful history is required, as some patients may not readily recall taking Flomax in the past. It may be useful to note the use of the other alpha-1 blockers also, because their use in conjunction with some other factor that increases cataract surgery risk may contribute to a milder form of IFIS. In my experience, the eyes most likely to experience IFIS are those that have poor dilation in the office with the usual dilating drop regimen. If the eyes dilate well, it seems to be less likely to develop.

Surgical Planning

The surgical plan should make note of the use of alpha-1 blockers. However, it does not seem to be helpful in preventing IFIS to have the patient discontinue Flomax preoperatively unless it was just recently started within the last few months. There are some surgeons who have recommended the use of Atropine 1% eye drops twice a day (BID) for 3 days prior to cataract surgery to increase the tone and rigidity of the iris.[2] Atropine may cause acute urinary retention in susceptible patients taking these medications and the patient must be warned to continue their alpha-1 blocker and call if they experience pain or reduced urinary frequency.

Surgical Techniques

I divide these eyes into two categories:

1. Mild to moderate risk for IFIS (eyes that dilate well in the office and preoperatively[3,4]): Maximal preoperative dilation using pledgets and/or intracameral epinephrine (preservative-free epinephrine 1:1000 mixed with balanced salt solution (BSS) in a 1:4 ratio) will help to increase iris rigidity. The use of dispersive viscoelastics such as Viscoat (Alcon, Fort Worth, TX) or Healon5 (Advanced Medical Optics, Santa Ana, CA) is imperative. Careful avoidance of iris manipulation or contact even with a fluid wave from a hydrodissection cannula will help to delay or minimize the onset of

the IFIS in borderline eyes. Careful efficient cataract surgery can often be accomplished and will often avoid iris billowing or constriction at least until near the conclusion of the case when it no longer presents difficulty.

2. Moderate to high risk for IFIS (dilates poorly, 5 mm or less, in the office and preoperatively):[3,4] In addition to intracameral epinephrine and dispersive viscoelastic, these eyes require the use of a pupil expansion device. Iris hooks or rings may be employed and should be placed prior to initiating the capsulorhexis. Manual iris stretching is to be avoided in these eyes. It will actually provoke the initiation of IFIS.

Small Pupils Associated with Narrow Angle Glaucomas

Eyes with a history of narrow angles or angle closure glaucoma will often present to the cataract surgeon with small pupil. These eyes have usually undergone treatment with a laser iridotomy or even a surgical iridectomy or trabeculectomy. The inflammation after laser, surgery, and/or an angle closure attack will often cause posterior synechiae to form, causing a small or irregular pupil. A prolonged angle closure attack may cause iris ischemia and may result in a thin or atrophic iris. In addition, eyes prone to narrow angles or acute angle closure commonly have a shallow anterior chamber and short axial length, increasing the complexity of the cataract surgery. The combination of a small or syneched pupil in the setting of a shallow anterior chamber can make surgical manipulation of the pupil more difficult.

Diagnostic Tips

Historical information about an angle closure attack and its duration before treatment may indicate a more severe condition of iris ischemia and shallow anterior chamber. Inspection of the eye for the location of the iridotomy may influence cataract incision placement. Documentation of the pupil shape and diameter following dilation will help to plan for synechialysis intraoperatively.

Surgical Planning

If pupil manipulation is planned, the surgeon may consider preoperative and postoperative treatment with NSAIDs, along with increased postoperative corticosteroids.

Surgical Techniques

In eyes that have not developed thin atrophic irides, simple release of posterior synechiae with a sweep of the viscoelastic cannula and placement of additional viscoelastic will often allow the iris to dilate adequately. It is important to not inject large boluses of viscoelastic beneath the iris at this stage. Even if the pupil seems large enough to complete it, posterior synechiae should be released prior to initiating the capsulorhexis. If not released, the synechiae can produce traction on the peripheral anterior capsule as the capsulorhexis is being performed and cause an uncontrolled tear toward the periphery.

If the iris seems thin and the pupil extremely small in addition to synechiae, the surgeon may need to manually stretch the pupil or use an expansion device. However, pupil expansion rings are quite difficult to use in eyes with shallow anterior chambers. If a device is used, iris retractors may be easier to use in these eyes. See also Chapter 18.

Small Pupils Associated with Prior Glaucoma Surgery

Prior intraocular glaucoma surgery may cause posterior synechiae. In eyes that have undergone filtration surgery, postoperative complications such as choroidal effusions or wound leak and associated hypotony may allow the development of a shallow anterior chamber. If the shallow anterior chamber is prolonged, posterior synechiae, anterior synechiae, or iridocorneal adhesions may develop. Glaucoma drainage implants with tubes in the anterior chamber may cause localized synechiae or cataract if the tube touches the iris or lens. Also, many eyes with tube implants have diminished endothelial cell counts and may be more prone to postoperative corneal edema. These factors may affect the surgical plan (see Chapter 17).

Diagnostic Tips

Often the exam notes from the postoperative period after filtration surgery are necessary to confirm the history of a shallow anterior chamber. However, iridocorneal adhesions in the presence of a filtration bleb almost certainly formed during a period of shallowness. Careful inspection of the location and position of tube implants should be performed, recognizing that the anterior chamber will become deeper following cataract removal.

Surgical Planning

The location of iridocorneal adhesions or tube implant may influence the placement of the cataract incision. Trabeculectomy blebs may fail after cataract surgery due to postoperative inflammation. Especially if iris manipulation is planned, the surgeon should be prepared to carefully monitor the filtration bleb, using 5-fluoruracil postoperatively if necessary. In some cases, if the bleb is marginal prior to cataract surgery, consideration should be given to performing a combined glaucoma and cataract surgery rather than a complex phacoemulsification alone. See also Chapter 16.

Surgical Techniques

Posterior synechiae are often easily released using a sweep of the viscoelastic cannula and additional viscoelastic. Iridocorneal adhesions can be left alone, or gently released with sweeping, taking care to avoid a large Descemet's detachment. Release of iridocorneal adhesions may cause bleeding and the surgeon should be prepared. Peripheral anterior synechiae in the angle may need to be released, but only if compromising the filtration bleb by obstructing the internal sclerostomy. If not, it is best to avoid additional iris trauma or bleeding to minimize postoperative inflammation in the setting of a functional filtration bleb.

Small Pupils Associated with Other Ocular Conditions

Pseudoexfoliation Syndrome and Pseudoexfoliation Glaucoma

Pseudoexfoliation (PXF) is an extremely common cause of poorly dilating pupils in glaucoma patients. Some, but not all, pseudoexfoliation patients will dilate poorly. The risk of having a complication during cataract surgery in PXF patients who dilate poorly is much higher. The small pupil may be a result of chronic injury to the pupillary sphincter as it chafes across the pseudoexfoliation material on the lens. Or there may be direct effects of pseudoexfoliation on the iris dilator muscle. In addition, poor dilation may be associated with severe PXF involvement of the zonules, weakening them. It is rare that the small pupil in PXF is associated with posterior synechiae. If the small pupil in PXF is also associated with a shallow chamber or narrow angle (that may or may not be asymmetric) or a previous laser iridotomy, then the surgeon needs to be prepared to encounter loose zonules during cataract surgery.

Diagnostic Tips

Careful inspection of the iris and dilated lens is important to detect subtle signs of PXF as a cause of small pupil. If the pupil dilates poorly and it is difficult to detect the PXF signs on the anterior capsule, sometimes there will be PXF material on the iris sphincter or even on the corneal endothelium. The surgeon should look for phacodenesis, which is sometimes present only before dilation because the cycloplegia can tighten the zonules enough to stabilize the lens. The eyes should also be examined by gonioscopy for the presence of narrow angles.

Surgical Planning

The size of the dilated pupil will determine the surgeon's approach to the cataract surgery.

Surgical Techniques

Any of the pupil expansion techniques can be used successfully to enlarge pupils in PXF patients.[5,6] In patients with dense cataracts and suspected zonular weakness, the surgeon may want to enlarge the pupil maximally with a device to provide optimal visualization during surgery. In addition, iris retractors can be modified to stabilize the capsular bag in the event of zonular dehiscence. PXF is discussed further in Chapter 15.

Uveitis

Patients with chronic uveitis often develop posterior synechiae leading to poorly dilating pupils. And of course, uveitis, cataract, and glaucoma can coexist. It is not uncommon to be faced with performing cataract surgery in these eyes.

Diagnostic Tips

Careful inspection for uveitis activity and the location and extent of posterior synechiae should be performed. It is also helpful to know the recent history of uveitis control. Patients with a history of herpes simplex keratouveitis are more at risk for postoperative reactivation of corneal involvement and also intraocular pressure control problems.

Surgical Planning

Uveitis activity should be well controlled for at least several months prior to elective cataract surgery. Sometimes the increased corticosteroids required to accomplish control will aggravate glaucoma control. It is best to see the patient frequently in the months preoperatively to monitor the IOP and consider if a combined filtration surgery and cataract operation is necessary. Perioperative treatment with antivirals, systemic or periocular corticosteroids, and NSAIDs should all be considered.

Surgical Techniques

In some eyes with chronic uveitis, there may be a fibrotic membrane encircling the pupillary sphincter. This can be carefully stripped with a capsulorhexis forceps prior to additional pupil expansion techniques. Any of the pupil expansion techniques can be successful in these eyes.

Congenital, Acquired, Traumatic, Surgically Altered Pupils

Eyes with congenital, acquired, traumatic, or surgically altered pupils may also develop glaucoma and present significant challenges during cataract surgery. Congenital abnormalities such as ectopia lentis et pupillae or traumatic pupil injury such as iridodialysis may also have weakened zonules or subluxed crystalline lenses.

Acquired iridoschisis occasionally has an associated angle closure glaucoma component and presents additional challenges with poor dilation and shallow anterior chambers. The anterior iris fibers in this condition are loose and prone to incarceration in the phacoemulsification and aspiration tips.

Iridocorneal endothelial (ICE) syndrome and Rieger's syndrome eyes often have eccentric pupils with atrophic irides. In ICE syndrome, however, the remaining iris can be rigid due to the overlying ICE membrane.

Diagnostic Tips

Conduct a careful inspection for phacodenesis, missing zonules, or lens subluxation. Extent and location of the iridoschisis should be noted. Correctopia and iris stretch holes in ICE and Rieger's may alter the surgical incision location.

Surgical Planning and Techniques

Surgical techniques chosen to be appropriate to the condition of the eye. Dispersive viscoelastics can be used to coat the iridoschisis fibers.[7] Iris retractors may be useful in containing the schisis fibers peripherally.[8] Pupil expansion rings may be particularly helpful to stabilize the iris and provide optimal visualization in these eyes.[9]

In addition to the cataract removal, the iris may need to be surgically repaired or altered in eyes with significant iris deformities.

General Concepts

Surgical Planning

Once the surgeon is faced with a poorly dilating pupil and understands the underlying etiology, he/she can develop the surgical plan for the cataract operation.

Preoperative planning always involves a detailed examination to evaluate and document conditions such as orbit depth, preexisting bleb or tube shunt, astigmatism, guttata, location of peripheral anterior synechiae, posterior synechiae, iridotomies, pupil size, and history of systemic and ocular medications. The density of the cataract, presence of pseudoexfoliation or zonular weakness should all be noted. Patient factors such as cooperation or lid squeezing will determine the choice of topical or local block anesthesia. To preserve conjunctiva, most glaucoma patients with cataract should undergo clear cornea cataract incisions whenever possible, but the location may need to be altered based on the status of the eye. When performing manual pupil stretching techniques, the paracentesis needs to be placed between 60° and 90° away from the main incision to allow room for movement of the intraocular iris manipulators.

Surgical Techniques

Anesthetics

Iris manipulation can be uncomfortable to some patients but excellent anesthesia can be accomplished with topical and/or intracameral preservative-free lidocaine 1%.[10] If the case is expected to be long or the patient is uncooperative, then any of the peribulbar or sub-Tenon's block techniques will be effective anesthesia. See also Chapter 2.

Dilating Agents

Topical dilating drops are especially effective in dilating the pupils if applied on a pledget in the preoperative area. The pledget allows for prolonged administration, undiluted by tearing or blinking. Intracameral administration of diluted epinephrine is also effective in providing maximal dilation quickly.[11,12] Preservative-free epinephrine is mandatory for intracameral use. Preserved epinephrine will cause corneal endothelial toxicity or even toxic anterior segment syndrome (TASS). Most US facilities have a ready supply of preservative-free 1:1000 epinephrine that can then be diluted 1:4 with balanced salt solution. Just a small bolus of 0.1–0.2 ml of the resulting dilution provokes rapid pupil dilation and may also increase rigidity of the iris in patients prone to IFIS.

Keep in mind that mechanically bound-down pupils will not respond even to intracameral epinephrine.

The use of preoperative NSAIDs has been shown to increase and maintain pupillary dilation during cataract surgery.[13,14]

Dispersive Viscoelastics

Dispersive viscoelastics, such as Viscoat (Alcon Laboratories Inc., Fort Worth, TX) or Healon5 (Advanced Medical Optics, Santa Ana, CA), are preferred for cataract surgery cases where iris manipulation is performed. They provide maximal retention of the anterior chamber depth, which allows more control when manipulating the iris. However, the surgeon should avoid injecting large boluses of viscoelastic beneath the iris, as it will cause forward bowing and stretching of the iris that may impair visualization.

In most cataract surgeries with small pupils, in addition to expanding the anterior chamber at the beginning of the case, additional viscoelastic will need to be instilled after or during iris expansion maneuvers, so it is helpful to have the necessary supply ready.

As always, it is imperative to remove all of the viscoelastic material, even from behind the intraocular lens (IOL), to help avoid a postoperative intraocular pressure spike.

Intraoperative Iris Expansion with Manual Technique

Using manual technique to stretch the pupil will oftentimes be sufficient for all but Flomax cases or extremely thick springy irides.[5,15,16] These maneuvers create small microtears in the iris sphincter, which allow the pupil to dilate further. The mechanism is not unlike older techniques where microscissors were used to make small radial cuts in the iris sphincter. However, stretching creates a more uniform series of microtears, which allow for a more normal appearing pupil postoperatively. There may be small hemorrhages

that form during stretching that are easily pushed away with additional viscoelastic.

Bimanual

In a bimanual technique, the surgeon uses two iris manipulators, such as Kuglen (Fig. 3.2a), collar button (Fig. 11.5), Connor wands, or Lester manipulators, placing one through the main incision and one through the paracentesis. The manipulators can be angled or straight instruments depending on the surgeon's preference. I prefer angled instruments. The paracentesis should be placed 60–90° away from the main incision to allow for appropriate spacing of the instruments. The hooks on the end of the manipulators are positioned to engage the iris sphincter at points 180° away from each other. The iris is then stretched into the far anterior chamber periphery, nearly to the angle, in both directions (Fig. 3.2b). The manipulators are repositioned 90° from the original stretch axis and an additional stretch is performed. Additional viscoelastic is instilled to push the iris sphincter open. The stretch may need to be repeated until adequate expansion is achieved.

Instrument-Assisted

The Beehler pupil dilator device (Moria, Antony, France) also stretches the pupil, but uses a special instrument that consists of three small hooks that retract into a shaft that has a small hook for the proximal iris (Fig. 3.3). The shaft of the instrument is inserted through the main incision; the hooks are pushed out partially and positioned to engage the iris sphincter. With a push of the plunger, the hooks move out peripherally simultaneously to create the stretch, allowing for a one-handed stretch. The plunger should be depressed very slowly to allow for a controlled, non-violent stretch of the iris.

Cautions

The bimanual technique requires surgeon comfort with bimanual intraocular manipulation, as both instruments must move in concert and precisely. Care must be taken to not engage the anterior capsule of the lens or the corneal endothelium. And the instruments should not actually touch the angle or peripheral iris to avoid lacerating the larger iris vessels.

Stretching is not effective in some very thick dark irides, and this will be readily apparent after the initial stretches

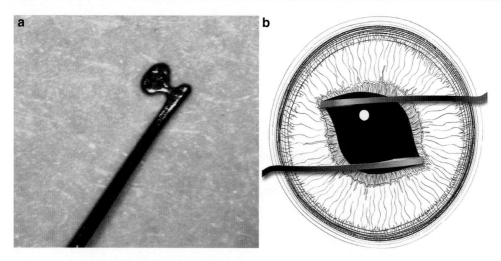

Fig. 3.2 (**a**) Kuglen iris manipulator tip. (**b**) Bimanual iris stretching technique, using Kuglen hooks

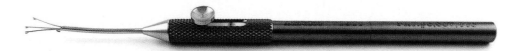

Fig. 3.3 Beehler pupil dilator device. Figure courtesy of Ambler surgical, Exton, PA

if the iris springs back into position. The surgeon can then move on to the use of an iris expansion device.

Stretching should be used with caution in fragile or atrophic irides where vigorous manipulation can rip through the sphincter and into the iris stroma creating an irregular pupil. By carefully watching the iris sphincter during a slow stretch maneuver, the surgeon can avoid this type of uncontrolled tear by stopping when the fine microtears of the sphincter have formed.

Stretching should not be used in patients with likely IFIS because it will precipitate pupil constriction in those eyes.

Advantages

Bimanual stretching is quicker to perform than inserting an iris expansion device, taking on average 1 minutes of surgical time.[5] Because no disposable device is used, it is less costly. Instrument-assisted stretching entails a one-time cost to purchase the instrument and also special care to clean and ensure smooth operation. Iris stretching techniques have been shown to cause minimal postoperative inflammation and no serious long-term consequences.[16]

Iris Expansion Retractors

Iris retractor hooks are available in 4-0 (Katena, FCI, and Oasis) and 6-0 (Alcon/Grieshaber) prolene. They come pre-

shaped and packaged in sets of five or six. Four or five hooks are placed through small, short, peripheral corneal stab incisions and then positioned to engage the iris sphincter. The hooks are then sequentially retracted to expand the iris[5,6,17–24] (Fig. 3.4). Each retractor has a small movable flange that is tightened once the hook is in position to maintain the hook's position and the pupil shape throughout the surgery. Once the IOL is in place, the hooks are disengaged from the iris sphincter and carefully removed. One version of the 4-0 prolene retractors is reusable, while the others are single-use.

Generally, viscoelastic and the main incision and paracentesis for the cataract surgery are placed prior to positioning the hooks. The preferred shape for the pupil is a diamond shape, where one of the hooks is placed beneath or just adjacent to the main incision. This shape prevents having the iris "bridge" anterior to the main incision, which can lead to iris prolapse during steps such as hydrodissection of the nucleus or viscoelastic instillation.

Cautions

Prior to placing the hooks, any posterior synechiae should be released by sweeping with a viscoelastic cannula. Care should be taken to avoid over-retracting the iris to avoid radial iris tears or reduction in pupil function.[25] Throughout the case, the hooks should be monitored to avoid engaging the anterior edge of the capsulorhexis.

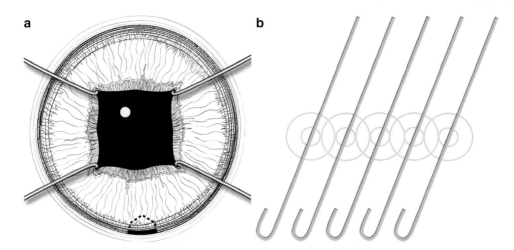

Fig. 3.4 (**a**) Iris retractors in place. (**b**) The appearance of iris retractors; FCI Ophthalmics IR-1005 iris retractors, courtesy of FCI Ophthalmics, Marshfield Hills, MA

Advantages

The surgeon has complete control over the size of the pupil expansion by adjustment of the retractors. This is not the case for the iris expansion rings that come in fixed diameters. Compared with the rings, retractors are less likely to cause corneal endothelial trauma and are easier to use in shallow anterior chambers or very small pupils. Retractors are an excellent choice for eyes with likely IFIS and are best placed prior to the development of the floppy iris and before the capsulorhexis. Retractors have been shown to take approximately 5 minutes to place, due to the need for multiple incisions, more than the time taken for the other techniques or devices.[5] Retractors are generally less expensive than rings, and one type can be reused.

Pupil Expansion Rings

There are several different designs of rings that can be placed to expand and retain the pupil throughout cataract surgery.[5,26–29] Most are best placed with an inserter, but some can be placed manually if desired. They differ in bulk, rigidity, and the amount of pupil expansion. See Table 3.2.

In general, the technique involves insertion of the inserter through the main incision and slow injection of the device engaging the distal pupil sphincter, taking care not to touch the corneal endothelium with the device. Usually a second instrument through the paracentesis is used to place the iris in the channel, arms, or rings of the device to allow for a round expansion of the pupil. The Morcher (Fig. 3.5a, b), Graether (Fig. 3.6a, b), and Perfect Pupil (Fig. 3.7a, b), due to their bulk, all have a gap in the ring that is placed at the main incision to allow for the phacoemulsification probe to travel unimpeded to the cataract. The Malyugin ring (Fig. 3.8a, b), made of thin 5-0 prolene, is less bulky and shaped in a continuous ring, so it needs to be placed in a diamond configuration to minimize iris prolapse. Except for the Malyugin ring, removal is performed manually.

Cautions

The rings can be bulky and difficult to use in relatively shallow anterior chambers or in very small pupils. Care

Table 3.2 Pupil expansion rings[5,26–29]

Pupil expansion ring	Material	Diameter of expansion	Inserter	Gap for phaco probe	Removal technique
Morcher 5S (FCI)	PMMA	5 mm	Optional Geuder injector, reusable	Gap	Manual removal, grasping tip
Graether pupil expander (Eagle Vision)	Silicone	6.3 mm	Disposable	Gap	Strap to enable removal
Perfect pupil (Miravella)	Polyurethane	8 mm	Disposable	Gap	With handle outside incision
Malyugin ring (MicroSurgical Technology)	5-0 prolene	Approx. 6 mm	Disposable	No gap	Use inserter to grasp and remove

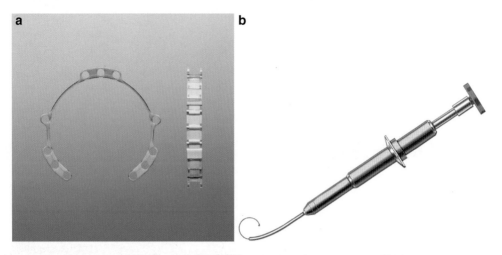

Fig. 3.5 (**a**) Morcher 5S pupil dilator and (**b**) Geuder pupil dilator injector. Figures courtesy of FCI Ophthalmics, Marshfield Hills, MA

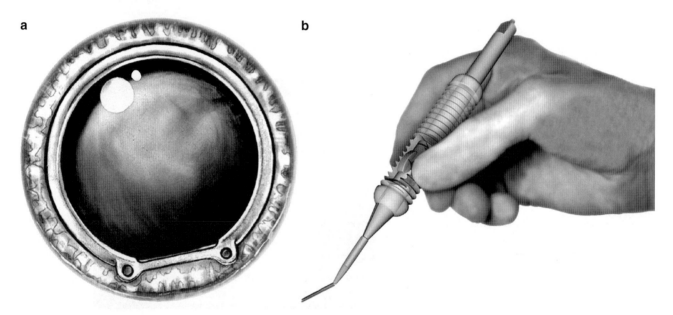

Fig. 3.6 (**a**) Graether 2000 pupil expander and (**b**) injector. Figures courtesy of Eagle Vision, Memphis, TN

must be taken to orient the rings properly to allow for the phacoemulsification probe. Corneal endothelial damage can occur from trauma, which can be minimized by careful handling and copious viscoelastic. Some of the devices produce an extremely large pupil dilation that, besides being unnecessary in most cases, can traumatize atrophic irides. Similar to iris retractors, the iris expansion rings should be placed prior to the capsulorhexis. The devices are not reusable and can be costly.

Advantages

No additional incisions are required. Once placed, the rings provide a very stable pupil expansion within the iris plane.

The flange of the rings protects the pupil margin from trauma by the phacoemulsification and aspiration tips. The Morcher 5S ring placement was shown to take approximately 3 miutes of surgical time, intermediate to manual stretching and iris retractor placement.[5]

Other Intraoperative Challenges in Eyes with Small Pupils

Iris Prolapse

Iris prolapse through the corneal incisions can be minimized by fashioning proper incision architecture. A too peripheral or too short corneal incision will be prone to iris prolapse.

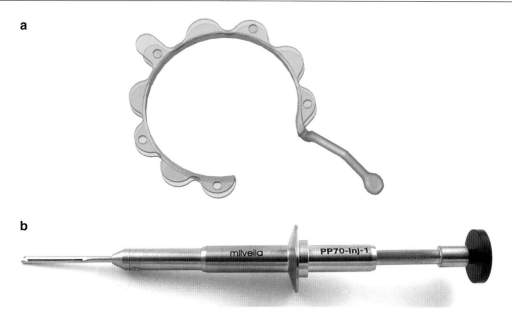

Fig. 3.7 (**a**) Perfect Pupil device and (**b**) injector. Figures courtesy of Ambler Surgical, Exton, PA

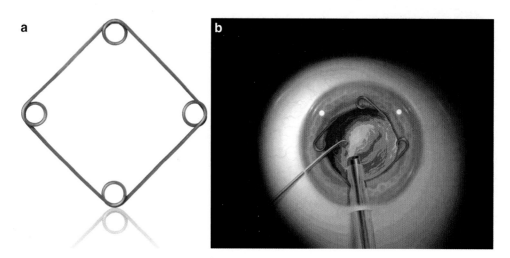

Fig. 3.8 (**a**) Malyugin ring and (**b**) inserted ring. Figures courtesy of MicroSurgical Technology (MST), Redmond, WA

However, fragile irides, after manual stretching or even in the presence of iris retractors or rings, may continue to prolapse. The surgeon should avoid overfilling with viscoelastic and gently perform hydrodissection to avoid prolapse during the initial stages of surgery. If prolapse does occur during the capsulorhexis, the surgeon may decide to complete the capsulorhexis while the visibility is still good and then proceed to managing the prolapse. The first maneuver to manage iris prolapse should be to decompress the anterior chamber by releasing viscoelastic by depressing the paracentesis. Once decompressed, if there is only a small amount of prolapse, massaging the cornea just anterior to the incision may allow the iris to spontaneously reposition itself. Otherwise, sweeping with a cannula from one side of the incision and gently repositing the iris will often be successful, as long as

the eye is soft. If this maneuver is unsuccessful, the surgeon may need to use an instrument or cannula inserted through the paracentesis and sweep the iris gently internally, taking extreme care to avoid an iridodialysis. Once the iris is safely inside the eye, a small bolus of dispersive viscoelastic can be placed just on top of the subincisional iris to allow the surgeon to move safely on to the next phase of the surgery. Refilling of the anterior chamber with viscoelastic will cause a recurrence of the iris prolapse, and the surgeon will have to repeat all the previous steps. Inserting the phaco tip bevel down, and subsequently the IOL cartridge bevel up, may minimize iris incarceration in the respective tips. Also, starting irrigation once the phaco tip is introduced into the anterior chamber may help avoid recurrent iris prolapse. The surgeon should carefully inspect the incisions at the conclusion of surgery to ensure that there are no strands of iris incarcerated in the wounds.

Cortex Removal

An iris manipulator instrument through the paracentesis can be used to retract the iris and inspect for residual nucleus or cortical remnants. Bimanual cortical removal instruments are useful for retrieving subincisional cortex.

Postoperative Care

Eyes that have undergone iris manipulation of any sort are more prone to postoperative inflammation and are therefore more at risk for developing cystoid macular edema (CME). Preoperative and postoperative NSAIDs can help reduce inflammation and the incidence of CME. Usually patients will require more frequent and longer duration postoperative corticosteroid dosing. Surgeons may consider using subconjunctival or intracameral steroids at the conclusion of surgery. If adequate postoperative treatment is used, it is rare to see these irides develop posterior synechiae to the capsule or IOL.

Postoperative intraocular pressure spikes may occur in any eye, but particularly in eyes with preexisting glaucoma, and in eyes with more intraocular manipulations. High-risk eyes may be treated with topical medications or systemic carbonic anhydrase inhibitors at the conclusion of surgery. Patients should be instructed to call with symptoms of headache, nausea, or vomiting. On the first postoperative day, the surgeon can perform a release of aqueous through the paracentesis in eyes with serious spikes.

Depending on the status of the sphincter and dilator muscle, the pupil may or may not dilate and constrict normally or pharmacologically postoperatively. However, if a radial iris tear past the sphincter has occurred, a permanently irregular pupil may result. Often the pupil will resume a normal round shape early postoperatively following the careful use of the above surgical techniques.

Summary

It is common to encounter poor pupil dilation in eyes with glaucoma and cataract. Small pupils increase the risk of surgical complications, but can be successfully managed with a variety of techniques. Careful preoperative assessment and planning by the surgeon will enhance the likelihood of success of the cataract surgery.

References

1. Chang DF, Campbell JR. Intraoperative floppy iris syndrome associated with tamsulosin. *J Cataract Refract Surg.* 2005;31: 664–673.
2. Bendel RE, Phillips MB. Preoperative use of atropine to prevent intraoperative floppy-iris syndrome in patients taking tamsulosin. *J Cataract Refract Surg.* 2006;32:1603–1605.
3. Chang DF, Osher RH, Wang L, Koch DD. Prospective multicenter evaluation of cataract surgery in patients taking tamsulosin (Flomax). *Ophthalmology.* 2007;114:957–964.
4. Manvikar S, Allen D. Cataract surgery management in patients taking tamsulosin: staged approach. *J Cataract Refract Surg.* 2006;32:1611–1614.
5. Akman A, Yilmaz G, Oto S, Akova Y. Comparison of various pupil dilatation methods for phacoemulsification in eyes with a small pupil secondary to pseudoexfoliation. *Ophthalmology.* 2004;111:1693–1698.
6. Goldman JM, Karp CL. Adjunct devices for managing challenging cases in cataract surgery: pupil expansion and stabilization of the capsular bag. *Curr Opinion Ophthalmol.* 2007;18:44–51.
7. Rozenberg I, Seabra FP. Avoiding iris trauma from phacoemulsification in eyes with iridoschisis. *J Cataract Refract Surg.* 2004;30:741–745.
8. Smith GT, Liu CSC. Flexible iris hooks for phacoemulsification in patients with iridoschisis. *J Cataract Refract Surg.* 2000;26: 1277–1280.
9. Auffarth GU, Reuland AJ, Heger T, Volcker HE. Cataract surgery in eyes with iridoschisis using the perfect pupil iris extension system. *J Cataract Refract Surg.* 2005;31:1877–1880.
10. O'Brien PD, Fitzpatrick P, William Power W. Patient pain during stretching of small pupils in phacoemulsification performed using topical anesthesia. *J Cataract Refract Surg.* 2005;31:1760–1763.
11. Lundberg B, Behndig A. Intracameral mydriatics in phacoemulsification cataract surgery. *J Cataract Refract Surg.* 2003;29: 2366–2371.
12. Lundberg B, Behndig A. Separate and additive mydriatic effects of lidocaine hydrochloride, phenylephrine, and cyclopentolate after intracameral injection. *J Cataract Refract Surg.* 2008;34: 280–283.
13. Thaller VT, Kulshrestha MK, Bell K. The effect of preoperative topical flurbiprofen or diclofenac on pupil dilatation. *Eye.* 2000;14:642–645.
14. Srinivasan R, Madhavaranga MS. Topical ketorolac tromethamine 0.5% versus diclofenac sodium 0.1% to inhibit miosis during cataract surgery. *J Cataract Refract Surg.* 2002;28:517–520.
15. Bacskulin A, Kundt G, Guthoff R. Efficiency of pupillary stretching in cataract surgery. *Eur J Ophthalmol.* 1998;8: 230–233.
16. Shingleton BJ, Campbell CA, O'Donoghue MW. Effects of pupil stretch technique during phacoemulsification on postoperative vision, intraocular pressure, and inflammation. *J Cataract Refract Surg.* 2006;32:1142–1145.
17. Mackool RJ. Small pupil enlargement during cataract extraction: a new method. *J Cataract Refract Surg.* 1992;18:523–526.
18. De Juan E, Hickingbotham D. Flexible iris retractor. *Am J Ophthalmol.* 1991;111:776–777.
19. Novak J. Flexible iris hooks for phacoemulsification. *J Cataract Refract Surg.* 1997;23:828–831.
20. Dada T, Sethi HS, Sharma N, Dada V. Using nylon hooks during small-pupil phacoemulsification. *J Cataract Refract Surg.* 2003;29:412–413.
21. Birchall W, Spencer AF. Misalignment of flexible iris hook retractors for small pupil cataract surgery: effects on pupil circumference. *J Cataract Refract Surg.* 2001;27:20–24.

22. Nichamin LD. Enlarging the pupil for cataract extraction using flexible nylon iris retractors. *J Cataract Refract Surg.* 1993;19:793–796.

23. Dupps WJ, Oetting TA. Diamond iris retractor configuration for small-pupil extracapsular or intracapsular cataract surgery. *J Cataract Refract Surg.* 2004;30:2473–2475.

24. Oetting TA, Omphroy LC. Modified technique using flexible iris retractors in clear corneal cataract surgery. *J Cataract Refract Surg.* 2002;28:596–598.

25. Yoguchi T, Oshika T, Sawaguchi S, Kaiya T. Pupillary functions after cataract surgery using flexible iris retractors in patients with small pupil. *Jpn J Ophthalmol.* 1999;43:2–24.

26. Kershner RM. Management of the small pupil for clear corneal cataract surgery. *J Cataract Refract Surg.* 2002;28:1826–1831.

27. Graether JM. Graether pupil expander for managing the small pupil during surgery. *J Cataract Refract Surg.* 1996;22:530–535.

28. Malyugin B. Small pupil phaco surgery: a new technique. *Ann Ophthalmol.* 2007;39:185–193.

29. Chang DF. Use of Malyugin pupil expansion device for intraoperative floppy-iris syndrome: results in 30 consecutive cases. *J Cataract Refract Surg.* 2008;34:835–841.

30. Blouin MC, Blouin J, Perreault S, Lapointe A, Dragomir A. Intraoperative floppy-iris syndrome associated with alpha1-adrenoreceptors: comparison of tamsulosin and alfuzosin. *J Cataract Refract Surg.* 2007;33:1227–1234.

31. Oshika T, Ohashi Y, Inamura M, et al. Incidence of intraoperative floppy iris syndrome in patients on either systemic or topical alpha(1)-adrenoceptor antagonist. *Am J Ophthalmol.* 2007;143:150–151.

32. Chadha V, Borooah S, Tey A, Styles C, Singh J. Floppy iris behaviour during cataract surgery: associations and variations. *Br J Ophthalmol.* 2007;91:40–42.

Chapter 4

Small Incision Cataract Surgery and Glaucoma

Brooks J. Poley, Richard L. Lindstrom, Thomas W. Samuelson, and Richard R. Schulze Jr.

Introduction and Pathogenesis

Ida Mann[1] completed her treatise on embryogenesis of the eye and the crystalline lens in 1957. She described the stages of development of the human lens as follows: "It will be seen that the first indication of its position is given by the thickening known as the lens plate, which soon develops the lens pit on its surface. This deepens to form the lens vesicle, at first attached to the surface by the lens stalk, but subsequently becoming separated. The cells of the anterior walls of the lens vesicle form the subcapsular epithelium, while those of the posterior wall elongate to form the primary lens fibers, which fill the cavity of the lens vesicle, and constitute the central region, recognized as the most translucent part of the adult lens and known to slit-lamp workers as the central dark interval. Growth of lens fibers does not cease by 25 years or so. Priestly Smith has shown indeed that it continues throughout life, even into old age."

Since lens cells are of ectodermal origin like skin cells, they continuously divide and cause the crystalline lens to slowly enlarge throughout life.

Francis Heed Adler[2] described lens growth in his Physiology of the Eye, Clinical Application in 1950. "In infancy and early childhood the lens grows like other structures associated with the nervous system, and after this early stage of rapid relative increment it enters a period of slow, steady growth, which continues throughout life. A loss of elasticity is associated with continued growth." Adler's graph shows that the emmetropic lens weight increases from 210 mg at the age of 20 years to 320 mg by the age of 84 years – an increase of 110 mg, or 52%. Another graph shows an increase in emmetropic lens thickness from 4.0 mm at the age of 20 years to 4.8 mm at the age of 65 years, an increase of 0.8 mm, or 20%.

The lens is essentially a dysfunctional organ within the eye at 60 years of age. As the lens ages, the following three changes occur:

- Lens cells are compressed, which causes hardening, so accommodation fails.
- Lens growth repositions the anterior lens capsule and the anterior uvea (iris and anterior ciliary body) forward, compressing the trabecular meshwork and the canal of Schlemm, so intraocular pressure (IOP) elevates.
- The lens begins to cloud causing decreased light transmission, so cataract begins.

Murray Johnstone[3,4] described a new aqueous outflow model involving a mechanical pump in 2004. In "A New Model Describes an Aqueous Outflow Pump and Explores Causes of Pump Failure in Glaucoma," he summarizes that "The aqueous outflow system is structurally organized to act as a mechanical pump. The aqueous outflow system is a part of a vascular circulatory loop. All other vascular circulatory loops return fluids to the heart by pumping action. The trabecular meshwork actively distends and recoils in response to IOP transients such as pulse, blinking, and eye movement. Trabecular meshwork flexibility is essential to normal function"[4] (Fig. 4.1).

Aqueous valves transfer aqueous from the anterior chamber to Schlemm's canal (SC). The valves are oriented circumferentially in SC, and their normal function requires that trabecular tissues retain their ability to recoil from the SC external wall. The aqueous pump provides a short-term pressure control by varying stroke volume in response to pressure changes. The aqueous pump provides long-term pressure control by modulating trabecular meshwork constituents that control stroke volume.

Johnstone describes pump failure because of SC apposition and trabecular stiffening. The trabecular meshwork (TM) stiffening is progressive and becomes irreversible. Clinically visible manifestations of pump failure are lack of pustule aqueous discharge into aqueous veins and gradual failure in the ability to reflux blood into SC.

B.J. Poley (✉)
Department of Ophthalmology, Volunteers in Medicine Clinic, Hilton Head Island, SC 29926, USA
e-mail: scbrooks@hargray.com

S.M. Johnson (ed.), *Cataract Surgery in the Glaucoma Patient*, DOI 10.1007/978-0-387-09408-3_4,
© Springer Science+Business Media, LLC 2009

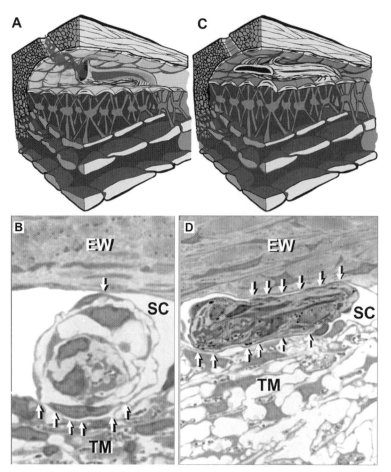

Fig. 4.1 Aqueous vein (70 long) with various degrees of compression against Schlemm's canal (SC) external wall (EW) by trabecular meshwork (TM) at IOP of 25 mmHg. *White arrows* designate areas of compression. Minimal compression (**a,b**). Marked compression with lumen closure (**c,d**). Reprinted from Johnstone[4] by permission of Springer Science + Business Media

This progressive change occurs as the crystalline lens enlarges with age, and its anterior surface moves forward within the eye's anterior segment, compressing the trabecular meshwork and SC. Johnstone further suggests SC lumen enlargement to correct pump failure should be targeted at the sclera spur and its ciliary body attachment without damaging the pump (trabecular meshwork). Cataract extraction by phacoemulsification with implantation of an intraocular lens (Phaco/IOL) accomplishes this by repositioning the anterior lens capsule rearward. This allows the ciliary body to rotate rearward, pivoting around the axis of the sclera spur. Phaco/IOL does not damage the pump. Rather, it allows the pump to re-expand, and regain its earlier function allowing a better facility of outflow.

Susan and Larry Strenk published information on in vivo magnetic resonance imaging (MRI) of the eye in 2006[5] and 2007.[6] Their 2007 publication shows composite images of a 25-year-old and a 49-year-old (Fig. 4.2), and both eyes of a 74-year-old with monocular intraocular artificial lens implantation (Fig. 4.3). Figure 4.2 shows that the anterior surface of the lens is rearward of the canal of Schlemm in a 25-year-old. Lens growth positions the anterior surface of

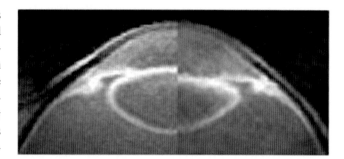

Fig. 4.2 In vivo composite image showing a 49-year-old (*left*) and a 25-year-old (*right*); lens growth displaces the uveal tract anteriorly with age. Figure courtesy of Strenk et al.[5] with permission from Elsevier

the lens to be well forward of the canal of Schlemm in the 74-year-old. The 74-year-old's zonules become lax, and the root of the iris compresses the TM and canal of Schlemm. Now, stiffening of the TM and collapse of the canal of Schlemm's lumen causes aqueous pump failure as described by Johnstone.[4] Higher IOP is the result.

Figure 4.3 shows rearward reorientation of the uveal tract when the enlarged crystalline lens is replaced by the thin

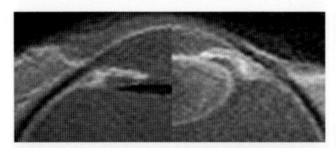

Fig. 4.3 In vivo composite image showing both eyes of a 74-year-old patient with a monocular implantation of the Alcon Acrysof; the uveal tract returns to an anterioposterior position of relative youth with IOL implantation. Figure courtesy of Strenk et al.[5] with permission from Elsevier

artificial lens. Now, the anterior surface of the lens capsule is well rearward of the canal of Schlemm. The iris root no longer compresses the trabecular meshwork and canal of Schlemm, and rearward tension of the zonules increases. The rearward traction of the zonules now expands the trabecular meshwork and the canal of Schlemm. The aqueous pump regains its ability to function properly, and lower IOP results.

The lens, as it ages, could be a major cause of ocular hypertension, a precursor to adult glaucoma. A continuum likely exists between having a normal crystalline lens early in life, and, at its most extreme maturation, developing phacomorphic glaucoma, which is classically defined as angle-closure glaucoma secondary to intumescence of the crystalline lens. See Chapter 20. The elevated IOP associated with the aging crystalline lens, as demonstrated in clinical studies,[7] represents a midpoint in this continuum. The definition of phacomorphic glaucoma could be broadened to recognize the slowly progressive effect the maturing lens may have on IOP. The term "phacomorphic glaucoma" in adults could subsume the traditional categories of open angle, narrow angle, and angle closure.

Phacomorphic ocular hypertension responds well to phacoemulsification with intraocular lens insertion, with benefits proportional to the magnitude of preoperative IOP. Clinical studies further demonstrate that eyes with preexisting glaucoma achieve a similar lowering of IOP with phaco/IOL. The benefit of phacoemulsification with intraocular lens insertion, classically indicated only for visually significant cataracts, may therefore be expanded as an early treatment for "phacomorphic" ocular hypertension and glaucoma (Fig. 4.3).

The Effect of Cataract Surgery on IOP and Anatomy

Hayashi et al. have published on the sustained increased anterior chamber depth and width following cataract surgery,

especially in angle-closure patients.[8] He studied 77 angle-closure eyes, 73 with open angle glaucoma, and 74 control eyes with Scheimpflug photography before and at various intervals following surgery. Steuhl had similar observations in his report on 33 patients with both open and narrow angle glaucoma who had anterior chambers measured by laser tomography.[9] His patients had reduction of IOP and glaucoma medications (Fig. 4.4a, b). There have been several reviews, to be discussed later, of the effect of cataract surgery on IOP in groups of non-glaucomatous and glaucomatous eyes. In one, Shingleton reviewed 297 eyes with pseudoexfoliation (PXF) with 427 eyes without PXF, with 2 years of follow-up.[10] Both groups of eyes experienced a decline of IOP with the PXF group experiencing a greater decrease. This review did not include patients with glaucoma. The authors further investigated this relationship between cataract surgery and IOP.

Surgical Technique

The authors employ small incision temporal clear cornea surgery. The temporal, corneal wound does not disrupt the conjunctiva in a glaucoma patient who may need future filtration surgery or who has already had filtration surgery. Meticulous removal of viscoelastic helps to prevent postoperative IOP elevation, especially important in eyes with compromised optic discs.[11-14]

The management of glaucoma medications preoperatively is discussed in Chapter 1. Many surgeons discontinue prostaglandin analogues and naturally discontinue any miotics that would impede dilation. Many surgeons administer glaucoma medications at the end of surgery and choose these based on their safety for a particular patient. Medications that may be administered at the end of cataract surgery include the following[15-20]:

- Oral or topical carbonic anhydrase inhibitors
- Brimonidine or apraclonidine
- Pilocarpine (or acetylcholine or carbachol intraoperatively)
- Beta blockers such as timolol
- Dorzolamide-timolol fixed combination.

Reviews of Long-Term IOP Reduction of Non-glaucoma and Glaucoma Eyes

Methods

Two retrospective chart reviews of cataract eyes operated with phaco/IOL are presented.[7]

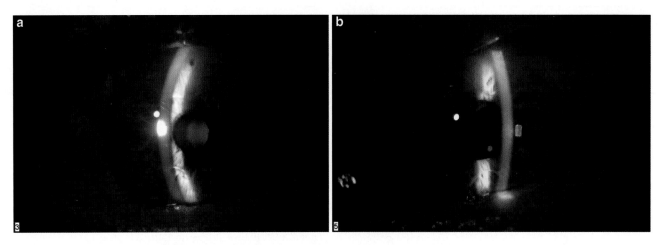

Fig. 4.4 These slit lamp photos are from the same patient. (**a**) Shows the anterior chamber preoperatively and (**b**) shows the deeper anterior chamber post-cataract surgery. The patient also reduced topical glaucoma medications

The first review was of 588 non-glaucomatous eyes[7]: 305 eyes from Minnesota Eye Consultants, Minneapolis, MN, and 283 eyes from Schulze Eye Surgery, Savannah, GA. Findings from these two practices were similar and the two groups were combined for analysis. This review included normotensive and ocular hypertensive (OHT) eyes only. The eyes had no previous glaucoma drops, glaucoma surgery (i.e., iridectomy or trabeculectomy), or laser trabeculoplasty/iridotomy.

The second review[7] included 124 eyes treated for glaucoma: 84 eyes from Minnesota Eye Consultants and 40 eyes from Schulze Eye Surgery. Findings from these two practices were similar and all eyes were combined for analysis. The eyes had glaucoma based on usage of glaucoma drops, and/or history of glaucoma surgery (i.e., iridectomy or trabeculectomy), and/or glaucomatous visual field loss.

Up to three measurements of each IOP were recorded, and the mean IOP of each eye was the IOP value used for Excel (Microsoft) spread sheet for analysis of the means and standard deviations of the grouped IOPs.

Data for each eye were recorded at the time of surgery, 1 year after surgery, and at the final visit. Table 4.1 shows the frequency of the number of eyes followed postoperatively < 1–10 years. Table 4.2 shows that the eyes were stratified and divided into five groups according to their presurgical IOPs. The presurgical IOP ranges of each group are shown.

Results for Non-glaucomatous and OHT Eyes

Table 4.3 and Fig. 4.5 show that the final mean IOP reduction of all 588 eyes without glaucoma was −1.6 mmHg/10%. However, stratifying the eyes according to their presurgi-

Table 4.1 Frequency of eyes in each postoperative year

PO years	Frequency	Percent	Cumulative percent
0	19	3.2	3.2
1	66	11.2	14.5
2	99	16.8	31.1
3	68	11.6	42.9
4	51	8.7	51.5
5	58	9.9	61.4
6	55	9.4	70.7
7	68	11.6	82.3
8	58	9.9	92.2
9	42	7.7	99.3
10	3	.7	100.0
Total	588	100.0	

Table 4.2 Range of presurgical IOPs

Range of presurgical IOPs in mmHg: high to low in each group	
Non-glaucoma eyes	Glaucoma eyes
31–23	29–23
22–20	22–20
19–18	19–18
17–15	17–15
14–9	14–5

cal IOPs revealed eyes with the highest IOP (i.e., range 23–31 mmHg) had the greatest final mean IOP reduction, −6.5 mmHg/27%. Eyes with the lowest preoperative IOP (range 9–14 mmHg) had insignificant final mean IOP elevation, +0.2 mmHg/0%. Figure 4.6 shows bar graphs of the presurgical mean IOPs and final mean IOPs of the eyes without glaucoma. It reveals that the two highest presurgical IOP groups were OHT eyes with mean IOPs of 24.5 and 20.9 mmHg. After surgery, these IOPs decreased, and the final mean IOPs were normotensive and measured 18.0 and

Table 4.3 Results: mean IOP reduction of all 588 non-glaucoma eyes

Non-glaucoma eyes sorted according to their presurgical IOP range in mmHg

Measure	IOP range	n	Mean Age years	PO years	IOP surgery	IOP 1 year	Change 1 year	IOP final	Change final (%)
	31–23	19	69.3	2.4	24.5	17.8	–6.7	18.0	–6.5/27
	22–20	62	70.9	4.6	20.9	15.8	–5.10	16.1	–4.8/22
	19–18	86	67.4	4.9	18.3	15.5	–2.8	15.8	–2.5/14
	17–15	223	71.2	4.7	15.9	14.6	–1.4	14.3	–1.6/10
	14–9	198	70.5	4.2	12.7	13.1	+0.4	12.9	+0.2/0
Total	31–9	588	70.3	4.5	16.0	14.5	–1.5	14.4	–1.6/10

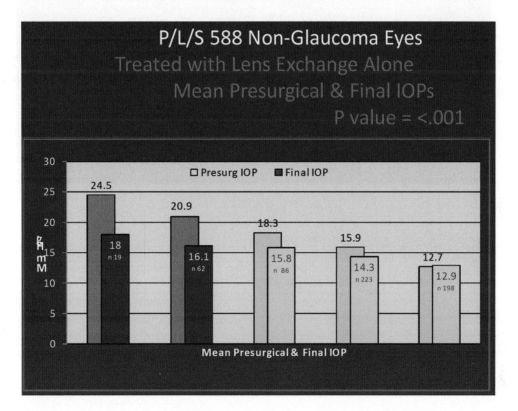

Fig. 4.5 Presurgical and final IOPs of the P/L/S study of 588 non-glaucoma eyes treated by lens exchange alone

16.1 mmHg, respectively. Eyes with the lowest presurgical mean IOP of 12.7 mmHg had a marginal mean IOP elevation to 12.9 mmHg after surgery.

Results for Eyes with Glaucoma

Table 4.4 shows that the final mean IOP reduction of the 124 eyes with glaucoma was –2.75 mmHg/15%, which is consistent with the data reported previously by Kim et al.[21] The Kim study reviewed 31 consecutive cataract surgeries in eyes with open angle glaucoma. The mean IOP change was –2.9 mmHg with a decrease in medications from a mean of 1.7 to a mean of 0.7, with a mean follow-up of 16.4 months. However, stratifying the eyes in our study according to their presurgical mean IOP revealed eyes with the highest IOP (23–29 mmHg) had the greatest final mean IOP reduction, –8.4 mmHg/34%. Eyes with the lowest preoperative IOP (5–14 mmHg) had final mean IOP elevation, +1.9 mmHg/15%. Figure 4.5 shows bar graphs of presurgical mean IOPs and final mean IOPs from the groups of eyes with glaucoma. It shows that two subsets of eyes with the highest presurgical IOP had presurgical mean IOPs of 24.7 and 20.7 mmHg. The presurgical IOPs of these subsets were recorded with the patients using maximal tolerated therapy of glaucoma drops, prior iridectomies/iridotomies, or even prior trabeculectomies. After surgery, their final mean IOP became 16.3 mmHg and 16.1 mmHg, respectively, and showed improved glaucoma control. Eyes with the lowest presurgical mean IOP of 11.6 mmHg had a mean IOP elevation to 13.4 mmHg. However, this final mean IOP level of 13.4 mmHg remained satisfactory for glaucoma control.

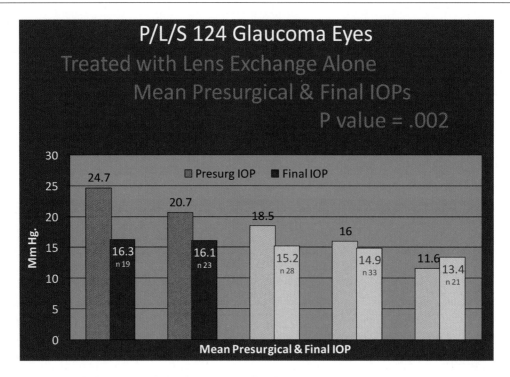

Fig. 4.6 Presurgical and final IOPs for a cohort of 124 glaucoma eyes of the P/L/S study treated by lens exchange alone

Table 4.4 Results: mean IOP reduction of all 124 glaucoma eyes

Glaucoma eyes sorted according to their presurgical IOP range in mmHg

	IOP range	n	Mean Age years	PO years	IOP surgery	IOP 1 year	Change 1 year	IOP final	Change final (%)
	29–23	17	73.3	5.8	24.7	18.7	–6.0	16.3	–8.4/34
	22–20	23	72.8	5.0	20.7	17.0	–3.7	16.1	–4.6/22
	19–18	28	75.4	4.6	18.5	15.8	–2.7	15.2	–3.3/18
	17–15	33	78.0	3.2	16.0	14.4	–1.6	14.9	–1.0/16
	14–5	23	76.3	4.6	11.6	12.9	+1.3	13.4	+1.9/16
Total		124	75.5	4.5	17.8	15.4	–2.4	15.1	–2.7/15

Medical Treatment of Glaucoma After Surgery

The mean number of drops was 1.3 before surgery and was 1.0 after surgery, representing a 23% reduction. No trabeculectomies, iridectomies/iridotomies, or laser trabeculoplasty procedures were done after phaco/IOL surgery.

Glaucoma Diagnosis

Table 4.5 shows mean IOP levels of eyes that had presurgical iridectomies, OAG eyes with no prior procedure, or presurgical trabeculectomies before phaco/IOL. Eyes with prior iridectomies/iridotomies were considered narrow angle glaucoma (NAG) types, while those without were considered open angle glaucoma (OAG) patients. NAG eyes had

a presurgical mean IOP of 20 mmHg and a mean IOP reduction of –6.2 mmHg (31%) to a final mean IOP of 13.8 mmHg. OAG eyes had a mean presurgical IOP of 18.1 mmHg and a mean IOP reduction of –2.4 mmHg (14%) to a final mean IOP of 15.7 mmHg. Eyes with prior trabeculectomies had a presurgical mean IOP of 14.3 mmHg and a mean IOP reduction of –0.3 mmHg (2%) to a final mean IOP of 14.0 mmHg.

Table 4.5 shows that NAG eyes had the highest presurgical mean IOP and the greatest mean IOP reduction to the lowest final mean IOP. POAG eyes had moderate mean presurgical IOP and moderate mean IOP reduction to the highest final mean IOP. Eyes with prior trabeculectomies had lowest presurgical mean IOP and essentially no mean IOP reduction. Table 4.6 shows IOP changes of eyes with trabeculectomies prior to phaco/IOL sorted according to their presurgical IOP. The three groups of eyes with the highest presurgical mean IOPs, from 18 mmHg to 24 mmHg, had mean IOP

Table 4.5 Mean IOP changes with iridectomies, iridotomies, or trabeculectomies

Mean IOP changes of eyes that had iridectomies/iridotomies or trabeculectomies before phaco/IOL

Event and condition	n	Age years	PO years	IOP surgery	IOP 1 year	Change 1 year	IOP final	Change final (%)
PI[a] NAG	12	76.3	5.2	20.0	16.0	−4.0	13.8	−6.2/31
None[b] POAG	91	74.5	4.0	18.1	15.7	−2.4	15.7	−2.4/14
Trabeculectomy	21	76.0	6.5	14.3	13.2	−1.1	14.0	−0.3/2
Total	124	75.5	4.5	17.8	15.4	−2.4	15.1	−2.7/15

[a]Eyes with prior iridectomy/iridotomy are considered narrow angle glaucoma.

[b]Eyes with no prior iridectomy/iridotomy are considered primary open angle glaucoma.

Table 4.6 Eyes with trabeculectomies before phaco/IOL

Eyes with trabeculectomies before phaco/IOL surgery sorted according to their presurgical IOP

IOP range	"n"	Age years	PO years	IOP surgery	IOP 1 year	Change 1 year	IOP final	Change final (%)
24	1	71	9.0	24.0	22	−2.0	18	−6.0/25
22–20	3	73	5.0	20.0	16	−4.0	15.3	−4.7/23
19–18	4	76	5.5	18.5	14.8	−3.7	13.5	−5.0/27
17–15	4	73	6.8	16.5	13.8	−2.7	15.5	−1.0/6
14–5	9	74	6.4	9.5	11.0	+1.5	12.6	+3.1/32
Total	21	76.0	6.5	14.3	13.2	−0.9	14.0	−0.3/2

reductions between −4.7 and −6.0 mmHg. The two groups of eyes with prior trabeculectomies with the lowest presurgical mean IOPs from 9.5 to 16.5 mmHg had a mean IOP reduction of −1.0 and a mean IOP elevation of +1.6 mmHg, respectively.

Discussion

In our case review, IOP reduction of non-glaucoma and glaucoma eyes following phaco/IOL surgery was proportional to their presurgical IOP as seen in Figs. 4.2 and 4.3.

Figures 4.7 and 4.8 show bar graphs of presurgical and final mean IOPs including multiple published studies of patients undergoing cataract surgery and our study (P/L/S).[7] The studies were reported as follows:

- Ge et al.[22] angle-closure glaucoma (ACG) eyes in 2001
- Euswas et al.[23] ACG eyes in 2005
- Hayashi et al. ACG[8] and open angle glaucoma (OAG) in 2001[24]
- Lai et al.[25] ACG in 2006
- Shingleton et al.[10] glaucoma eyes in 2006
- Mathalone et al.[26] OAG in 2005, and
- Tham et al.[27] chronic angle-closure glaucoma (CACG) – medically controlled in 2008.
- Suzuki et al.[28] eyes without glaucoma in 1997
- Tong et al.[29] eyes without glaucoma in1999
- Tennen[30] eyes without glaucoma in 1996
- Issa[31] eyes without glaucoma in 2005.

The five groups of P/L/S eyes were sorted according to their presurgical mean IOPs and were inserted between the bar graphs of the data from earlier reports, also arranged according to their presurgical IOP levels. Figure 4.7 shows the bar graphs for the patients in each study that did not have glaucoma. They are arranged by preoperative IOP from highest to lowest.

In Fig. 4.8 there are six bar graphs of eyes with presurgical mean IOPs greater than 20 mmHg. Four bar graphs represent data from earlier reports and two are of P/L/S's groups of eyes. All have mean IOP reductions and final IOPs were 12.0, 16.3, 17.1, 15.0, 16.1, and 16.4 mmHg. The eyes from earlier reports and P/L/S's glaucoma eyes with marginal IOP control with mean IOPs greater than 20 mmHg before surgery became eyes with improved IOP control after surgery with mean IOP less than 19 mmHg.

The three bar graphs of the earlier reports with the highest presurgical mean IOPs were ACG eyes.[8,22,23] ACG eyes have the largest crystalline lenses and/or smaller crowded anterior segments. We conclude that these enlarged lenses cause the shallowest anterior chambers, compressed trabecular meshwork, and collapsed canals of Schlemm.[7] It is hypothesized that, since the outflow channels are most compressed by these large lenses, these outflow facilities are the most compromised and this compression causes the high presurgical pressures.[32] Since phaco/IOL allows the anterior uveal tissue to return to a rearward position of its former youth,[32] we conclude that compression of the outflow channels is relieved.[7] The facility of outflow improves, and the greatest IOP reductions occur, allowing normotensive IOPs to be maintained thereafter.[31] The predominant factor determining the amount of IOP reduction after phaco/IOL is the presurgical IOP, which could be related to the size of the "phacomorphic" crystalline lens.[7] This is also supported by the series by Hayashi where the effect of cataract surgery was compared between ACG and OAG cohorts.[8] Hayashi

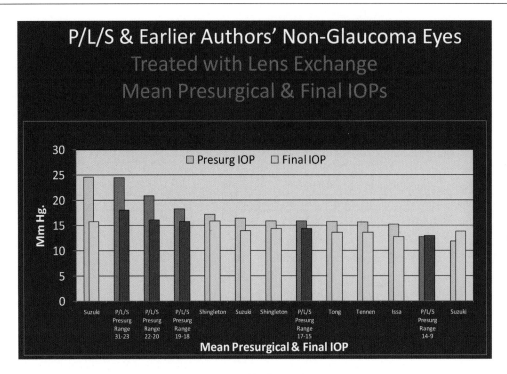

Fig. 4.7 Combined studies showing IOPs of non-glaucoma eyes treated by lens exchange

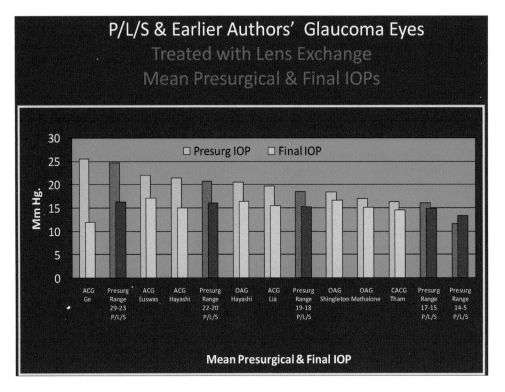

Fig. 4.8 Presurgical and Final Mean IOP from other studies and the authors' P/L/S study

has also reported on the effect of cataract surgery on a cohort of angle closure (ACG) and open angle glaucoma (OAG) patients. The mean preoperative IOP level was the same for each group, with a larger standard deviation in the OAG group (3.9 versus 5.4). Both groups experienced a decrease in mean IOP and number of medications, but the mean decrease in IOP and percentage of IOP reduction was greater in the ACG group. After 2 years of follow-up, the ACG cohort had a better survival probability of almost 92% versus the 72% in the OAG group. Over 40% of the ACG group had IOP control without medications versus 19% in the OAG.[24] Cataract surgery in ACG is discussed further in Chapter 18.

Long-Term Effect of Cataract Surgery on IOP

Figure 4.9 shows that the mean IOP of the group of eyes without glaucoma was decreased 1 year after phaco/IOL surgery and at the final IOP measurement (1–10 years post-op, average 4.5 years) compared to the preoperative mean IOP. Again, eyes with the highest presurgical IOP range (23–31 mmHg) had the greatest mean IOP reductions (–6.0 mmHg at 1 year and –6.5 mmHg/27% at final measurement). Eyes with the lowest presurgical IOP range (14–9 mmHg) had slight mean IOP elevations (+0.4 mmHg at 1 year, and +0.2 mmHg/0% at final measurement). Figure 4.10 shows mean IOP changes 1 year after phaco/IOL surgery for eyes with glaucoma and at the final IOP measurement (1–10 years post-op, average 4.5 years). Eyes with the lowest presurgical IOP range (5–14 mmHg) had mean IOP elevations (+1.3 mmHg at 1 year and +1.9 mmHg/16% at final measurement). Eyes with the highest presurgical IOP range (23–29 mmHg), mean of 24.7 mmHg, had the greatest mean IOP reductions: –6.0 mmHg at 1 year and –8.4 mmHg/34% at the final measurement, with a range of –2 to –16 mmHg. This is depicted in Table 4.7 where the results for these 19 eyes are listed individually.

Figures 4.9 and 4.10 show that in eyes with and without glaucoma the mean long-term IOP change after phaco/IOL surgery were essentially the same. IOP reductions achieved at 1 year were maintained for up to 10 years of the study. In the long term, the same trend continued with IOP reductions after surgery being proportional to the presurgical IOPs. Eyes with the highest presurgical IOPs had the greatest IOP reductions. There is always a concern over loss of IOP con-

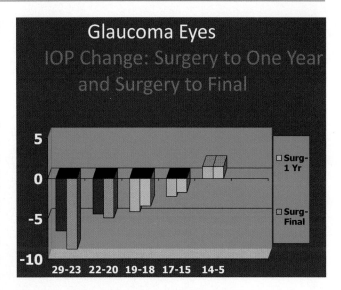

Fig. 4.10 Mean IOP change at 1 year and at final reading for eyes with glaucoma

trol following cataract surgery, and Tables 4.8 and 4.9 show that all eyes with IOP above 23 mmHg had IOP reductions, none elevated.

Figure 4.11 shows the mean IOP reduction of 34 eyes 1 year post-op, and the mean IOP reductions 6 through 10 years post-op of the same eyes. Eyes were again sorted according to their presurgical mean IOPs. The eyes with the highest preoperative IOP levels showed mean IOP reduction of –7.3 mmHg 6 through 10 years post-op. Figure 4.11 shows that the mean IOP reductions of eyes in the highest presurgical IOP group were greater in the sixth through tenth year post-op than they were in their first year post-op.

Table 4.8 shows the frequency of OHT eyes (defined as IOP 20 mmHg and higher) pre-surgery, at 1 year, and at the final visit. There were 81 eyes with IOP 20 mmHg or over preoperatively, 24 at 1 year, and 21 at the final reading of IOP. The highest IOP before surgery was 31, and after surgery the highest was 24 mmHg. Table 4.9 shows the frequency of glaucoma eyes with IOPs ≥20 mmHg: 40 before surgery, 12 at 1 year after surgery, and 9 at the final measurement. Highest IOP before surgery is 29 mmHg. Highest IOP after surgery is 23 mmHg.

Phaco/IOL kept the number of OHT eyes from increasing over the 10 years of the study; 60 of 81 OHT eyes (74%) with IOPs ≥20 mmHg before surgery converted to normotensive eyes with IOPs ≤19 mmHg after surgery at the final measurement. This is likely due to the restoration of the anatomy of the eye's anterior segment to a position of its former youth[32] as discussed previously. The improvement in the anterior segment anatomy has been shown in angle-closure eyes by Nonaka et al.[33] using ultrasound bimicroscopy (UBM) and as discussed previously by Hayashi[8] using Scheimpflug videophotography and Steuhl using laser tomography.[9]

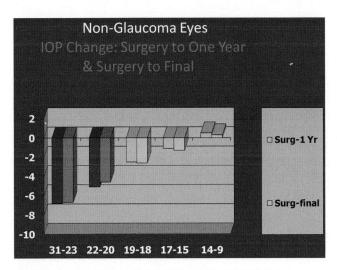

Fig. 4.9 One year IOP change for eyes without glaucoma

Table 4.7 IOP reductions in glaucoma eyes following phaco/IOL

Glaucoma eye's IOP reductions following phaco/IOL surgery

Eyes sorted according to their presurgical IOP: range 29–23 mmHg, $n = 19$

	Age years	Years PO	IOP surgery	IOP 1 year	Change 1 year	IOP final	Final change
	76	6	29	16	−13	13	−16
	76	9	27	13	−14	18	−9
	80	11	27	15	−12	16	−11
	53	5	27	24	−3	14	−13
	80	7	25	22	−3	23	−2
	68	2	25	27	+2	21	−4
	69	8	25	23	−2	21	−4
	68	3	25	19	−6	18	−7
	66	9	25	20	−5	11	−14
	71	9	24	22	−2	21	−3
	71	9	24	22	−2	18	−6
	78	5	24	16	−2	17	−7
	64	3	24	22	−2	16	−8
	87	1	24	16	−8	16	−8
	76	9	24	12	−12	12	−12
	70	4	23	22	−1	21	−2
	84	8	23	19	−4	16	−7
	81	5	23	13	−10	13	−10
	76	6	23	13	−10	9	−14
Mean	73.1	6.3	24.7	18.7	−6.0	16.3	−8.4

Table 4.8 Frequency of presurgical IOPs 20 mmHg and higher in OHT eyes

Frequency of OHT eyes with presurgical IOPs 20 mmHg and higher

	IOP frequencies (n)		
Presurgical IOP mmHg	No. of presurgical eyes	No. of eyes at 1 year	No. of eyes at final
20	25	12	12
21	19	5	5
22	18	3	1
23	9	2	1
24	4	2	2
25	2		
27	3	1	
31	1		
No. of OHT eyes	81/100%	24/30%	21/26%
No. of OHT Eyes Become Normotensive		57/70%	60/74%

Table 4.9 Presurgical IOPs 20 mmHg and higher in glaucoma eyes

Frequency of glaucoma eyes with presurgical IOPs 20 mmHg and higher

	IOP frequencies (n)		
Presurgical IOP mmHg	No. of presurgical eyes	No. of eyes at 1 year	No. of eyes at final
20	12	2	5
21	5	2	3
22	6	6	
23	4		1
24	6	1	
25	4		
27	2	1	
29	1		
Total no of eyes	40/100%	12/33%	9/22%
After surgery: no. of eye's IOPs become ≤ 19 mmHg		28/70%	31/78%

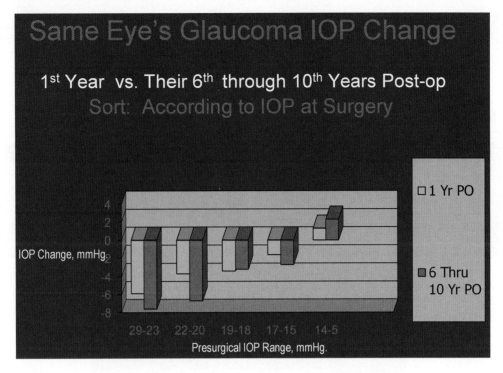

Fig. 4.11   IOP changes for the same glaucoma eyes at 1 year, and 6 through 10 years following surgery

Phaco/IOL also helped 31 of 40 glaucoma eyes (78%) with IOPs ≥20 mmHg before surgery to become eyes with IOPs ≤19 mmHg after surgery, at the final measurement. Detailed history of glaucoma medication use was not included in the study. Phaco/IOL has the same effect on the IOP of glaucoma eyes after surgery as it has the IOP of OHT eyes after surgery. There were 26 and 22% of eyes with IOP that remained over 20 in the glaucoma and OHT groups, respectively.

Effect of Age on IOP Control with Cataract Surgery

Figure 4.12 a, b, and c show 1-year and final IOP changes following phaco/IOL of three age groups segregated by decade: 80 years and older, 70–79 years, and 69 years and younger. Figure 4.12 a, b, and c showed IOP reductions following phaco/IOL were essentially the same for eyes of all three age groups. The effect of cataract surgery on IOP for racial differences was not assessed.

Decision Trees

Proposed decision tree for phaco/IOL to treat OHT eyes to prevent adult glaucoma OHT eyes are currently identified during routine eye examinations. If the IOP is

≥24 mmHg, and an additional risk factor exists, consider earlier phaco/IOL for treatment of the OHT and the vision if there is cataract present and visual impairment for the patient.

Additional glaucoma risk factors to consider would include the following:

- Anatomy with decreased central corneal thickness, enlarged cup-to-disc ratio
- Family history of glaucoma
- Shallow anterior chamber
- Poor patient glaucoma drop compliance.

Proposed decision tree for phaco/IOL to better control the IOP of glaucoma eyes

- If the IOP is marginally controlled (i.e., ≥24 mmHg) consider phaco/IOL in the treatment plan of early to moderate glaucoma, especially if additional risk factors exist and there is a component of narrow angle. The likelihood of IOP reduction is about 78% and likely to be a larger decrease if there is a narrow angle.
- Additional risk factors are the same for glaucoma and OHT eyes.
- If a target IOP of 18 mmHg is adequate for the control of the glaucoma, treat with phaco/IOL. If a lower target is required for adequate glaucoma control, (i.e., 14 mmHg) consider a combined procedure or a trabeculectomy.

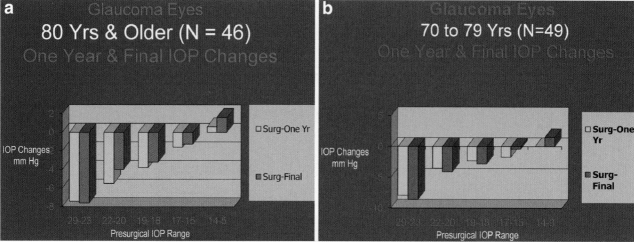

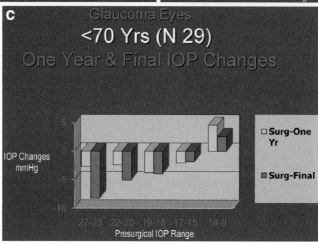

Fig. 4.12 One year and final IOP changes for glaucoma eyes for patients (**a**) 80 years and older, (**b**) 70–79 years, and (**c**) younger than 70 years

- A new baseline visual field should be obtained following cataract surgery due to the effects cataract may have on the test, as discussed in Chapter 1.
- Trabeculectomy or other filtration procedure can be done at a later time if the patient is in the 20–25% of patients who continue with marginal control based on our data. A deeper anterior chamber established by the cataract extraction may be of benefit in the postoperative filtered eye.

Advantages of phaco/IOL versus glaucoma drops for treating OHT and glaucoma are listed in Figs. 4.13 and 4.14.[34–37] Phaco/IOL still entails more risk than glaucoma drops. Endophthalmitis and retinal detachment, although rare, still occur. Moshifar et al. reported the incidence of endophthalmitis following phaco/IOL in 20,013 cases was 0.1% for eyes treated with moxifloxacin and 0.06% for eyes treated with gatifloxacin.[38]

Russell et al. reported that the incidence of rhegmatogenous retinal detachment after uncomplicated phacoemulsification cataract surgery was 1.17% after 10 years.[39]

Trabeculoplasty can be used as an adjunct to medications, until a patient's cataract is bothersome to the patient and surgery is pursued.[40,41] Treatment plans for glaucoma and OHT should include early phaco/IOL as a contribution to improved IOP control to help avoid later trabeculectomy.

Summary

In summary, these studies show IOP reduction following phaco/IOL surgery is proportional to the eye's IOP preoperatively and greater for angle closure versus open angle types of glaucoma. The higher the mean presurgical IOP, the greater the mean IOP reduction. IOP reductions achieved 1 year after surgery were maintained up to the 10 years of the study. IOP reduction was the same for the three decades of age studied. One hundred percent of eyes with OHT or glaucoma with presurgical IOPs ≥23 mmHg achieved IOP reduction after phaco/IOL surgery. Seventy-four percent of OHT eyes with

ISSUE	Phaco/IOL vs.	Glaucoma Drops
Patient compliance	Eliminated	Unsolvable problem
IOP reduction sustained	For 10 Yrs of study	Only when on glaucoma drops
IOP reduction stabilized	For 10 Yrs of study	IOP creeps up, need additional glaucoma drops
Visual Acuity	Maximized	No improvement
Cost	< 65 Yrs- $ 5,000/eye ≥ 65 Yrs Medicare	$1,000/ eye every Yr $1,000/eye every Yr
Adverse reactions	Minimal to none	Ocular & Systemic
Risk	Minimal	Minimal

Fig. 4.13 Comparison of the benefits of phaco/IOL alone versus glaucoma drops for eyes with OHT or glaucoma

ISSUE	PHACO/IOL VS.	TRABECULECTOMY
Complications	Minimal	Numerous
Long Term Failure	Minimal to None	25-40%
Vision Reestablished	One week	Three months
Vision Quality	Maximum	Unchanged or Decreased
Post OP Care	Minimal 3 Visits/ 6 Weeks	Extensive 8-12 visits/ 3 Months
IOP Reduction	Adequate If IOP Target =18	Greatest IOP Reduction IOP Target Low as 8
Cataract Removed	Yes	No
Skilled Surgeons	All Phaco Surgeons	Primarily Glaucoma Surgeons

Fig. 4.14 Comparison of the benefits of phaco/IOL versus trabeculectomy for glaucoma eyes

IOP ≥20 mmHg converted to normotensive eyes with IOP ≤19 mmHg after phaco/IOL surgery. Seventy-eight percent of glaucoma eyes with IOP ≥20 mmHg converted to eyes with IOP ≤19 mmHg after phaco/IOL surgery.

Our studies and earlier studies of non-glaucoma eyes appear to support the proposition that phaco/IOL in OHT eyes lowers the IOP. Adult glaucoma becomes an avoidable disease in some individuals when their OHT eyes are treated with phaco/IOL, as elevated IOP is an important risk factor for the disease.[42]

Our studies and earlier studies suggest phaco/IOL can be an effective treatment for glaucoma eyes if a target IOP of 18 mmHg following surgery is deemed adequate. However, if a lower target IOP is needed (i.e., 14 mmHg) for more advanced glaucoma, then a trabeculectomy before cataract surgery or combined procedure would be advisable.[43,44]

References

1. Mann I. *Developmental abnormalities of the eye*. Philadelphia: J P Lippincott; 1957:298–299.

2. Adler FH. *Physiology of the eye, clinical application*. St Louis: CV Mosby; 1950:247–253.

3. Johnstone MA. The aqueous outflow system as a mechanical pump: evidence from examination of tissue and aqueous movement in human and non-human primates. *J Glaucoma*. 2004;13:421–438.

4. Johnstone MA. A new model describes an aqueous outflow pump and explores causes of pump failure in glaucoma. In: Grehn F, Stampler R, eds. *Glaucoma*. Berlin Heidelberg: Springer-Verlag; 2006:3–34.

5. Strenk SA, Strenk LM, Guo S. Magnetic resonance imaging of aging, accommodating, phakic, and pseudophakic ciliary muscle diameters. *J Cataract Refract Surg*. 2006;32:1792–1798.

6. Strenk SA, Strenk LM. In vivo MRI…visualizing the haptics. *Eye World*. 2007;September:49–52.

7. Poley BJ, Lindstrom RL Samuelson TW. Long-term effects of phacoemulsification with intraocular lens implantation in normotensive and ocular hypertensive eyes. *J Cataract Refract Surg*. 2008;34:735–742.

8. Hayashi K, Hayashi H, Nakao F, Hayashi F. Changes in the anterior chamber angle width and depth after intraocular lens implantation in eyes with glaucoma. *Ophthalmology*. 2000;107:698–703.

9. Steuhl KP, Marahrens P, Frphn C, Frohn A. Intraocular pressure and anterior chamber depth before and after extracapsular cataract extraction with posterior chamber intraocular lens implantation. *Ophthalmic Surg*. 1992;23:233–237.

10. Shingleton BJ, Pasternack JJ, Hung JW, O'Donoghe MW. Three and five year changes in intraocular pressures after clear corneal phacoemulsification in open angle glaucoma patients, glaucoma suspects and normal patients. *J Glaucoma*. December 2006;15:494–498.

11. Berson FG, Patterson MM, Epstein DL. Obstruction of aqueous outflow by sodium hyaluronate in enucleated human eyes. *Am J Ophthalmol*. 1983;95:668–672.

12. Storr-Paulsen A. Analysis of the short-term effect of two viscoelastic agent on the intraocular pressure after extracapsular cataract extraction. Sodium yaluronate 1% vs hydroxypropyl methylcellulsose. *Acta Ophthalmol*. 1993;71:173–176.

13. Fry LL. Postoperative intraocular pressure rises: a comparison of Healon, Amvisc, and Viscoat. *J Cataract Refract Surg*. 1989;15:415–420.

14. Lehmann R, Brint S, Stewart R, et al. Clinical comparisons of Provisc and Healon in cataract surgery. *J Cataract Refract Surg*. 1995;21:543–547.

15. West DR, Lischwe TD, Thompson VM, Ede Ch. Comparative efficacy of the B-blockers for the prevention of increased intraocular pressure after cataract extraction. *Am J Ophthamol*. 1988;106:168–173.

16. Gupta A, Bansal RK, Grewal SPS. Natural course of intraocular pressure after cataract extraction and the effect of intracameral carbachol. *J Cataract Refract Surg*. 1992;18:14–19.

17. Feist RM, Palmer DJ, Fiscella R, et al. Effectiveness of apraclonidine and acetazolamide in preventing postoperative intraocular pressure spikes after extracapsular cataract extraction. *J Cataract Refract Surg*. 1995;21:191–195.

18. Rainer G, Menapace R, Findl O, et al. Effect of a fixed dorzolamide-timolol combination on intraocular pressure after small-incision cataract surgery with Viscoat. *J Cataract Refract Surg*. 2003;29:1748–1752.

19. Rainer G, Menapace R, Findl O, et al. Randomised fellow eye comparison of the effectiveness of dorzolamide and apraclonidine on intraocular pressure following phacoemulsification cataract surgery. *Eye*. 2000;14:757–760.

20. Zohdy GA, Rogers ZA, Lukaris A, Sells M, Roberts-Harry TJ. A comparison of the effectiveness of dorzolamide and acetazolamide in preventing post-operative intraocular pressure rise following phacoemulsification surgery.

21. Kim DD, Doyle JW, Smith MF. Intraocullar pressure reduction following cataract extraction by phacoemulsification with posterior chamber lens implantation in glaucoma patients. *Ophthal Surg Lasers*. 1999;30:37–40.

22. Ge J, Guo Y, Liu Y. Preliminary clinical study on the management of angle closure glaucoma by phacoemulsification with foldable posterior chamber intraocular lens implantation. *ZhonghuaYan Ke Za Zhi*. 2001;37:355–358.

23. Euswas A, Warrasak S. Intraocular pressure control following phacoemulsification in patients with chronic angle closure glaucoma. *J Med Assoc Thai*. 2005;88:S121–S125.

24. Hayashi K, Hayashi H, Nakao F, Hayashi F. Effect of cataract surgery on the intraocular pressure control in glaucoma patients. *J Cataract Refract Surg*. 2001;27:1779–1786.

25. Lai JS, Tham CC, Chan JC. The clinical outcomes of cataract extraction by phacoemulsification in eyes with primary angle-closure glaucoma (PACG) and coexisting cataract: a prospective case history. *J Glaucoma*. 2006;15:47–52.

26. Mathalone N, Hymas M, Neiman S, Buckman G, Hod Y, Geyer O. Long-term intraocular pressure control after clear corneal phacoemulsification in glaucoma patients. *J Cataract Refract Surg*. 2005;31:479–483.

27. Tham CY, Kwong YY, et al. Phacoemulsification versus combined phacotrabeculectomy in medically controlled chronic angle closure glaucoma with cataract. *Ophthalmology*. 2008;115:2167–2173.

28. Suzuki R, Kuroki S, Fujiwara N. Ten year follow up of intraocular pressure after phacoemulsification and aspiration with intraocular lens implantation performed by the same surgeon. *Ophthalmology*. 1997;211:79–83.

29. Tong JT, Miller KM. Intraocular pressure change after sutureless phacoemulsification with foldable posterior chamber lens implantation. *J Cataract Refract Surg*. 998;24:1560.

30. Tennen DG, Masket S. Short and long term effect of clear corneal incisions on intraocular pressure. *J Cataract Refract Surg*. 1996;22(5):568–570.

31. Issa SA, Pacheco J, Mahmood U, Nolan J, Beatty S. A novel index for predicting intraocular pressure reduction following cataract surgery. *Br J Ophthalmol*. 2005;89:543–546.

32. Strenk SA, Strenk LM, Koretz J. The mechanism of presbyopia. *Prog Retin Eye Res*. 2005;24:379–393.

33. Nonaka A, Kondo T, et al. Cataract surgery for residual angle closure after peripheral laser iridotomy. *Ophthalmology*. 2005;112:974–979.

34. Doyle JW, Smith F, Tierney JW. Glaucoma Medical Treatment-2002: does yearly cost now equal the year. *Optom Vis Sci*. 2002;79:489–492.

35. Cantor LB, Katz JW, Cheng JW, et al. Economic evaluation of medication, laser trabeculoplasty and filtering surgeries in treating patients with glaucoma in the US. *Curr Med Res Opoin*. 2008;24:2905–2918.

36. Rylander NR, Vold SD. Cost analysis of glaucoma medications. *Am J Ophthalmol*. 2008;145:106–113.

37. Haynes WL, Alward WL. Control of intraocular pressure after trabeculectomy. *Surv Ophthalmol*. 1999;43:345–355.

38. Moshirfar M, Feiz V, Vitale AT, Wegelin JA, Basavanthappa S, Wolsey DH. Endophthalmitis after uncomplicated cataract surgery with the use of fourth generation fuuroquinolones, retro-

spective observational case series. *Ophthalmology*. 2007;114: 686–691.

39. Russell M, et al. Pseudophakic retinal detachment after phacoemulsification cataract surgery: ten year retrospective review. *J Cataract Refract Surg*. March 2006;32(3): 442–445.

40. Damji KF. Selective laser trabeculoplasty: a better alternative. *Surv Ophthalmol*. 2008;53:646–651.

41. Pham H, Mansberger S, Brandt J. Argon laser trabeculoplasty. The gold standard. *Surv Ophthalmol*. 2008;53:641–646.

42. Gordon MO, Beiser JA, Brandt JD, et al. OHTS:Baseline factors that predict the onset of primary open-angle glaucoma. *Arch Ophthalmol*. 2002;120:714–720.

43. AGIS: the advanced glaucoma intervention study (AGIS) 7. The relationship between control of intraocular pressure and visual field deterioraton. The AGSI Investigators. *Am J Ophthalmol*. 2000;130:429–440.

44. Musch DC, Gillespie BW, Lichter PR, et al. Visual field progression in the collaborative initial glaucoma treatment study. *Ophthalmololgy*. 2009;116:200–207.

Chapter 5

Elevated Intraocular Pressure After Cataract Surgery

Parag A. Gokhale and Emory Patterson

Introduction

The phenomenon of elevated intraocular pressure (IOP) following cataract surgery has been documented since the 1950s. In 1976, a review of 630 cases of cataract extraction with lens implant concluded that elevated IOP was a transient and benign occurrence.[1] In nearly all patients, pressures returned to baseline with or without treatment. Some individuals, however, may experience pain, corneal edema, glaucomatous nerve damage, or anterior ischemic optic neuropathy.[2] It is therefore important to continue monitoring the effect of new cataract surgical techniques on postoperative IOP, as well as the impact of increased IOP on visual outcomes.

Elevated pressure is the most frequent postoperative complication demanding treatment following phacoemulsification.[3] As many as 18–45% of patients may experience an IOP greater than 28 mmHg following phacoemulsification, but most pressures will return to normal by 24 h postoperatively.[1] The peaks most commonly occur 8–12 h after surgery, and only 1.3–10.0% of cases measure an IOP higher than 30 mmHg 24 h postoperatively. After uneventful phacoemulsification in eyes without glaucoma, however, IOP spikes may even reach 68 mmHg.[3]

As previously mentioned, in most patients, postoperative increases in IOP are transient and benign.[1] In individuals without glaucoma, no visual field defects were evident once the IOP returned to normal.[1] Although patients without optic nerve damage seem to tolerate transient increases in IOP without problems, glaucoma patients do not. The latter individuals may experience further visual field loss and/or a loss of fixation.[1] Glaucoma patients are also more likely to experience pressure spikes following cataract extraction.[1]

Surgeons therefore must be keenly aware of a glaucoma patient's risk for postoperative IOP spikes and understand the various treatment options for elevated pressure when it does occur.

Etiology

The causes of the elevated IOP are likely multifactorial. Major factors include preexisting compromise of outflow facility and retained ophthalmic viscosurgical devices (OVDs). Surgical trauma, watertight wound closure, retained lenticular debris, the release of iris pigment, hyphema, and inflammation are also thought to contribute to elevations in IOP.[3] The skillfulness of the surgeon has been implicated as well. Increased surgical experience is correlated with a decreased risk for ocular hypertension following cataract extraction.[3]

A review of 2727 phacoemulsification procedures over a 2-year period demonstrated that the most frequent complication of posterior capsular rupture ($n = 45$) was raised IOP. Nine eyes (20%) had an IOP exceeding 30 mmHg 1 day after surgery despite prophylactic acetazolamide. Five of the nine eyes had sustained vitreous loss requiring an anterior vitrectomy.[4]

The Role of Ophthalmic Viscosurgical Devices

In 1983, Berson et al. reported that sodium hyaluronate caused a substantial decrease (55–60%) in the outflow of aqueous humor when injected into the anterior chamber.[5] Subsequently, it has become well accepted that retained viscoelastic materials inhibit aqueous outflow and result in increased IOP.

Ophthalmic viscosurgical devices (OVDs) are generally classified according to their molecular weight and viscosity. Cohesive agents are more viscous than dispersive OVDs,

P.A. Gokhale (✉)
Department of Ophthalmology, Virginia Mason Medical Center, Seattle, WA 98115, USA
e-mail: ophpag@vmmc.org

and they have higher molecular weights and longer molecular chains. These properties make cohesive OVDs an excellent choice for maintaining space, stabilizing tissues, and opposing the posterior pressure that occurs during cataract extraction.

The particles of low-viscosity OVDs are considered dispersive because they do not adhere to one another like they do in high-viscosity OVDs. Dispersive viscoelastics are better able than high-viscosity OVDs to protect individual structures in the anterior chamber such as the corneal endothelium.[6] Because of their dispersive nature, however, low-viscosity OVDs are generally more difficult to completely remove from the eye.

According to Arshinoff et al.[6] high-viscosity OVDs are associated with higher postoperative IOPs (although not necessarily above 21 mmHg), compared with lower viscosity OVDs. He asserted that retained viscoelastic and patients' predispositions (e.g., trabecular insult or undiagnosed glaucoma) are the main causes of postoperative rises in IOP above 21 mmHg.

Healon 5 (Advanced Medical Optics, Santa Ana, CA) is a newer OVD that can be classified as a viscoadaptive OVD. It acts as a high-viscosity OVD under low shear but becomes pseudodispersive with high turbulence.[6,7] If retained, it is more likely to cause a rise in IOP as compared to Healon and other viscoelastics.[6–8] It did not lead to more frequent IOP elevations when compared to Viscoat (a medium viscosity dispersive) but the maximum IOPs were higher with Healon 5.[9] In early use, it was more difficult to remove from the eye than other OVDs and therefore caused IOP elevation.[10] A newer technique of irrigating and aspirating behind the intraocular lens was recommended for its removal.[11] Arshinoff found that if adequately removed there were no more IOP elevations than there were with Healon.[6]

Arshinoff has published multiple studies comparing different viscoelastic materials.[6,12] He concluded that, if not completely removed, all OVDs cause postoperative increases in IOP. If no OVD is retained in the anterior segment, however, then increases in IOP following cataract extraction is of no greater severity or duration than if no OVD had been used at all.

Elevated IOP in Glaucoma

Although increases in IOP after cataract surgery are usually benign, they can lead to further loss of retinal ganglion cells in patients whose optic discs have already been compromised. Studies comparing patients with and without glaucoma have routinely revealed a difference in their postoperative rises in IOP. Shingleton et al. reported a maximum increase in IOP to 44 versus 32 mmHg in patients with and

without glaucoma, respectively, 24 h after cataract surgery.[13] Another study found a mean IOP of 29.9 mmHg, 8 h after cataract surgery, in patients with glaucoma compared with a mean IOP of 22.2 mmHg 12 h postoperatively in patients without glaucoma. Seven of the thirteen eyes in the glaucoma group had peak IOPs that were greater than 35 mmHg.[1] In their study, Arshinoff et al. discovered that 8 of 40 patients with elevated IOP had glaucoma, were glaucoma suspects, or were steroid responders. Subsequently, the investigators realized that higher IOP spikes correlated directly with glaucoma risk. Eight of forty patients with a pressure greater than 21 mmHg in either eye were found to fit into one of the glaucoma groups.[12]

Presentation

A patient with elevated intraocular pressure often will present with headache, nausea, and vomiting. On clinical exam, there is often blurred vision and microcystic edema of the cornea. Viscoelastic may be visible in the anterior chamber.

Medical Treatment

Pharmaceuticals

Although several drugs lower IOP after cataract surgery, none of them consistently prevents increases in pressure from occurring. The classes of drugs used to treat postoperative increases in IOP are listed in Table 5.1. Acetazolamide has been used for many years to treat IOP increases following cataract extraction and has proven moderately successful. This carbonic anhydrase inhibitor was more effective than topical apraclonidine, an alpha agonist, in a head-to-head trial.[14] Another comparative study showed that subjects' mean IOP in the first 24 h following cataract extraction was greater than 21 mmHg in the acetazolamide group and less than 21 mmHg in the dorzolamide group. Both groups, however, had an equal number of patients with an IOP greater than 30 mmHg 4 h following surgery.[15] A study comparing

Table 5.1 Medications to lower postoperative IOP

- Carbonic anhydrase inhibitors (acetazolamide, dorzolamide, and brinzolamide)
- Alpha agonists (apraclonidine and brimonidine)
- Prostaglandin analogs (latanoprost and travoprost)
- Beta blockers (timolol and levobunolol)
- Miotics (intracameral carbachol, pilocarpine, and intracameral acetylcholine)

acetazolamide and brinzolamide found that the drugs were equally effective at 4–6 h after cataract surgery, but that only brinzolamide produced a statistically significant decrease in IOP at 24 h.[16]

Rainer et al. compared dorzolamide and latanoprost, a prostaglandin analog. Both drugs produced a clinically significant reduction in IOP 6 h after cataract surgery, but only dorzolamide was effective at 24 h.[16] Neither drug prevented elevations in IOP greater than 30 mmHg from occurring. A comparison of travoprost and brinzolamide showed that both produced a clinically significant decrease in IOP 6 and 24 h postoperatively. Neither, however, was always able to prevent a spike greater than 30 mmHg.[2]

Tests of apraclonidine to prevent postoperative increases in IOP have been inconsistent in their results. The explanation may be differences in surgical technique, surgeons' experience, the OVD used, or the administration of the IOP-lowering agents. Most recently, Kasetti et al. found no benefit with apraclonidine versus placebo to reduce postoperative IOP and prevent pressure spikes.[14]

The alpha 2 agonist brimonidine 0.2% dosed twice the day before and the day after cataract surgery was more effective than placebo at reducing postoperative IOP. The mean IOP in the brimonidine group was significantly lower than in the placebo group at most time points. At 6 h postoperatively, one patient in the brimonidine group and six in the placebo group experienced an IOP spike greater than 10 mmHg over baseline. No patients treated with brimonidine had a peak IOP exceeding 30 mmHg.[17] In other studies in which subjects received one drop of brimonidine 0.2% 1 h before surgery or just after cataract extraction, the drug did not produce a significant decrease in IOP compared to placebo.[18,19]

In another study, timolol but not latanoprost was effective in reducing postoperative IOP. In fact, patients receiving one drop of timolol at the end of surgery had a mean decrease in IOP of 4.77 and 2.99 mmHg at 4 and 24 h, respectively.[20]

Rainer et al. compared a fixed dorzolamide-timolol combination with latanoprost. The fixed combination reduced postoperative IOP more effectively, and it prevented any increase in IOP to greater than 30 mmHg.[21] Another study comparing a dorzolamide-timolol combination to placebo found that the fixed combination produced a clinically significant reduction in postoperative IOP. The agent, however, did not completely prevent pressure spikes greater than 30 mmHg.[22]

A 1992 report concluded that intracameral carbachol intraocular solution 0.01% (Miostat, Alcon, Fort Worth, TX) was the most effective medication to control IOP following extracapsular cataract extraction. Timolol, acetazolamide, pilocarpine, and levobunolol also produced a clinically significant reduction in IOP but were less effective.[23]

In addition, carbachol was more effective than acetylcholine (Miochol-E, Novartis, East Hanover, New Jersey) when both drugs were administered intracamerally.[9]

Decompression of the Anterior Chamber

Another proposed method of controlling IOP after cataract surgery is decompressing the anterior chamber. In 2003, Hildebrand et al. found that decompression effectively corrected 11 consecutive cases of severely increased IOP.[3] Pressure decreased from a range of 40–68 mmHg to a mean of 4.73 ± 3.00 mmHg immediately after decompression. The IOP, however, rapidly rose to greater than 30 mmHg and 38.5 mmHg 30 and 60 minutes after decompression. Hildebrand et al., therefore, concluded that this measure provides only a transient benefit and that additional treatment is necessary in high-risk eyes.[3] Arshinoff recommended multiple attempts at sideport drainage (Fig. 5.1, Table 5.2). He proposed decompressing the anterior chamber hourly for 3 h in combination with the administration of one drop each of pilocarpine 2% and latanoprost four times a day for 2 days postoperatively.[7] The paracentesis can usually be opened for 48 h following its creation and, if need be, a new one can be created at the slit lamp, using sterile technique.

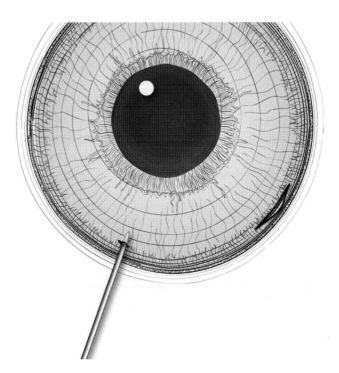

Fig. 5.1 The bevel up needle is used to depress the posterior lip of the paracentesis

Table 5.2 Anterior chamber decompression

- Topical anesthetic
- Prophylactic antibiotic drops pre and post
- Betadine 5% cleansing of the lid margin and a drop in the inferior fornix
- Tb syringe with needle for depressing at paracentesis site
- Repeat maneuver at 10-minutes intervals, lowering IOP about 10 mmHg per depression, to avoid a single large drop in IOP
- Dose glaucoma medications at the end of the procedure

Proposed Guidelines

Ophthalmologists must recognize the potential for postoperative increases in IOP and IOP spikes following uncomplicated phacoemulsification, know the risk factors for this complication, and be comfortable with a variety of treatment options. In patients with known outflow obstruction or optic nerve damage or in those who are already being treated for increased IOP, we recommend the following:

- Prophylactic treatment both before and after surgery.
- Aggressive removal of OVDs from the eye.
- Injection of carbachol intracamerally at the end of surgery.
- Aggressive treatment to lower the IOP postoperatively if a posterior capsular rupture occurs intraoperatively.

The medications used will depend on the patient's tolerance (e.g., due to allergy and systemic conditions).

Summary

We recommend the following approach for patients with high-risk eyes if they tolerate the medications. Surgeons should administer a fixed combination of timolol and dorzolamide along with brimonidine at the end of the case, and patients should instill these drugs at their usual scheduled time. Depending on the patient's level of risk for postoperative IOP spikes and the status of the optic nerve at the time of surgery, it may be prudent to see the patient later on the operative day to perform serial paracenteses if the IOP is elevated. If paracenteses are required, surgeons can consider prescribing prostaglandins and/or cholinergics up to qid for 2 days after surgery. If the patient is at high risk, then performing combined cataract and glaucoma surgery or glaucoma surgery alone before cataract surgery may be in the patient's best interest.

Acknowledgments Adapted with permission from Gokhale et al.[24] Bryn Mawr Communications LLC.

References

1. Tranos P, Bhar G, Little B. Postoperative intraocular pressure spikes: the need to treat. *Eye*. 2004;18:673–679.
2. Ermis SS, Ozturk F, Inan UU. Comparing the effects of travoprost and brinzolamide on intraocular pressure after phacoemulsification. *Eye*. 2005;19:303–307.
3. Hildebrand GD, Wickremasinghe SS, Tranos PG, et al. Efficacy of anterior chamber decompression in controlling early intraocular pressure spikes after uneventful phacoemulsification. *J Cataract Refract Surg*. 2003;29:1087–1092.
4. Ang GS, Whyte IF. Effect and outcomes of posterior capsule rupture in a district general hospital setting. *J Cataract Refract Surg*. 2006;32:623–627.
5. Berson FG, Patterson MM, Epstien DL. Obstruction of aqueous outflow by sodium hyaluronate in enucleated human eyes. *Am J Ophthalmol*. 1983;96:668–672.
6. Arshinoff S, Albiani DA, Taylor-Laporte J. Intraocular pressure after bilateral cataract surgery using Healon, Healon 5, and Healon GV. *J Cataract Refract Surg*. 2002;28:617–625.
7. Zetterstrom C, Wejde G, Taube M. Healon5: comparison of 2 removal techniques. *J Cataract Refract Surg*. 2002;28:1561–1564.
8. Holzer MP, Tetz MR, Auffarth GU, Welt R, Volcker HE. Effect of Healon5 and 4 other viscoelastic substances on intraocular pressure and endothelium after cataract surgery. *J Cataract Refract Surg*. 2001;27:213–218.
9. Arshinoff S. Postoperative intraocular pressure spikes. *J Cataract Refract Surg*. 2004;30:733–734.
10. Shingleton BJ, Gamell LS, O'Donoghue MW, et al. Long-term changes in intraocular pressure after clear corneal phacoemulsification: normal patients versus glaucoma suspect and glaucoma patients. *J Cataract Refract Surg*. 1999;25:885–890.
11. Kasetti SR, Desai SP, Sivakumar S, Sunderraj P. Preventing intraocular pressure increase after phacoemulsification and the role of perioperative apraclonidine. J Cataract Refract Surg. 2002;28:2177–2180.
12. Dayanir V, Ozcura F, Kir E, et al. Medical control of intraocular pressure after phacoemulsification. *J Cataract Refract Surg*. 2005;31:484–488.
13. Rainer G, Menapace R, Schmetterer K, et al. Effect of dorzolamide and latanoprost on intraocular pressure after small incision cataract surgery. J Cataract Refract Surg. 1999;25:1624–1629.
14. Katsimpris JM, Dimitrios S, Konstas AGP, et al. Efficacy of brimonidine 0.2% in controlling acute postoperative intraocular pressure elevation after phacoemulsification. *J Cataract Refract Surg*. 2003;29:2288–2294.
15. Cetinkaya A, Akman A, Akova YA. Effect of topical brinzolamide 1% and brimonidine 0.2% on intraocular pressure after phacoemulsification. *J Cataract Refract Surg*. 2004;30:1736–1741.
16. Rainer G, Menapace R, Findl O, et al. Effect of topical brimonidine on intraocular pressure after small incision cataract surgery. *J Cataract Refract Surg*. 2001;27:1227–1231.
17. Lai JSM, Chua JKH, Leung ATS, et al. Latanoprost versus timolol gel to prevent ocular hypertension after phacoemulsification and intraocular lens implantation. *J Cataract Refract Surg*. 2000;26:386–391.
18. Rainer G, Menapace R, Findl O, et al. Intraindividual comparison of the effects of a fixed dorzolamide-timolol combination and latanoprost on intraocular pressure after small incision cataract surgery. *J Cataract Refract Surg*. 2001;27:1227–1231.
19. Rainer G, Menapace R, Findl O, et al. Effect of a fixed dorzolamide-timolol combination on intraocular pressure after small incision cataract surgery with Viscoat. *J Cataract Refract Surg*. 2003;29:1748–1752.

20. Fry LL. Comparison of the postoperative intraocular pressure with Betagan, Betoptic, Timoptic, Iopidine, Diamox, Pilopine Gel, and Miostat. *J Cataract Refract Surg*. 1992;18:14–19.

21. Ruiz RS, Rhem MN, Prager TC. Effects of carbachol and acetylcholine on intraocular pressure after cataract extraction. *Am J Ophthalmol*. 1989;107:7–10.

22. Tetz MR, Holzer MP, Lundberg K, Auffarth GU, Burk RO, Kruse FE. Clinical results of phacoemulsification with the use of Healon5 or Viscoat. *J Cataract Refract Surg*. 2001 March;27(3): 416–420.

23. Dada T, Muralidhar R, Jhanji V. Intraocular pressure rise after use of Healon5 during extracapsular cataract surgery. *Can J Ophthalmol*. 2007 April; 42(2):338.

24. Gokhale PA, Patterson E. Elevated IOP after cataract surgery. *Glaucoma Today*, May/June 2007;5:19–22.

Chapter 6

Combined Cataract and Trabeculectomy Surgery

Sandra M. Johnson

Introduction

When the decision has been made to perform cataract surgery in a glaucoma patient, the options of cataract surgery alone or combined with glaucoma surgery (glaucoma triple procedure) are available to the surgeon. Trabeculectomy is the glaucoma procedure that has been most frequently and for the longest time combined with cataract surgery, to assist in the control of intraocular pressure (IOP). Other combined procedures are discussed in Chapter 14 and elsewhere in the text. As discussed throughout the text, cataract and glaucoma often present in the same patient and are common comorbidities.

The presence of a cataract may drive the decision for combined surgery, and on the other hand, a need for lower intraocular pressure (IOP) may drive the decision for a combined procedure. If the surgeon deems it is likely that the patient will need to return to the operating room for a cataract surgery, following the trabeculectomy, it may be best to perform both surgeries at the same operative session. Progression of cataract is a known complication of trabeculectomy.[1,2] One surgical experience may be the best for a patient, depending on their health status and socioeconomic concerns.

The status of the glaucoma and the target intraocular pressure are the important factors to consider in deciding to pursue a combined cataract extraction and glaucoma procedure versus a cataract procedure alone.[3] The patient is likely to have more IOP lowering with a combined versus a cataract extraction alone.[4,5] This has been shown since the initiation of the combined procedure.

Trabeculectomy was originally combined with extracapsular cataract extraction (ECCE) with a 11-mm wound, as studied by Bobrow in 1999. He was able to follow 35 patients for at least 80 months. He found the eyes with trabeculectomy combined with cataract surgery versus those that underwent cataract surgery alone had an IOP reduction of 8.2 ± 4.6 mmHg versus 4.4 ± 3.3 mmHg. Medications were reduced by 1.76 ± 0.82 versus 1.28 ± 0.86, respectively.[6]

The surgeon should carefully review the visual field status, level of IOP control and how maximal the therapy is, and the status of the optic disc and/or retinal nerve fiber layer (Figs. 6.1, 6.2, and 6.3). General principles to consider are as follows:

1. A patient with advanced visual field loss and disc damage who is not likely to withstand any elevated postoperative IOP, due to the risk of further damage, is less likely to have elevated IOP following a combined procedure.[7,8]
2. A patient who cannot tolerate medical therapy due to drop allergies, cost, or compliance issues such as dementia or tremor will likely lessen the burden of medical

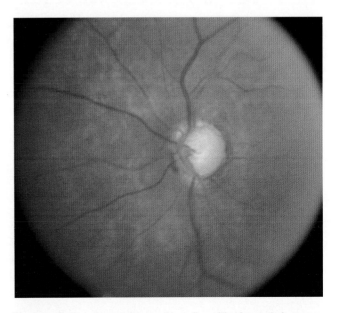

Fig. 6.1 Fundus photo demonstrating a disc with advanced glaucomatous damage

S.M. Johnson (✉)
Department of Ophthalmology, University of Virginia School of Medicine, Charlottesville, VA 22908, USA
e-mail: catglaubk@gmail.com

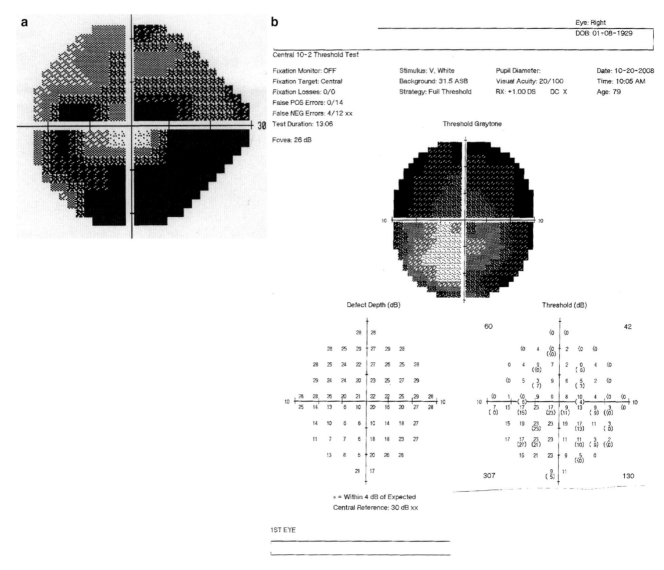

Fig. 6.2 (**a**) Visual field grayscale image of a left eye with a dense inferior nasal step and field loss superior near fixation. (**b**) A 10° visual field demonstrating advanced visual field loss

therapy more so with a combined procedure, although compliance with drops is essential during the postoperative period.

3. A patient who is on maximal medical therapy and has no further options for escalation of therapy for loss of IOP control post cataract surgery may be better served with a combined procedure.

4. A narrow angle patient with poor IOP control and permanent synechial angle closure will be easier to manage postoperatively if the chamber is deepened with concurrent cataract surgery at the time of filtration surgery. There will be the added option of YAG laser capsulotomy and laser to the anterior hyaloid face, should aqueous misdirection present.

5. As noted previously, if a patient is undergoing a trabeculectomy for loss of IOP control and there is a significant or near significant cataract present, then a combined should be considered, as cataracts often progress post trabeculectomy.[9–11] There may be some added lowering of IOP by removing a cataract with pseudoexfoliation (PXF) present.[12–14] or for an angle-closure patient (see Chapters 15 and 18).

A two-staged procedure, with a cataract extraction later, may be pursued if the IOP is very high and the risk of suprachoroidal hemorrhage is elevated, as it may be more likely to occur intraoperative with a more prolonged surgery.[15] In these instances, it is best to gain control of the IOP initially and then pursue visual rehabilitation with a later cataract surgery. See Chapter 16.

Disadvantages of a combined surgery are listed in Table 6.1.

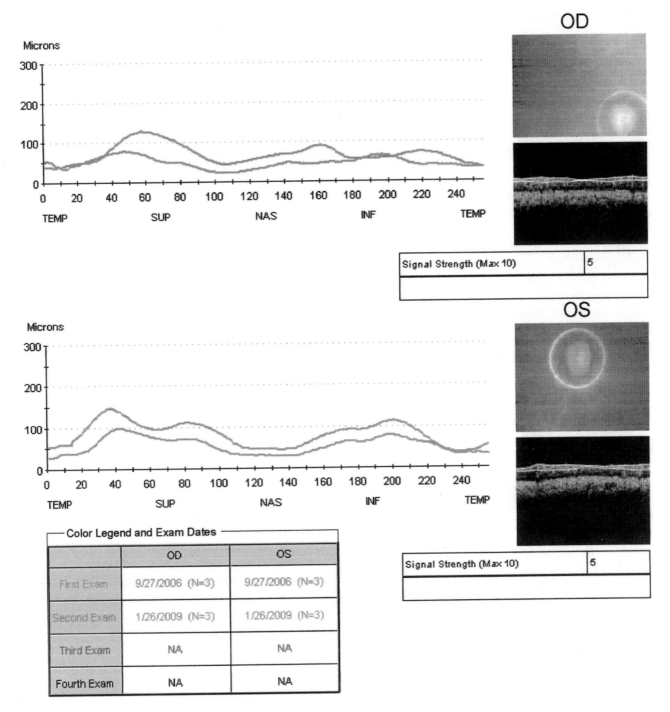

Fig. 6.3 Retinal nerve fiber (RNFL) assessment by ocular coherence tomorgraphy (Zeiss Meditec, Dublin, CA). Note the decreased RNFL in one eye versus the other consistent with a more advanced glaucoma status. Image courtesy of Lloyd Situkali, ophthalmic photography, UVA.

Preoperative Assessment

As for any pre-surgical patient, a history of systemic medications including anticoagulants is essential, and the patient should be current with their surveillance of his/her anticoagulation status if on warfarin. If the patient is hyper-tensive, blood pressure should be in good control as well as any tachycardia. The current eye medications should be reviewed. As discussed in Chapter 1, the surgeon may want to discontinue prostaglandin analogues if there is a concern for postoperative inflammation. Miotics must be discontinued to allow for maximal pupil dilation. If there is conjunctival inflammation secondary to drops, the surgeon

Table 6.1 Disadvantages of combined surgery versus cataract surgery alone

- Longer operating room time for procedure
- More complex postoperative care
- Slower visual recovery
- Possibly less IOP control versus trabeculectomy alone
- Possibly more astigmatism or myopic shift
- Long-term bleb problems

must decide on whether to discontinue topical medications for a quieter eye and weigh this against performing surgery on an eye with higher intraocular pressure. The patient may need to be instructed on the cessation of oral carbonic anhydrase inhibitors postoperatively. Older patients should be counseled about their increased risk of choroidal effusions.[10,16,17]

A complete eye exam should be done to assess for conditions such as those listed in Table 6.2. This will assist the surgeon in anticipating complications and to prepare adequately.

Table 6.2 Preoperative ocular assessment

- Blepharitis
- Conjunctival inflammation
- Prior conjunctival incisions
- Corneal guttatae
- Pupillary dilation
- Pseudoexfoliation
- Vitreous in the anterior chamber
- Gonioscopy
- Retinal conditions

Surgical Evolution

Incision Size

Simmons et al. and Hurvitz reported similar outcomes in similar case reviews of large-incision ECCE.[18,19] The Simmons report reviewed 75 cases of ECCE combined with trabeculectomy and mean IOP was decreased 3.6 mmHg at 12 months with 1.5 less medications. Shingleton et al. reviewed 35 eyes that underwent a planned extracapsular cataract extraction (ECCE) with an 11-mm incision and 37 that underwent a phacoemulsification procedure with a 6-mm incision. At 1 year, the mean IOP decrease was 5 mmHg for the 6-mm incision group versus 3 mmHg for the ECCE group. The preoperative IOP was slightly higher in the phacoemulsification group, but otherwise the groups were similar.[20] Stewart et al. reported on a group of 18 ECCE cases versus 16 phacoemulsification cases combined with trabeculectomy, and at 1 year the eyes in the phacoemulsification group had a mean lower IOP of 2.3 mmHg and a trend toward less glaucoma medications.[21] Wishart et al.

reported similar findings in a comparison of phacoemulsification versus ECCE.[22] The final IOP at 1 year or more was controlled with no medications for 79% of the phacoemulsification patients and 53% of the ECCE patients. There was more astigmatism in the ECCE group and 32% had some pupillary capture of the intraocular lens. Pupillary capture can result from a multiple puncture/can opener style anterior capsulotomy when an anterior chamber shallows with filtration. This type of capsulotomy maintains the intraocular lens position less compared to a continuous curvilinear capsulorhexis that is fashioned to be slightly smaller than the optic of the IOL implanted. In a report by Tous et al., reviewing 475 consecutive cases, there were more complications in the ECCE group (80 eyes) versus the phacoemulsification group (395) with a minimum follow-up of 12 months.[23]

Lyle and Jin studied 216 patients who had undergone combined surgery of which 104 had 3-mm incisions and 112 had a 6-mm incision.[24] Follow-up was for a minimum of 6 months with a mean of 18 months, with longer follow-up for the 6-mm incision group. The smaller incision group had faster visual rehabilitation and less need for any medications at 1 year; 78% versus 68%. At 6 months, the IOP decrease was close to 7 mmHg in the 6-mm incision group and nearly 9 mmHg in the smaller incision group. Several years later, Stewart et al. reported a similar study and found no difference in IOP control at 1 year.[25] A report from Vyas et al. compared 3.5 and 5.2 mm incisions and found no difference in IOP control at 1 year or difference in astigmatism.[26]

Incision sizes have further decreased with the development of the foldable intraocular lens. In one early study of this technology, 49 eyes underwent small incision phacoemulsification with foldable intraocular lens implantation and trabeculectomy. At a mean follow-up of 31.5 months, all patients had IOP control with 80% on no medications and 16% on fewer medications than preoperatively. Mean postoperative IOP was 14.2 ± 3 compared to 22.3 ± 4.3 mmHg preoperative.[27] The literature supports better IOP control with smaller incision cataract surgery; however, there are some reports that do not support this when 6 mm versus 3 mm incisions are compared, and the difference may not be as pronounced as decreasing the incision size from 11 to 6 mm. Six millimeter incisions are still used in countries where there is no access to phacoemulsification and/or foldable IOLs (see Chapter 7).

Antimetabolites

There have been several reports assessing the effect of 5-fluorouracil (5-FU) augmented trabeculectomy combined with phacoemulsification cataract extraction and posterior chamber intraocular lens (PCIOL). In 1993, O'Grady et al. reported no effect from 5-FU augmentation versus no 5-FU used for glaucoma triple procedure in a randomized study of 74 patients.[28] The 5-FU was delivered subconjunctival for a mean of five 5 mg injections, and the surgery was a single site procedure with a 6-mm incision. On the other hand, in a retrospective study, Cohen reported better IOP control in a group of patients receiving postoperative injections of 5-FU (mean of 4.5 injections/mean 17.3 mg given) as compared to a group that did not receive 5-FU. His surgery was done through a single site with a 6-mm incision and there were 22 eyes in each group. Mean follow-up was short – less than 6 months in the 5-FU group – as compared to over 1 year for the O'Grady groups.[29] Gandolphi, in 1997, reported a greater success of combined surgery utilizing 5-FU injections with a two-site technique in a prospective randomized trial with a 1 year follow-up.[30] Likewise, Donoso and Rodriquez were able to control the IOP in 22 patients who underwent a combined surgery with intraoperative 5-FU and showed survival curves with maintenance of IOP at 20 mmHg or less. The mean preoperative IOP was 19.8 mmHg and postoperative the mean was 12.2 mmHg on no medications. They found similar IOP control with a comparison group of patients undergoing phacoemulsification, following a prior trabeculectomy with intraoperative 5-FU.[31] Chang et al. did a retrospective review of 5-FU trabeculectomy versus the results of 5-FU trabeculectomy combined with phacoemulsification and PC IOL.[32] The study found similar mean IOP levels for both groups with 3 years or more follow-up, although the trabeculectomy group had higher preoperative IOP. The 5-FU was given intraoperatively and then postoperative as needed. More combined procedure eyes required postoperative 5-FU, suture lysis or release, and bleb needling. An evidence-based review published in 2002 concluded that there was not evidence for a benefit from the use of 5-FU for glaucoma triple procedure and that there was a small benefit for the use of MMC.[33]

Mitomycin C (MMC) augmented trabeculectomy has been studied more than 5-FU, likely due to the greater ease of administration. It has improved the outcome of trabeculectomy alone.[34] It has been adopted by many surgeons for use in the glaucoma triple procedure and good outcomes have been reported.[35–40] In a report by Carlson, a randomized study on 29 patients undergoing glaucoma triple procedure with or without MMC was done.[41] The MMC group had an IOP that was 3 mmHg lower on no medications with a mean follow-up of 20 months. The global use of MMC has been questioned by Shin and coauthors who initially found no difference in IOP control in primary triple procedures with and without augmentation with MMC, unless certain factors were present.[42,43] The factors identified as benefiting from the use of MMC were African ancestry, preoperative IOP of 20 mmHg or more, or two or more preopera-

tive medications. In a further study, prior failed trabeculectomy was added to the list of factors.[44] In a later study of 203 eyes that had undergone primary glaucoma triple procedure with 124 receiving MMC, Shin evaluated the results at 36 months. With this review, he concluded that the MMC group had more stable visual fields, less medication use, and lower IOPs.[45] Chapter 8 summarizes and reviews the use of antimetabolites.

Surgical Approach

Various studies have reviewed one-site combined surgery and/or two-site combined surgery. One-site is where both procedures are done superiorly in a quadrant through one incision. Two-site surgery involves two separate surgical procedures on the same day, where a trabeculectomy is done superior and a temporal approach is used for cataract extraction.[36,37] In either approach, there is a choice in how to create the conjunctival incision.[46–48] There have been some reports of greater vitreous loss from a one-site procedure with a limbal-based conjunctival flap.[8,49] There is likely less maneuverability of the instrumentation for cataract surgery working under conjunctiva and a fornix-based flap is the preferred approach for a one-site procedure. In another report, more wound leaks were reported in eyes with a one-site approach that included a limbal-based conjunctival flap versus a fornix-based.[50] The authors hypothesized that the greater manipulation of the conjunctiva led to the wound leaks.

Initially, studies suggested that a two-site approach yields a better IOP result. One of these was a randomized study by Wyse and coauthors who studied 33 patients and their follow-up went beyond 3 months.[51] The two-site group required more medications for the same IOP outcome. The evidence-based review by Jampel in 2002, which assessed effect of technique, concluded that two-site surgery resulted in slightly lower IOPs.[33] However, multiple other studies have shown no difference.[52,53] More recently a randomized, prospective study comparing one-site versus two-site phacotrabeculectomy has shown that the IOP control is similar in both groups.[54] This study randomized 80 eyes and had follow-up for 24 months. In addition, the authors reported that the two-site approach is more time consuming and that although it seems to lead to a more pronounced endothelial cell loss at 3 and 12 months, there is no significant difference in this parameter 24 months after surgery. Endothelial cell loss with two-site versus one-site surgery has also been reported in another study with 12 months follow-up.[55] Cotran has also shown that both surgical approaches were equally effective at lowering IOP over a 3-year follow-up in a randomized study.[56] Again, there was longer operative time in the two-site procedures and he reported higher post-op day one IOPs. His one-site group had more early leaks with a rate of 6 in 44 eyes.

Intraocular Lens Choice

Tezel and coauthors reviewed the results of glaucoma triple procedure with MMC done with foldable versus rigid intraocular lens placement. The study reviewed 103 eyes with a rigid lens and 112 with a foldable silicone lens. At a minimum follow-up of 12 months, the IOP was less than 20 mmHg without medications in 52% and 67% of eyes in the respective groups.[57] Alzafiri and Harasymowycz reviewed the results of eyes with MMC-augmented glaucoma triple procedure with either a rigid PMMA lens (19 eyes) or a foldable acrylic lens (41 eyes). The IOP control was comparable and the visual rehabilitation was faster in the acrylic foldable lens group.[58]

In another study of glaucoma triple procedure with MMC, the results with foldable silicone lenses were compared with foldable acrylic lenses. The authors reported lower IOP in the first 2 months in the silicone group and more flap suture release in the acrylic group. At the last follow-up over 12 months, the IOPs were not statistically different between the two groups.[59] Another study reported inflammatory membranes on silicone IOLs in 33% of a group of eyes that had undergone phacotrabeculectomy.[60] Serpa compared 124 eyes that had glaucoma triple procedure with a PMMA lens, a silicone foldable, or an acrylic foldable lens. The IOP lowering was the same in all groups. They also reported fibrin deposits in eyes that had silicone IOLs.[61]

Surgical Technique

The author favors a one-site approach. Topical anesthetic, 0.75% preservative-free bupivacaine applied every 15 minutes for 3–4 doses while the patient is preparing for surgery, is used to initiate the case. An inferior traction suture is placed through the inferior peripheral cornea for rotation of the globe downward. A 6-0 Vicryl on an S-29 needle is usually used (Ethicon, Johnson & Johnson, New Brunswick, NJ). Some surgeons employ a similar suture through the superior peripheral cornea, but care should be taken not to abrade the cornea, which would impair visualization during the cataract surgery and cause the patient discomfort postoperative (Fig. 11.11).

A limbal conjunctival peritomy, 5–6 mm, is fashioned with a Westcott scissor and a conjunctival forceps in one superior quadrant (Figs. 6.4 and 6.5a). The conjunctiva and

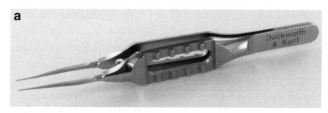

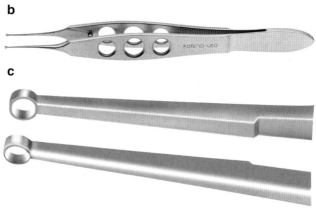

Fig. 6.4 Conjunctival forceps designed not to tear the delicate conjuctival tissue. (**a**) Duckworth and Kent DK 2-100 forceps. Image courtesy of Duckworth and Kent Ltd., Herts, England. (**b**) Fechtner K5-1820 conjunctival forceps with (**c**) close-up of Fechtner forceps. Part figures (**b**) and (**c**) courtesy of Katena Products Inc, Denville, NJ.

Tenon's are undermined in each direction to anticipate the broad application of MMC. This leaves a quadrant for a subsequent filtering procedure if needed in the future. Additional bupivacaine and/or preservative-free 1% lidocaine is injected into the quadrant with a sub-Tenon's cannula, such as the Connor cannula for deeper anesthesia, and this can be supplemented with intracameral 1% preservative-free lidocaine (see Chapter 2). Cautery is used to blanch but not char the episclera.

A scleratome blade is used to fashion a partial thickness scleral flap 3–4 mm at its base, at least $\frac{1}{2}$ thickness of the sclera (Figs. 6.5b and 6.6). To avoid premature entry into the anterior chamber, which would make the use of MMC risky, the author stops before reaching the limbus and applies pieces of (Merocil® or Weckcel®, Medtronics, Minneapolis, MN) cellulose sponges with MMC 0.4 mg/ml under the Tenon's layer, in a broad area for 3 minutes, taking care not to treat the limbus or the conjunctival wound edge (Fig. 6.7). After irrigation of the MMC treated area, with 30 cc of balanced salt solution (BSS), the scleral flap is continued into the peripheral cornea and, if needed for a non-foldable intraocular lens or ECCE, a scleral groove is made to one side (Fig. 6.8). A keratome is used to enter the anterior chamber under the flap creating a two-plane hinged incision for the phacoemulsification (Fig. 6.9). Viscoelastic is injected, taking care not to overly elevate the intraocular pressure, espea   b

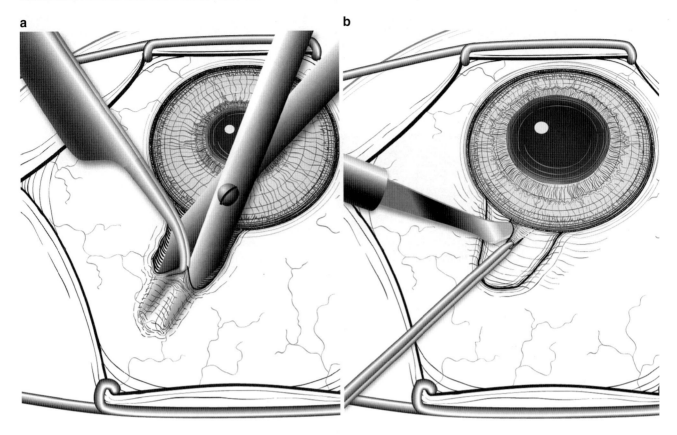

Fig. 6.5 Diagram of the conjunctival incision

cially if there is significant glaucoma damage. A paracentesis is fashioned for the surgeon's use of a second instrument and for injection of BSS as needed.

Once the cataract surgery is complete and the intraocular lens has been placed, the author does not remove residual viscoelastic, to help maintain the globe. The author uses a foldable acrylic IOL. Acetylcholine chloride intraocular solution (Miochol-E, Novartis, East Hanover, NJ) is injected to constrict the pupil. A Kelly punch is used to create a sclerostomy under the scleral flap with a minimum of 1 mm of flap maintained on each side of it (Fig. 6.10). A jeweler's forceps and Vaness scissor are used to create a peripheral iridectomy (Fig. 6.11). The necessity of this has been questioned in a report by Shingleton.[62] A 23-gauge cautery tip is used for any bleeders in the sclerostomy site. Once it is ensured there is no bleeding from the sclerostomy or iridectomy, the scleral flap is closed with two interrupted or releasable 10-0 nylon sutures, near the base of the flap (Fig. 6.12). The anterior chamber is deepened with BSS through the paracentesis and the eye observed to ensure that the anterior chamber is deep, the eye not hard, and that there is some flow of fluid from beneath the flap. Flow toward the 12 o'clock limbus and posterior is preferred over flow toward the palpebral fis-

sure. Additional sutures are placed as needed. Releasables are used if a laser is not readily available postoperative and for patients with conjunctival melanosis that will interfere with laser suture lysis (see Chapter 10).

The limbal epithelium is abraded with a Tooke knife and the conjunctiva brought up to the limbus (Fig. 6.13). It is secured tightly to its original position with interrupted 8-0 Vicryl sutures on a TG 140 or BV 130 needle. Again the anterior chamber is formed and the wound observed for any leaks and need for reinforcement. A Seidel test can be done (Fig. 9.4). Viscoelastic can be left in the anterior chamber as long as the tactile IOP is not too high for the patient. The fixation suture is removed. Subconjunctival injections of a steroid and antibiotic are given in the inferior fornix. The eye is patched with a combination steroid antibiotic ointment for 24 h.

A technique popularized by Khaw is the Moorfield's safe surgery technique, which is described briefly in Chapter 9 and reviewed in Chapter 8. The surgical principals involve the diversion of filtration posterior and over a wide area avoiding filtration along the limbus anterior to the insertion of Tenon's and very localized filtration. These principals help to avoid a focal ischemic bleb prone to

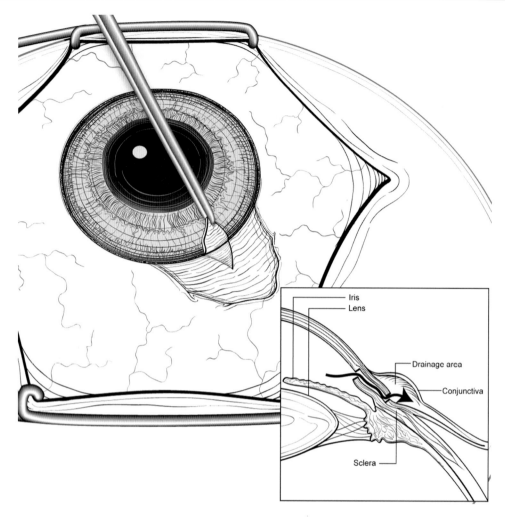

Iris
Lens
Drainage area
Conjunctiva
Sclera

Fig. 6.6 Diagram of the scleral flap fashioned after the conjunctival incision. Profile of the scleral flap dissection

dysfunction years postoperative.[63,64] The technique also discusses alternate closure of the conjunctiva to help avoid leaks. Chapter 14 reviews a conjunctival incision that is several millimeters posterior to the limbus that leaves a skirt of conjunctiva that can be sutured in a running fashion for a tight closure.

Surgeons who are not adept at a superior approach to phacoemulsification or who have a preference for a limbal-based trabeculectomy often prefer a two-site approach. The surgeon's standard phacoemulsification is done, the temporal wound sutured, and viscoelastic left in the eye, taking care not to over pressurize the eye. A standard superior trabeculectomy is then completed. A limbal-based trabeculectomy is likely to have less risk of postoperative wound leak and can endure earlier laser suture lysis due to this.[56] It has been reported to take longer than a fornix-based approach. Typical instruments used in a combined surgery are listed in Table 19.4 and Chapter 19 includes a review of two-site surgery.

Postoperative Care

The patient is seen on postoperative day 1, then about day 5, then 7 days later, then 7–10 days later, and so forth. A broad-spectrum antibiotic such as Vigamox (Alcon, Fort Worth, TX) is used for the first 10–14 days as prophylaxis against infection. The author uses prednisolone acetate 1% drops initially four times a day, then increases this to six times or more at the second visit, to allow some conjunctival healing before the use of aggressive anti-inflammatory drops.

If there is a wound leak on postoperative day 1, it is treated conservatively with a bandage contact lens. Leaks detected or persisting after that are generally sutured closed due to the possible increased risk of bleb failure.[65] Steroids are tapered over 6–8 weeks, as directed by intraocular and bleb inflammation.

Laser suture lysis or release of releasable sutures is done as needed to preserve bleb function, as well as supplemental 5-FU injections. Decision for suture release is usually made

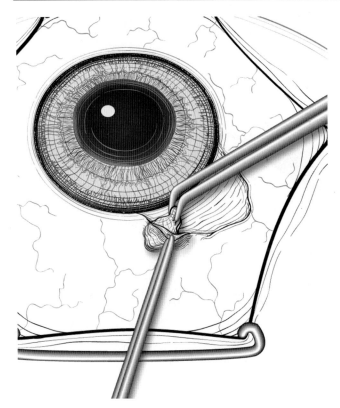

Fig. 6.7 Scleral groove adjacent to scleral flap if needed for IOL insertion

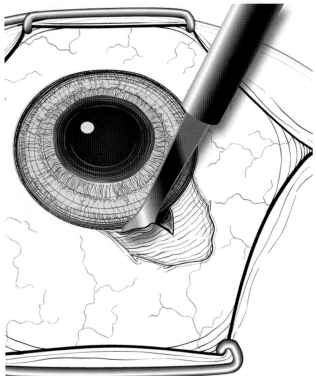

Fig. 6.8 Sponges with MMC placed under the conjunctiva with avoidance of the wound edges

in the second or later postoperative week (see Chapter 10). Predictors of suture release were assessed in one report by Shin et al. African-American ancestry, more than two medications preoperative, and pressure of 14 or over in the first week were found to be predictors of need for suture release.[66] The authors pursued suture release when digital pressure did not result in increased filtration.

Fundus exams are done to ensure that there are no significant choroidal effusions, especially if there is marked shallowing of the anterior chamber or hypotony. They are managed as needed to preserve integrity of the cornea, prevent posterior anterior synechiae (PAS), and to maintain bleb function (see Chapter 12). Results from the Advanced Glaucoma Intervention Study (AGIS) versus the Collaborative Initial Glaucoma Treatment Study (CIGITS) suggest that older patients are more likely to develop choroidal effusions following a filtration procedure.[10,16]

Outcomes

In the report by Buys, the mean preoperative IOP was over 17 mmHg on a mean of three medications. At 2 years follow-up, the mean IOP was between 12 and 13 mmHg and mean

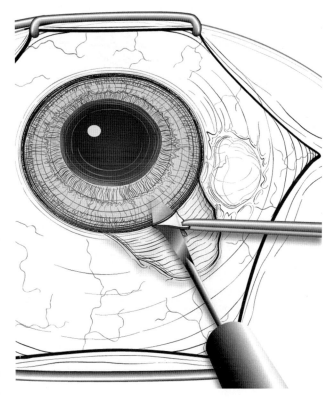

Fig. 6.9 Keratome incision under the scleral flap

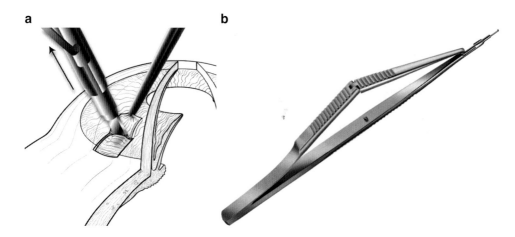

Fig. 6.10 (**a**) Kelly Descemet's Punch. Figure courtesy of Bausch & Lomb, Rochester, NY. (**b**) The punch is used to create the sclerostomy

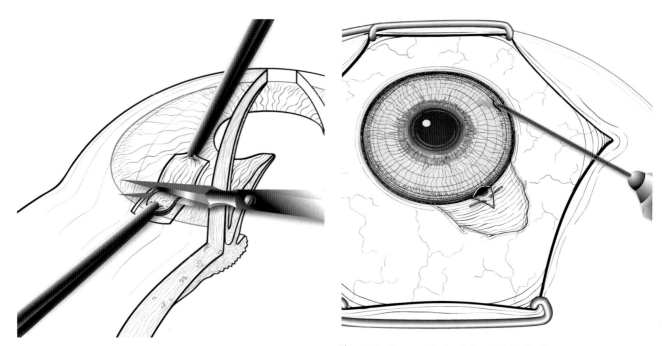

Fig. 6.11 Iridectomy

Fig. 6.12 Closure of scleral flap with 10-0 nylon sutures.

medications were under 0.5 for 76 of the 80 patients enrolled in the study.[54] In the study by Cotran, 74 of 90 eyes were studied at 3 years of follow-up. Mean preoperative medications were 2.3 to 2.5 ± 0.9 and less than 0.5 ± 1 at 3 years. Mean preoperative IOP decreased from 20.1 ± 3.8 and 19.5 ± 5.3 to 12.6 ± 4.8 and 11.7 ± 4 mmHg at 3 years for the two groups.[56] Both of these studies used MMC 0.4 mg/ml for 2 minutes. They also used acrylic IOLs.

Figure 6.14a–c illustrates an eye postoperative a one-site combined surgery. Hong reported on a Korean population that included 540 triple procedures followed up to 15 years, with a minimum of 3.[67] The mean preoperative IOP was about 20 ± 12.6 and the mean last mean IOP was 12.5 ± 2.61 mmHg. The IOP mean was quite stable from 1 to 15 year. Less than 3% of patients required a second trabeculectomy procedure. Laser suture lysis was required in 32% of the patients.

Refractive Outcomes

Several studies have reviewed astigmatism associated with glaucoma triple procedure with 6-mm incisions and found that less astigmatism was induced with the cataract procedure done temporal.[51,68,69] In more recent years, biometry has changed from a contact examination to non-contact with the technology of the IOL Master (Zeiss-Humphrey,

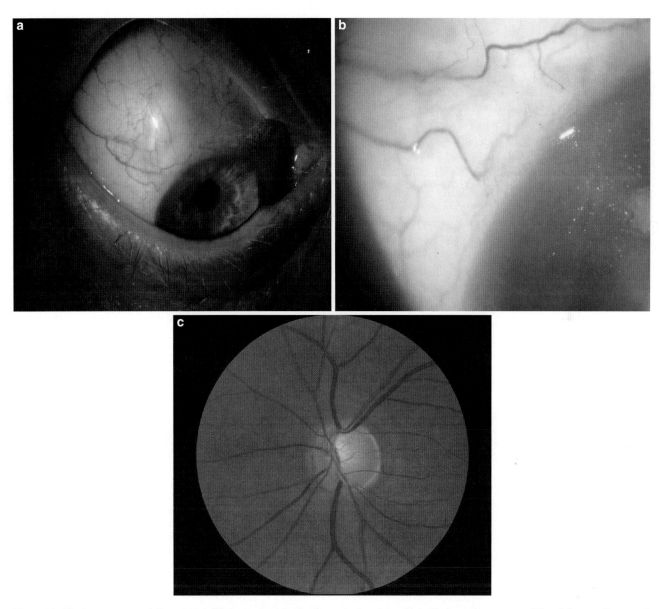

Fig. 6.13 Storz EO390 Tooke knife. Courtesy of Bausch & Lomb, Rochester, NY

Fig. 6.14 Final appearance of the eye; (**a**) Slit lamp photograph of a diffuse bleb following a combined procedure. At 1 year of follow-up, IOP was remained 10–12 mmHg without medications. (**b**) Close-up of the low lying bleb. Photograph courtesy of Tom Monego, Dartmouth Hitchcock Medical Center (DHMC), Lebanon, NH. (**c**) Fundus photo of the disc of the patient. Photograph courtesy of Tom Monego at DHMC

Dublin, CA). It uses the principal of partial coherence interferometry. Caprioli and authors reviewed the predicted and actual refractive outcomes in 24 eyes that had undergone a glaucoma triple procedure with a comparison group who had undergone phacoemulsification alone. Their measurements confirmed an overall with the rule astigmatism and shortening of the axial length in eyes following glaucoma triple procedure, using a two-site technique. The spherical equivalents of the postoperative refractions did not differ significantly from predicted refraction.[70] Care should be taken in surgery to not induce astigmatism with overly tight sutures and aggressive cautery. The change in axial length can manifest as a myopic shift as reported by Chan and coauthors. They studied 90 consecutive patients, 25 of whom had undergone glaucoma triple procedure. They conclude that the postoperative change in anterior chamber depth is responsible for the myopic shift in patients who have trabeculectomy at the time of cataract surgery.[71] Interestingly, Shin has noted decreased posterior capsular opacification in eyes status post glaucoma triple procedure with MMC.[43]

Complications

Besides complications related to cataract extraction in general, a glaucoma triple procedure is subject to the same complications as any filtering procedure, as listed in Table 6.3. Most complications are self limited and treated conservatively, but complications requiring invasive intervention may occur. In the Cotran study, there was one case of hypotony maculopathy that required surgery in one group and one patient in the other group developed corneal edema related to shallow anterior chamber and subsequently underwent penetrating keratoplasty. Two late wound leaks developed in the two-site group and one developed blebitis. Both underwent bleb revision.[56] In the Buys study, one patient underwent bleb needling.[54] In the Hong study, there were more bleb leaks, hyphema, and endophthalmitis in the triple-procedure group compared to a trabeculectomy-alone group, which had more hypotony.[67]

Table 6.3 Complications associated with glaucoma triple procedure with MMC[35,36,54,5,6]

- Choroidal detachment and/or hemorrhage
- Hypotony: shallow anterior chamber, maculopathy
- Hyphema
- Wound leaks
- Blocked sclerostomies
- Late endophthalmitis
- Astigmatism

Summary

As cataract incisions have gotten smaller, the results of combined surgery have improved. For incisions of 6 mm and under, the effect of the incision length on IOP outcomes does not appear to be as significant, although the globe remains better formed in surgery with a smaller incision. MMC has assisted in the success of the procedure, even including surgery with larger incisions for ECCE. A capsulorhexis, smaller than the size of the IOL optic, helps to prevent IOL capture should the anterior chamber shallow in the postoperative period. The impact on refractive error has also lessened with the adoption of smaller incision cataract procedures combined with glaucoma surgery.[36,70,71]

Ophthalmologists should consider combined surgery in patients with low target IOP, complex medical regimens, and advanced glaucoma. The surgical approach should be chosen that best suits the surgeon's skills and preferences, taking into consideration the possible adverse effect that a two-site procedure may have on the corneal endothelium and the longer surgical time it entails, and balance this against increased risk of wound leak with a one-site approach. The surgeon should be prepared for the more complex postoperative management dictated by the trabeculectomy (Table 6.4) and counsel the patient regarding a less predictable refractive outcome versus cataract alone. Management of the bleb is discussed in Chapter 9 and choroidal effusions are discussed in Chapter 12.

Table 6.4 Common minor procedures post trabeculectomy

- Anterior chamber injection: viscoelastic,[72] TPA
- Bleb needling
- Postoperative subconjunctival 5-FU injections
- Treatment of wound leaks: sutures or other
- Bandage contact lenses for over filtration or leaks
- Palmberg sutures
- Suture lysis or release
- YAG capsulotomy/anterior hyaloidectomy for malignant glaucoma
- Reversal of blocked sclerostomy
- IOL repositioning for pupil capture

References

1. Lichter PR, Musch DC, Gillespie BW, et al. Interim clinical outcomes in the collaborative initial glaucoma treatment study comparing initial treatment randomized to medications or surgery. *Ophthalmololgy.* 2001;108:1943–53.
2. CNTGSG. Comparisons of glaucomatous progression between untreated patients with normal tension glaucoma and patients with therapeutically reduced pressure. *Am J Opthalmol.* 1998;126: 487–97.
3. The AGIS Investigators. The advanced glaucoma intervention study (AGIS) 7. The relation between control of intraocular pressure and visual field deterioration. *Am J Ophthalmol.* 2000;130:429–40.
4. Yu CBO, Chong NHV, Caeser RH, et al. Long term results of combined cataract and glaucoma surgery versus trabeculectomy alone in low-risk patients. *J Cataract Refract Surg.* 1996;22: 352–7.
5. Friedman DS, Jampel HD, Lubomski LH, et al. Surgical strategies for coexisting glaucoma. An evidence-based update. *Ophthamology.* 2002;109:1902–13.
6. Bobrow JC. Prospective intrapatient comparision of extracapsular cataract extraction and lens implantation with and without trabeculectomy. *Am J Ophthamol.* 2000;129:291–6.
7. Krupin T, Feitl ME, Bishop KI. Postoperative intraocular pressure rise in open angle glaucoma patients after cataract or combined cataract filtration surgery. *Ophthalmology.* 1989;96:579–84.
8. Murchison JF, Shields MB. An evaluation of three surgical approaches for coexisting cataract and glaucoma. *Ophthalmic Surg.* 1989;20:393–8.

9. The AGIS Investigators. AGIS 8. Risk of cataract formation after trabeculectomy. *Arch Ophthalmol*. 2001;119:1771–80.

10. Lichter PR, Musch DC, Gillespie BW, et al. Interim clinical outcomes in the collaborative initial glaucoma treatment study comparing initial treatment randomized to medications or surgery. *Ophthalmology*. 2001;108:1943–53.

11. Hylton C, Congdon N, Griedman D, et al. Cataract after glaucoma filtration surgery. *Am J Ophthalmol*. 2003;135:231–2.

12. Merkur A, Damji KF, Mintsioulis G, Hodge WG. Intraocular pressure decrease after phacoemulsification in patients with pseudoexfoliation syndrome. *J Cataract Refract Surg*. 2001;27:528–32.

13. Damji KF, Konstas AG, Liebmann JM, et al. Intraocular pressure following phacoemulsification in patients with and without exfoliation syndrome: a two year prospective study. *Br J Ophthalmol*. 2006;90:1014–8.

14. Shingleton BJ, Heltzer J, O' Donoghue MW. Outcomes of phacoemulsification in patients with and without pseudoexfoliation syndromes. *J Cataract Refract Surg*. 2003;29:1080–6.

15. Jeganathan VSE, Ghosh S, Ruddle JB, et al. Risk factors for delayed suprachoroidal haemorrhage following glaucoma surgery. *Br J Ophthalmol*. 2008;92:1393–6.

16. The AGIS Investigators. AGIS 11. Risk factors for failure of trabeculectomy and argon laser trabeculoplasty. *Am J Ophthalmol*. 2002;134:481–98.

17. Jampel HD, Musch DC, Gillespie BW, et al. Perioperative complications of trabeculectomy in the collaborative initial glaucoma treatment study (CIGITS). *Am J Ophthalmol*. 2005;140:16–22.

18. Simmons ST, Litoff D, Nichols DA, et al. Extracapsular cataract extraction and posterior chamber intraocular lens implantation combined with trabeculectomy in patients with glaucoma. *Am J Ophthalmol*. 1987;104:465–70.

19. Hurwitz LM. 5-FU-supplemented phacoemulsification, posterior chamber intraocular lens implantation and trabeculectomy. *Ophthalmic Surg*. 1993;24:674–80.

20. Shingleton BJ, Jacobson LM, Kuperwaser MC. Comparison of combined cataract and glaucoma surgery using planned extracapsular and phacoemulsification techniques. *Ophthalmic Surg Lasers*. 1995;26:414–9.

21. Stewart WC, Crinkley CMC, Carlson AN. Results of trabeculectomy combined with phacoemulsification versus trabeculectomy combined with extracapsular cataract extraction in patients with advanced glaucoma. *Ophthalmic Surg*. 1994;25:621–7.

22. Wishart PK, Austin MW. Combined cataract extraction and trabeculectomy: phacoemulsification compared with extracapsular technique. *Ophthalmic Surg*. 1993;24:814–21.

23. Tous HM, Nevarez J. Comparison of outcomes following combined ECCE-trabeculectomy versus phacoemulsification-trabeculectomy. *PR Health Sci J*. 2006;25:319–23.

24. Lyle WA, Jin JC. Comparison or a 3- and 6-mm incision in combined phacoemulsification and trabeculectomy. *Am J Ophthalmol*. 1991;111:189–96.

25. Stewart WC, Sine CS, Carlson AN. Three-millimeter versus 6-mm incisions in combined phacoemulsification and trabeculectomy. *Ophthalmic Surg Lasers*. 1996;27:832–8.

26. Vyas AV, Bacon PJ, Pervical SPB. Phacotrabeculectomy: comparision of results from 3.5- and 5.2-mm incisions. *Ophthalmic Surg Lasers*. 1998;29:227–33.

27. Wedrich A, Menapace R, Radax U, Papapanos P. Long-term results of combined trabeculectomy and small incision cataract surgery. *J Catract Refract Surg*. 1995;21:49–54.

28. O'Grady JM, Juzych MS, Shin DH, et al. Trabeculectomy, phacoemulsification, and posterior chamber lens implantation with and without 5-fluorouracil. *Am J Ophthalmol*. 1993;116:594–9.

29. Cohen JS. Combined cataract implant and filtering surgery with 5-fluorouracil. *Ophthalmic Surg*. 1990;21:181–6.

30. Gandolfi SA, Vecchi M. 5-fluorouracil in combined with trabeculectomy and clear-cornea phacoemulsification with posterior chamber intraocular lens implantation. A one-year randomized controlled clinical trial. *Ophthalmology*. 1997;104:181–6.

31. Donoso R, Rodriguez A. Combined versus sequential phacotrabeculectomy with intraoperative 5-fluorouracil. *J Cataract Refract Surg*. 2000;26:71–4.

32. Chang L, Thiagarajan M, Moseley M, et al. Intraocular pressure outcome in primary 5-FU phacotrabeculectomy compared with 5-FU trabeculectomies. *J Glaucoma*. 2006;15:475–81.

33. Jampel HD, Friedman DS, Lubomski LH, et al. Effect of technique on intraocular pressure after combined cataract and glaucoma surgery. *Ophthalmology*. 2002;109:2215–24.

34. Reibaldi A, Uva MG, Longo A. Nine-year follow-up of trabeculectomy with or without low-dosage mitomycin-C in primary open angle glaucoma. *Br J Ophthalmol*. 2008;92:1666–70.

35. Rockwood EJ, Larive B, Hahn J. Outcomes of combined cataract extraction, lens implantation, and trabeculectomy surgeries. *Am J Ophthalmol*. 2000;130:704–11.

36. Belyea DA, Dan JA, Lieberman MT, Stamper RL. Midterm follow-up results or combined phacoemulsification, lens implantation and mitomycin-C trabeculectomy procedure. *J Glaucoma*. 1997;6:90–8.

37. Jin GJC, Crandall AS, Jones JJ. Phacetrabeculectomy: assessment of outcomes and surgical improvements. *J Cataract Refract Surg*. 2007;33:1201–8.

38. Lederer CM. Combined cataract extraction with intraocular lens implant and mitomycin-augmented trabeculectomy. *Ophthalmology*. 1996;103:1025–34.

39. Munden PM, Alward WLM. Combined phacoemulsification, posterior chamber intraocular lens implantation and trabeculectomy with mitomycin C. *Am J Ophthalmol*. 1995;119:20–9.

40. Scott IU, Greenfield DS, Schiffman J, et al. Outcomes of primary trabeculectomy with the use of adjunctive mitomycin. *Arch Ophthalmol*. 1998;116:286–91.

41. Carlson DW, Alward WLM, et al. A randomized study of mitomycin augmentation in combined phacoemulsification and trabeculectomy. *Ophthalmology*. 1997;104:719–24.

42. Shin DH. Simone PA, Song MS, et al. Adjunctive subconjunctival mitomycin C in glaucoma triple procedure. *Ophthalmology*. 1995;102:1550–8.

43. Shin DH, Ren J, Juzych MS, et al. Primary glaucoma triple procedure in patients with primary open angle glaucoma: The effect of mitomycin C in patients with and without prognostic factors for filtration failure. *Am J Ophthalmol*. 1998;125:346–52.

44. Shin DH, Kim YY, Sheth N, et al. The role of adjunctive mitomycin C in secondary glaucoma triple procedure as compared to primary glaucoma triple procedure. *Ophthalmology*. 1998;105:740–5.

45. Shin DH, Iskander NG, Ahee JA, et al. Long-term filtration and visual field outcomes after primary glaucoma triple procedure with and without mitomycin C. *Ophthalmology*. 2002;109:1607–11.

46. Tezel G, Kolker AE, Kass MA, Wax MB. Comparitive results of combined procedures for glaucoma and cataract: II. Limbus-based versus fornix-based conjunctival flaps. *Ophthalmic Surg Lasers*. 1997;28:551–7.

47. Shingleton BJ, Chaudhry IM, O'Donoghue MW, et al. Limbus-based versus fornix-based conjunctival flaps in fellow eyes. *Ophthalmology*. 1999;106:1152–5.

48. Kozobolis VP, Siganos CS, Christodoulakis EV, et al. Two-site phacotrabeculectomy with intraoperative mitomycin-C: fornix-versus limbus-based conjunctival opening in fellow eyes. *J Cataract Refract Surg*. 2002;28:1758–62.

49. Berestka JS, Brown SVL. Limbus- versus fornix-based conjunctival flaps in combined phacoemulsification and mitomycin C trabeculectomy surgery. *Ophthalmology*. 1997;104:187–96.

50. Lemon LC, Shin DH, Kim C, et al. Limbus-based versus fornix-based conjunctival flap in combined glaucoma and cataract surgery with adjunctive mitomycin C. *Am J Ophthalmol*. 1998;125:340–5.

51. Wyse T, Meyer M, Ruderman JM, et al. Combined trabeculectomy and phacoemulsification: a one-site versus a two-site approach. *Am J Ophthalmol*. 1998;125:334–9.

52. El Sayyad F, Helal M, el Maghraby A, et al. One-siet versus two-site phacotrabeculectomy: a randomized study. *J Catract Refract Surg*. 1999;25:77–82.

53. Borggefe J, Lieb W, Grehn F. A prospective reandomized comparison of two techniques of combined cataract-glaucoma surgery. *Graefes Arch CLin Exp Ophthalmol*. 1999;237:887–92.

54. Buys YM, Chipman ML, Zack B, et al. Prospective randomized comparison of one-versus tow site phacotrabeculectomy two year results. *Ophthalmology*. 2008;115:1130–3.

55. Nassiri N, Nassiri N, Rahnavardi M, Rahmani L. A comparison of corneal endothelial cell changes after 1-site and 2-site phacotrabeculectomy. *Cornea* 2008;27:889–94.

56. Cotran PR, Roh S, McGwin G. Randomized comparison of 1-site and 2-site phacotrabeculectomy with 3-year follow-up. *Ophthalmology*. 2008;115:447–54.

57. Tezel G, Kolker AE, Kass MA, Wax MB. Comparative results for combined procedures for glaucoma and cataract: I. Extracapsular cataract extraction versus phacoemulsification and foldable versus rigid intraocular lenses. *Ophthalmic Surg Lasers*. 1997;28:539–50.

58. Alzafiri Y, Harasymowycz P. Foldable acylic versis rigid polymethylmethacrylate intraocular lens in combined phacoemulsification and trabeculectomy. *Can J Ophthalmol*. 2004;39:609–13.

59. Lemon LC, Shin DH, Song MS, et al. Comparatvie study of silicone versis acrylic foldable lens implantation in primary glaucoma triple procedure. *Ophthalmology*. 1997;104:1708–13.

60. Friedrich Y, Raniel Y, Lubovsky E, Friedman Z. Late pigmented-membrane formation on silicone intraocular lenses after phacoemulsification with or without trabeculectomy. *J Catraract Refract Surg*. 1999;25:1220–5.

61. Serpa E, Wishart PK. Comparison of PMMA, foldable silicone and foldable acrylic hydrophobic intraocular lenses in combined phacoemulsification and trabeculectomy. *Arq Bras Oftalmol*. 2005;68:29–35.

62. Shingleton BJ, Chaudhry IM, O'Donoghue MW. Phacotrabeculectomy: peripheral iridectomy or no peripheral iridectomy. *J Catract Refract Surg*. 2002;28:998–1002.

63. Jones E, Clarke J, Khaw PT. Recent advances in trabeculectomy technique. *Curr Opin Ophthalmol*. 2005;16:107–13.

64. Stalmans K, Gillis A, Lafaut AS, Zeyen T. Safe trabeculectomy technique: long term outcome. *Br J Ophthalmol*. 2006;90:44–7.

65. Parrish RK, Schiffman JC, Feuer WJ, Heuer DK. Fluorouracil filtering surgery study group. Prognosis and risk racotrs for early postoperative wound leaks after trabeculectomy with and without 5-fluorouracil. *Am J Ophthalmol*. 2001;132:633–40.

66. Morris DA, Peracha MO, Shin DHH, et al. Risk factors for early filtration failure requiring suture release after primary glaucoma triple procedure with adjunctive mitomycin. *Arch Ophthalmol*. 1999;117:1149–54.

67. Hong S, Park K, Ha SJ, et al. Long-term intraocular pressure control of trabeculectomy and triple procedure in primary open angle glaucoma and chronic primary angle closure glaucoma. *Ophthamologica*. 2007;221:395–401.

68. Gayton JL, Van Der Karr MA, Sanders V. Combined cataract and glaucoma procedures using temporal cataract surgery. *J Catract Refract Surg*. 1996;22:1485–91.

69. Hong YJ, Choe CM, Lee YG, et al. The effect of mitomycin C on postoperative corneal astigmatism in trabeculectomy and a triple procedure. *Ophthalmic Surg Lasers*. 1998;29:484–9.

70. Law SK, Mansury AM, Vasudev D, Caprioli J. Effects of combined catraract surgery and trabeculectomy with mitomycin C on ocular dimensions. *Br J Ophthalmol*. 2005;89:1021–5.

71. Chan JC, Lai JS, Tham CC. Comparison of postoperative refractive outcome in phacotrabeculectomy and phacoemulsification with posterior chamber intraocular lens implantation. *J Glaucoma*. 2006;15:26–9.

72. Osher RH, Cionni RJ, Cohen JS. Re-forming the flat anterior chamber with Healon. *J Cataract Refract Surg*. 1996;22:411–5.

Chapter 7

Managing Cataract and Glaucoma in the Developing World – Manual Small Incision Cataract Surgery (MSICS) Combined with Trabeculectomy

Rengaraj Venkatesh, Rengappa Ramakrishnan, Ramasamy Krishnadas, Parthasarathy Sathyan, and Alan L. Robin

Introduction

There is a strong interrelation between surgical management of glaucoma and cataract. Performing cataract surgery alone can lower the intraocular pressure, by about 4–6 mmHg. Glaucoma and cataract are diseases whose prevalence increases with advancing age. People living in developing countries have the highest risk of developing blindness from glaucoma.[1] Angle-closure glaucoma predominates in some parts of East Asia, whereas in most of the Indian subcontinent, Africa, and in Hispanic populations, open angle forms are more common.[2] Treatments for glaucoma vary depending on the type of glaucoma and the setting. Glaucoma filtration surgery also has a higher risk of inducing operable cataracts, especially with the addition of antimetabolites such as mitomycin C or if shallow anterior chamber or persistent choroidal detachments occur.[3]

Patients usually perceive the benefits of cataract surgery, through increased vision, leading to improved quality of life. The advent of small incision cataract surgery and intraocular lens implantation has greatly increased patients' satisfaction with surgical interventions. In contradistinction, most perceive a worsening of their well-being after glaucoma surgery due to invariable loss of a few lines of visual acuity. In a developed nation, this concept may be difficult to convey to a patient. In a developing nation, the magnitude of this negative social marketing may increase manyfold and even convince an entire village not to come for routine eye care. Individuals may perceive that the doctors are diminishing good vision rather than preserving vision. Thus balancing the benefits of glaucoma surgery against the risk of cataract formation is dependent on the socioeconomic background in which glaucoma occurs.

Access to eye care is important, and as most tertiary care ophthalmology services are in urban centers, people often have to travel far to receive good quality services. Accessibility and distance to healthcare are critical factors associated with utilization of services as well as compliance in developing countries.[4] Good quality care for cataract is definitely available but can vary greatly depending upon the location. Good surgical treatment for glaucoma in the developing world is much less readily available and most disease remains undetected.[5,6] This is partly due to an emphasis primarily on training to detect and treat cataracts, which is the leading cause of reversible visual disability, and the relative lack of specialized glaucoma training. Drugs for glaucoma are also relatively expensive, difficult to obtain, and the quality of the generics may vary. Manpower and equipment for glaucoma care is limited. Thus, persistence with medical therapy is low and inclination to perform surgery before medical treatment is much higher, in contrast to the developed world, where surgery is usually performed later in the course of treatment.

Cataract is the most common cause of surgically reversible blindness worldwide, and cataract formation as a complication of trabeculectomy adds to the burden of preventable lost sight. People are less likely to return for further surgery if they do not perceive a benefit, especially if treatment for glaucoma makes their vision worse. The high cost of present methods for glaucoma screening is a barrier to the identification of people at high risk for glaucoma blindness. In essence, surgery has the potential to fulfill many features of an ideal approach to reduce intraocular pressure (IOP) compared with medications. It can lower the IOP to low teens, achieve long-term IOP reduction, minimize IOP fluctuations, lower the long-term cost, and minimize systemic side effects. The major drawbacks, though, are the potentially devastating, but rare, ocular side effects such as endophthalmitis, suprachoroidal hemorrhage, and corneal decompensation.

Trabeculectomy combined with cataract surgery is considered safe and effective in the management of cataract associated with glaucoma. It prevents early intraocular pressure

R. Venkatesh (✉)
Department of Glaucoma, Aravind Eye Hospital, Pondicherry, 605007, India
e-mail: venkatesh@pondy.aravind.org

S.M. Johnson (ed.), *Cataract Surgery in the Glaucoma Patient*, DOI 10.1007/978-0-387-09408-3_7,
© Springer Science+Business Media, LLC 2009

spikes responsible for visual field "wipe out" in eyes with advanced glaucoma undergoing cataract surgery and provides beneficial visual rehabilitation with long-term IOP control.[7] The use of phacoemulsification and wound-healing modulators have improved the results of combined cataract and glaucoma surgery with intraocular lens implantation (glaucoma triple surgery). Reports suggest that IOP control is superior to standard extracapsular cataract surgery combined with filtering surgery.[8,9] Smaller wounds in eyes undergoing phacoemulsification have several advantages in addition to IOP control. These include less surgically induced astigmatism, earlier visual rehabilitation, and decreased hospital stay.[10] The advantage of phacoemulsification is related to the smaller incision. But phacoemulsification has a relatively steep learning curve and is costly in terms of fixed and consumable equipment. Phacoemulsification requires constant power, good maintenance, and immediate service if the instruments or hand piece are damaged. It is technically more difficult and carries a higher risk of complications in brunescent hard cataracts that typically occur more frequently in underserved populations.[11] Extracapsular cataract extraction (ECCE) may be associated with problems related to wound suturing and greater astigmatism. Manual Small Incision Cataract Surgery (MSICS) is an inexpensive alternative to phacoemulsification; it also achieves better uncorrected visual acuity compared to ECCE.[12]

With MSICS, high-volume and cost-effective surgery is possible without compromising quality.[13] Randomized controlled trials have proven the safety and efficacy of MSICS as compared to phacoemulsification in terms of visual recovery as well as intraoperative complications, depending on the surgical expertise.[14,15] With MSICS, any type of cataract can be tackled with ease and the timing of surgery is not altered by the density of cataract, in contrast to phacoemulsification. In the developing world, patients present later for surgery and present with more advanced cataracts. They often assume that loss of vision is a normal consequence of aging, are unable to come for routine eye care, or do not have the support system to easily bring them in for cataract surgery. The difference in the prevalence of advanced cataracts can be seen in multiple studies[16] and patients with these often visit the hospital through outreach eye camps, and may be found to have elevated intraocular pressure and compromised optic nerves simultaneously. We therefore need a cost-effective and highly productive surgical technique to tackle both cataract and glaucoma. If a manual small-incision technique is used for the cataract surgery, the small-incision advantage should theoretically still be applicable for performing a combined surgery. Such a technique is called Manual Small Incision Cataract Surgery Combined with Trabeculectomy (MSICS-Trab).

Procedure

General Principles

Anesthesia

Local anesthesia with either retrobulbar and facial block, or a peribulbar block is generally used. Sub-Tenon's anesthesia is also an option. See Chapter 2.

Bridle Suture

A 4/0 silk bridle suture is placed beneath the tendon of the superior rectus muscle to facilitate the creation of a superior scleral tunnel. Advantages of a bridle suture are as follows:

- To maneuver the globe and to fixate it during the steps of surgery like fashioning the scleral tunnel incision and suturing.
- It provides counter traction during procedures like nucleus removal and epinucleus delivery, thereby making these procedures easier and less traumatic.

Cataract Surgery

Conjunctival Flap and Scleral Dissection

Initial Incision

A fornix-based conjunctival flap at the limbus with a chord length of approximately 6.5 mm is made (Fig. 7.1). After Tenon's capsule is carefully dissected, light cautery is applied. Mitomycin C, 0.4–0.5 mg/ml, is applied to a broad area with a cellulose sponge(s) for approximately 3 minutes and then the area copiously irrigated with balanced salt solution. Care is taken not to treat the conjunctival wound edge. A one-third to one-half-thickness external scleral groove parallel to limbus, around 6–6.5 mm in width, is made 3 mm posterior to the surgical limbus (Fig. 7.2a, b).

Sclerocorneal Tunnel

The actual scleral tunnel is fashioned by gentle side-to-side motion of the bevel-up crescent blade along the tunnel toward the limbus. The posterior margin of the incision may be held and slightly elevated and the crescent blade

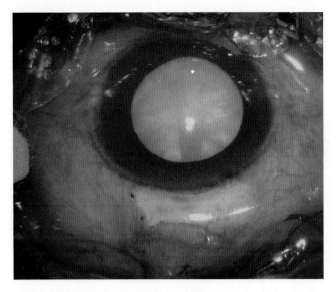

Fig. 7.1 Fornix-based 6.5 mm conjunctival flap

Creating a Side Port Entry

One side port entry is usually made using a 15° super blade at the 10 o'clock position and perpendicular to the tunnel in the clear cornea adjacent to the limbus. It is useful for the following:

1. Injection of viscoelastics to prevent the keratome from accidentally injuring the anterior lens capsule
2. To aspirate residual subincisional superior cortex at the end of irrigation and aspiration
3. To refill the anterior chamber at the end of the procedure, to ensure that the rate of fluid flow under the flap is not too great as this could cause a flat chamber.

wiggled back and forth gradually coming closer to the limbus. The roof of the tunnel should be uniform in thickness and the tunnel should extend up to 1.5 mm into the clear cornea along the entire width of the incision. This maneuver will prevent the tearing of the wound lips. The surgeon should keep in mind that the scleral tunnel is not a direct tunnel toward the inside of the eye but rather goes upwards along the curve of the globe. During tunneling forward one should raise the tip and depress the heel of the blade to prevent premature entry into the anterior chamber (Fig. 7.3).

Internal Corneal Incision

This is done using a sharp 3.2 mm angled keratome. The heel of the keratome is raised until the blade becomes parallel to the iris plane resulting in a dimple in Descemet's layer. The keratome is then advanced anteriorly in the same plane until the anterior chamber is entered and the internal wound is visualized as a straight line (Fig. 7.4). During extension of the incision, care should be taken to keep it in the same plane. The anterior chamber is totally reformed with viscoelastic (hydroxyl propyl methyl cellulose, HPMC) before extending the incision.

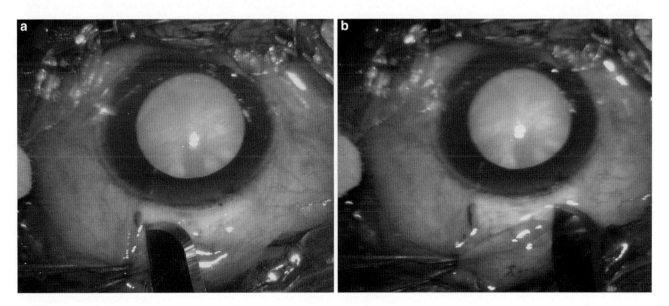

Fig. 7.2 (**a**) Shows construction of a partial thickness limbus parallel external scleral groove (**b**) of around 6–6.5 mm in width made 3 mm from the surgical limbus

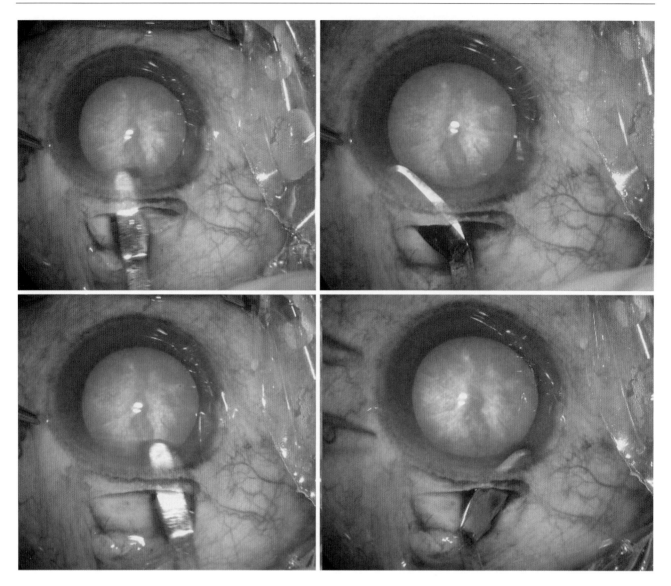

Fig. 7.3 Counterclockwise from top right, shows wriggling and swiping moment of the bevel up crescent blade along the tunnel in either direction

Capsulotomy

One of the significant advantages of MSICS over standard phacoemulsification is that it can be performed with any form of capsulotomy. Continuous curvilinear capsulorhexis (CCC) may be the ideal choice in view of the good centration of the intraocular lens (IOL) it provides. The diameter of the CCC is determined by the anticipated size of the endonucleus and it should have a minimum diameter of 5 mm to enable easy prolapse of the endonucleus into the anterior chamber. Capsular staining with 0.1 ml of 0.06% trypan blue is helpful in cases with white and dense brown nuclei where a good red reflex is not visible (Fig. 7.5 and Table 20.5). The capsular staining helps in making the difficult step of nucleus prolapse through an intact capsulorhexis safe and effortless, as the dye-stained capsular rim is distinctly visible all throughout the surgery. If the CCC created is smaller than desired, it is safer to make relaxing incisions and convert it to a can-opener style capsulotomy. In brown and black cataracts with much denser and larger nuclei, a can-opener capsulotomy is preferred, as it may facilitate a more effortless prolapse of the hard nucleus into the anterior chamber. Multiple confluent small tears (approximately 15–20 punctures per quadrant) are preferred to avoid capsular tags.

Hydrodissection

Hydrodissection is performed after removal of viscoelastic in the anterior chamber, using a 27-gauge bent tip cannula

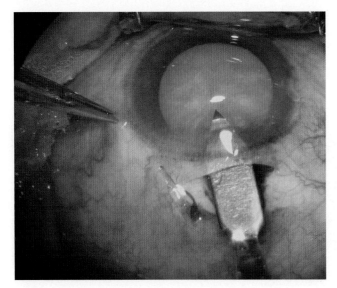

Fig. 7.4 Anterior chamber entry using a beveled down 3.2 mm keratome with internal wound visualized as a straight line

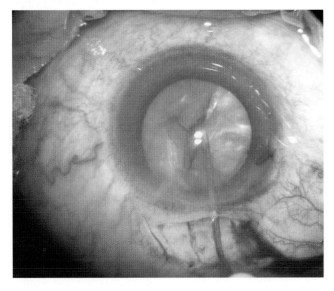

Fig. 7.5 *Trypan blue* assisted continuous curvilinear capsulorhexis in a mature white cataract

attached to a syringe filled with balanced salt solution (BSS). In the presence of capsulorhexis, this procedure can be completed in one smooth step by very gently injecting the fluid beneath the anterior capsular rim. A fluid wave can be appreciated when fluid is injected in the right plane. Tenting up the edge of the anterior capsulorhexis and injecting fluid ensures cortical cleaving hydrodissection. In the presence of a can-opener capsulotomy, small amounts of fluid can be injected in multiple quadrants to "unshackle" the nucleus from the confines of the cortex. At the end, a complete hydrodis-section should be confirmed by ability to freely rotate the

endonucleus within the capsular bag. Rotation of the nucleus also polishes the epithelial cells from the equator and may play a role in reducing posterior capsular opacification rates.

Prolapse of Nucleus into the Anterior Chamber

Hydroprolapse

Hydrodissection is usually done at the 9 or 3 o' clock position and the fluid wave is allowed to continue without decom-pressing the bag (as opposed to phacoemulsification), until one part of the equator of the nucleus is forced out of the cap-sulorhexis/capsulotomy. Continued injection of fluid slowly and gently increases the hydrostatic pressure within the bag to gently prolapse the nucleus. Once part of the equator is anterior to the capsulorhexis, stop the hydroprolapse. Inject viscoelastic slowly beneath the exposed equatorial region. Then introduce a Sinskey hook through the scleral tunnel to rotate the nucleus in a tire rolling fashion either clockwise or anticlockwise to elevate the entire nucleus into the anterior chamber.

Mechanical Method

This method can be used in cases of white or hard cataracts, whose nuclei are difficult to prolapse following hydrodissec-tion. In such cases, where the nucleus is hard and bulky, it is difficult to prolapse a pole out of the capsular bag by mere hydrostatic pressure created during hydrodissection. In addition, the posterior capsule in such cases is thinned, making it to prone to posterior capsular tear and nucleus drop if hydrostatic pressure builds within the capsule· during forceful hydrodissection (intraoperative capsular block syn-drome). The nucleus can be levered out of the bag using a Sinskey hook, even without hydroprocedures as if the nuclear attachment with the cortex may be almost nonexistent. In hypermature morgagnian cataracts with liquefied milky cor-tex, it is worthwhile to wash away some of the milky cortical matter, using a Simcoe cannula through a small opening cre-ated in the anterior lens capsule. This reduces intralenticular pressure and provides easy access to rotate the nucleus within the capsular bag before it is prolapsed. In cases with compro-mised zonules, a second instrument (cyclodialysis spatula) is passed between the hooked nuclear pole and the posterior capsule through a side port and the nucleus is rotated out using the support provided by the second instrument, reduc-ing stress on the zonules (Fig. 7.6a, b).

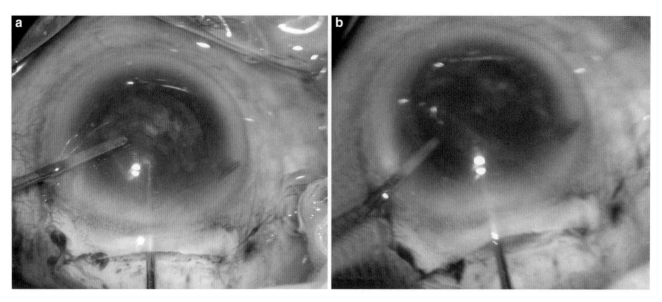

Fig. 7.6 (**a**) A second instrument (cyclodialysis spatula) is passed between the nucleus and the posterior capsule through a side port and (**b**) the nucleus is rotated out using the support provided by the second instrument, reducing stress on the zonules

Nucleus Extraction

Table 7.1 shows the four techniques for extracting the nucleus.

Table 7.1 Methods of nucleus extraction in MSICS

- Irrigating vectis technique
- Phacosandwich technique
- Modified blumenthal technique
- Fish hook technique

Irrigating Vectis Technique

This technique is a combination of mechanical and hydrostatic forces to express the nucleus. After the nucleus is prolapsed into the anterior chamber, viscoelastics are liberally but gently injected, first above and then below the nucleus. The upper layer shields the endothelium, while the lower layer pushes the posterior capsule and iris diaphragm posteriorly. This maneuver creates adequate space in the anterior chamber for atraumatic nuclear delivery. A good superior rectus bridle suture is necessary for the success of this step. The bridle suture is held loosely in one hand. After checking the patency of the ports (Fig. 7.7a), the vectis is now inserted beneath the nucleus with concave side up with the fellow hand. If it is an immature cataract, one will be able to see the margins of the vectis under the nucleus in place. As the superior rectus bridle suture is pulled tight, the irrigating vectis is slowly withdrawn without irrigating, until the superior pole of the nucleus is engaged in the tunnel (Fig. 7.7b).

Irrigation is then started and the vectis is slowly withdrawn, while pressing down the posterior scleral lip until the entire nucleus is expressed out of the section (Fig. 7.7c).

The force of irrigation has to be reduced when the maximum diameter of the nucleus just crosses the inner lip of the tunnel to help prevent the nucleus from being forcibly expelled with consequent sudden anterior chamber decompression and shallowing.

Phacosandwich Technique (an Assistant Is Required to Hold the Bridle Suture)

This technique is employed in cases with a hard nucleus, as sandwiching the nucleus with the help of two instruments can help to deliver the nucleus without enlarging the tunnel. In this technique, a Sinskey hook is used in addition to the vectis to sandwich the nucleus. The nucleus should be sufficiently dense to prevent cheese wiring of the two instruments engaging it. The key requisite is an adequately filled anterior chamber with viscoelastics to avoid endothelial damage by the second instrument and sufficient space for sliding the vectis beneath the nucleus. A curved vectis measuring approximately 4 mm at its greatest width and 8 mm in length is then introduced underneath the nucleus. The vectis should be allowed to find its own plane and this should not require any force for positioning. Once the vectis is placed beneath the nucleus, the Sinskey hook is carefully introduced and placed on top of the nucleus, sandwiching it between the vectis and the Sinskey hook. The tip of the Sinskey hook is placed beyond (inferior to) the central portion of the lens to get a better grip using a two-handed technique. With the

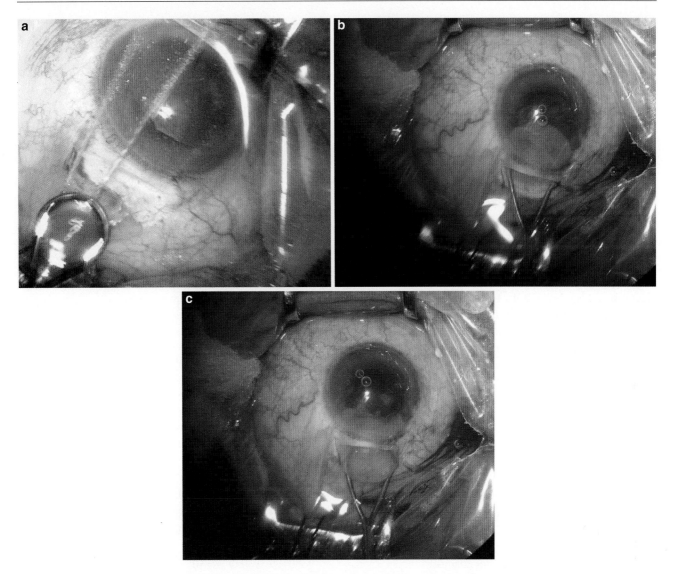

Fig. 7.7 (**a**) Irrigating vectis under the nucleus; (**b**) engaging the width of the tunnel; (**c**) nucleus expressed out of the tunnel

Sinskey hook in the dominant hand and vectis in the other, the nucleus is sandwiched and extracted, being slowly pulled toward the wound. While extracting the nucleus, an assistant should pull the superior rectus suture and at the same time should pull the globe down by grasping the conjunctiva at the 6 o' clock position near the limbus with the help of the toothed forceps. The outer portion of the nucleus, the epinucleus, and a portion of the cortex will be sheared off in this technique and can be removed with the irrigating vectis after nucleus delivery.

Modified Blumenthal Technique

This technique differs in that it requires an "anterior chamber maintainer," which is a hollow tube with 0.9 mm outer diameter and 0.65 mm inner diameter attached to a

BSS bottle, suspended approximately 50–60 cm above the patient's eye.

Two small beveled entries are made in the cornea; one is 1.5 mm long, placed between 5 and 7 o'clock position for connecting the anterior chamber maintainer. The other port is 1 mm wide, placed at the 11 o'clock position for the entry of various instruments. The fluid flow from the anterior chamber maintainer is stopped only during the capsulotomy. The bottle height is maintained at 50–60 cm above the patient's head. After a good hydrodissection, the nucleus is prolapsed into anterior chamber with mechanical nudging. The free nucleus in the deep anterior chamber is ready to be propelled out by the hydropressure generated by the anterior chamber maintainer system.

A plastic glide 3–4 mm wide, 0.3 mm thick, and 3 cm long is inserted under the nucleus for a distance of one-third to one-half of the width of the nucleus. Now the bottle height is raised between 60 and 70 cm and slight pressure is applied over the lens glide on the scleral side. Intermittent pressure will engage more and more nucleus out of the tunnel's mouth. Subsequently, a few more taps to open the scleral tunnel valve with the glide will enable the epinucleus and cortex to flow out of the anterior chamber.

Fish Hook Technique

After making the scleral tunnel of adequate length, a side port opening is made with a 15° blade and the anterior chamber is filled with viscoelastics. The anterior chamber is entered with a slit knife, and extended. A linear capsulotomy or an envelope capsulotomy is made. In a linear or envelope capsulotomy, a linear incision is made into the anterior lens capsule using a bent 26G needle, from 2 to 10 o' clock, extending across the pupil, in a well-dilated eye. Then Vannas scissors is used to cut either end in a curvilinear fashion toward 6 o'clock. The capsular flaps thus created on either side are joined using Utrata's capsule-holding forceps. After a thorough hydrodissection, the anterior chamber is filled with viscoelastics and only the superior pole of the nucleus is brought into the anterior chamber. Inject viscoelastic both in front and behind the nucleus again. Introduce a 30G needle with its tip modified as a fish hook into the anterior chamber, oriented sideways to prevent endothelial injury. It is then maneuvered behind the nucleus to hook the undersurface of the nucleus. Viscoelastics can be reinjected if there is difficulty in traversing the fish hook. Once the nucleus is hooked, slide it out with slight pressure by the hook on the posterior lip of the tunnel. The nucleus is thus delivered without performing extensive maneuvers in the anterior chamber.

Epinucleus Removal, Cortex Aspiration, and IOL Implantation

After the extraction of endonucleus from the anterior chamber, a mixture of epinucleus and viscoelastics materials remains in the anterior chamber. It is easier to remove this mixture with the help of an irrigating vectis. It can be removed by either of the following methods:

1. It can be flipped out of the bag by introducing the Simcoe cannula under the anterior capsular rim and lifting out the epinucleus in toto into the anterior chamber. The prolapsed epinucleus can then be extracted by depressing the inferior scleral lip with the Simcoe cannula and pulling the superior rectus bridle suture at the same time.

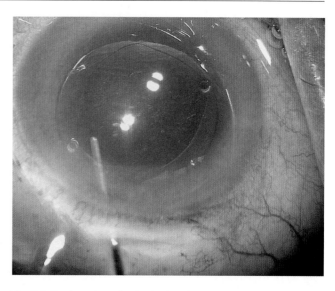

Fig. 7.8 Implantation of a single-piece lens

2. The epinucleus can also be manipulated using viscodissection. A significant amount of epinucleus can be retained within the bag, especially in cases of soft cataracts with corticocapsular adhesions. It becomes difficult to find a cleavage plane between the capsule and the epinucleus. Resistant epinuclear plates can be quite unnerving for the surgeon. If such a scenario arises, viscoelastics material can be injected under the capsular rim, between the capsule and epinucleus and the latter is lifted out of the bag into the anterior chamber and extracted through the tunnel. The residual cortical matter can then be aspirated using a Simcoe cannula. As the size of the wound is at least 6 mm, it is preferable to place a 6 mm optic rigid three-piece PMMA IOL if a can-opener capsulotomy has been made. A single-piece lens can be implanted in the bag in cases where a capsulorhexis has been made (Fig. 7.8).

Trabeculectomy

Perform the trabeculectomy after the nucleus and cortex is removed by excising a block of 2 mm by 1 mm trabecular tissue from the posterior lip of the scleral tunnel incision using a Kelly's Descemet's membrane punch (cutting backwards) (Fig. 7.9a, b). Alternatively, the 15-degree blade can be used to cut the sides of a sclerectomy and the anterior edge grasped with a toothed forceps like a 0.12 and a Vaness scissor used to cut across, parallel to the limbus, to connect the two incisions made by the super sharp blade and completing the small sclerectomy.

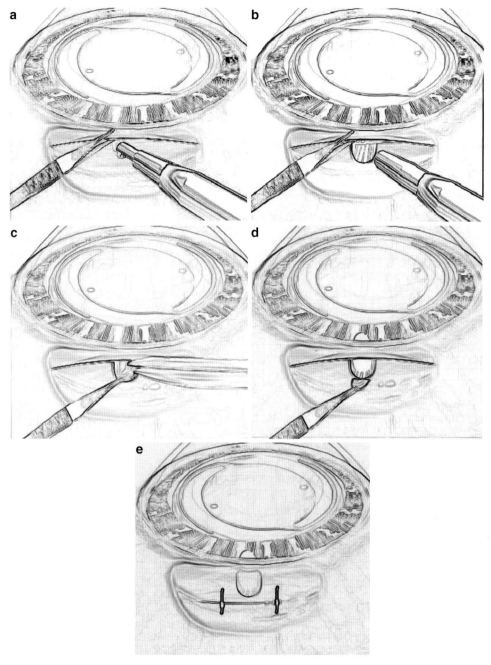

Fig. 7.9 (**a**) Initiation of punching in the posterior lip of the scleral tunnel. (**b**) Punching in progress in the posterior lip of the scleral tunnel. (**c**) Initiation of iridectomy through the punched area. (**d**) Completion of iridectomy. (**e**) Good tight closure of the scleral tunnel with two 10-0 nylon sutures on either side of the punched site

The goal is to excise a block with at least 1.0 mm overlap by the scleral flap, on three sides. Perform a peripheral iridectomy through the sclerostomy/trabeculectomy (Fig. 7.9c, d).

The scleral tunnel is well approximated and closed with two interrupted 10-0 nylon sutures on either side of the punched area, until there is a good approximation of the anterior and posterior scleral flaps (Fig. 7.9e).

A surgeon can also use releasable sutures to approximate the scleral tunnel. See Chapter 10. The conjunctival flap is closed with 8-0 braided dyed (violet) polyglactin 910 (Vicryl®) suture in a watertight manner. Test the patency of trabeculectomy by injecting Ringer's lactate or BSS through the side port and watch fluid gently seep through the wound edges under the conjunctiva. A bleb should form with a maintained anterior chamber and no detectable leaks in the conjunctival closure.

Postoperative Protocol

Postoperatively, place the patient on a tapering course of antibiotic and steroid eye drops, such as 0.3% ofloxacin with 0.1% dexamethasone, for a period of 6 weeks. Homatropine is recommended twice daily for a period of 2 weeks and ketorolac four times daily for 4 weeks in order to prevent cystoid macular edema. Discontinue any preoperative glaucoma drugs in the immediate postoperative period and assess the need for restarting them at each follow-up visit. Discharge the patient on the second postoperative day, with follow-up on postoperative days 7 and 28 if surgery and postoperative course are uneventful. Thereafter, follow-up is scheduled at 3-months intervals for 1 year, then every 6 months, as a preferred practice pattern. In case of postoperative complications like hypotony and choroidal detachments, torpedo patching is done for 3 days postoperatively or until the anterior chamber forms well. In case of iridocorneal touch due to hypotony, reform the anterior chamber with viscoelastic. In case of raised intraocular pressure, perform laser suture lysis or pull releasable sutures after 3 weeks postoperatively.

Results and Outcomes

Unpublished data of a retrospective analysis of mitomycin C augmented trabeculectomy combined with single site MSICS show that a significant reduction in IOP levels to 16.59 ± 4.01 mmHg at 6 months follow-up ($P = 0.035$) compared to the preoperative IOP of 30.4 ± 10.3 mmHg, irrespective of the type of glaucoma.

References

1. Chen PP. Risk factors for blindness from glaucoma. *Curr Opin Ophthalmol*. 2004;15:107–11.
2. Thomas R, Chandra Sekhar G, Kumar RS. Glaucoma management in developing countries: medical, laser, and surgical options for glaucoma management in countries with limited resources. *Curr Opin Ophthalmol*. 2004;15:127–31.
3. Robin AL, Ramakrishnan R, Krishnadas R, et al. A long-term dose response study of mitomycin C in glaucoma filtration surgery. *Arch Ophthalmol*. 1997;115:969–74.
4. Lee BW, Sathyan P, John RK, Singh K, Robin AL. Predictors of barriers associated with poor follow-up in patients with glaucoma in South India, *Arch Ophthalmol*. In press.
5. Nirmalan PK, Katz J, Robin AL, et al. Utilisation of eye care services in rural South India: the Aravind comprehensive eye survey. *Br J Ophthalmol*. 2004;88:1237–41.
6. Robin AL, Nirmalan PK, Krishnadas R, et al. The utilization of eye care services by persons with glaucoma in rural South India. *Trans Am Ophthalmol Soc*, 2004;102:47–56.
7. Hopkins JJ, Apel A, Trope GE, et al. Early intraocular pressure after phacoemulsification combined with trabeculectomy. *Ophthalmic Surg Lasers*. 1998;29:273–79.
8. Carlson DW, Alward WL, Barad JP, et al. A randomized study of mitomycin augmentation in combined phacoemulsification and trabeculectomy. *Ophthalmology*. 1997;104:719–24.
9. Kosmin AS, Wishart PK, Ridges PJ. Long-term intraocular pressure control after cataract extraction with trabeculectomy: phacoemulsification versus extracapsular technique. *J Cataract Refract Surg*. 1998;24:249–55.
10. Chia WL, Goldberg I. Comparison of extracapsular and phacoemulsification cataract extraction techniques when combined with intra-ocular lens placement and trabeculectomy: short-term results. *Aust N Z J Ophthalmol*. 1998;26:19–27.
11. Bourne RR, Minassian DC, Dart JK, Rosen P, Kaushal S, Wingate N. Effect of cataract surgery on the corneal endothelium: modern phacoemulsification compared with extracapsular cataract surgery. *Ophthalmology*. 2004;111:679–85.
12. Muralikrishnan R, Venkatesh R, Prajna VN, Frick KD. Economic cost of cataract surgery procedures in an established eye care centre in Southern India. *Ophthalmic Epidemiol*. 2004;11:369–80.
13. Venkatesh R, Muralikrishnan R, Balent LC, Prakash SK, Prajna NV. Outcomes of high volume cataract surgeries in a developing country. *Br J Ophthalmol*. 2005;89:1079–83.
14. Gogate P, Deshpande M, Nirmalan PK. Why do phacoemulsification? manual small-incision cataract surgery is almost as effective, but less expensive. *Ophthalmology*. 2007;114:965–68.
15. Ruit S, Tabin G, Chang D, Bajracharya L, et al. A prospective trial of phacoemulsification versus manual sutureless small-incision extracapsular cataract surgery in Nepal. *Am J Ophthalmol*. 2006;143:32–38.
16. Ruit S, Robin AL, Pokhrel RP, Sharma A, DeFaller J. Extracapsular cataract extraction in Nepal: 2-year outcome. *Arch Ophthalmol*. 1991;109:1761–63.

Chapter 8

Antimetabolite-Augmented Trabeculectomy Combined with Cataract Extraction for the Treatment of Cataract and Glaucoma

Sumit Dhingra and Peng Tee Khaw

Introduction

Cairns first described glaucoma filtration surgery for the treatment of glaucoma in 1968.[1] The main aim of the operation, as he described it, was to improve the drainage of aqueous into the canal of Schlemm, hence the name trabeculectomy. Interestingly, the formation of a drainage bleb following the surgery was initially regarded as a failure. It was not until subsequent studies showed improved effectiveness in the presence of a drainage bleb[2] that the idea of surgically creating a diversion of aqueous to the sub-Tenon's space became the goal of the procedure.

It was soon realized that following a successful trabeculectomy excessive postoperative scarring was the most common cause of failure, particularly when combined with cataract surgery. Over the years, improvements in the surgical technique in combination with agents to modulate this wound-healing response have been developed. One of the major advances is the use of antimetabolites. These agents may interfere with cellular processing at any stage of the wound-healing process. The two most commonly used antimetabolites are 5-fluorouracil (5-FU) and mitomycin C (MMC). Prospective studies have clearly shown that the application of antimetabolites improves the survival outcome of trabeculectomy surgery.[2,3]

The antimetabolite 5-fluorouracil was first used to treat scarring in an experimental model of proliferative vitreoretinopathy following retinal detachment.[4] Subsequently, its use was adapted for glaucoma filtration surgery by administrating it as postoperative subconjunctival injections. They achieved markedly improved surgical outcomes in eyes that had a poor surgical prognosis, including those that had had previous cataract surgery.[5] Although 5-FU injections

postoperatively are still used safely today, it may also be given as a single intraoperative sponge.[6] The latter method is simpler and less uncomfortable to the patient. Both these delivery methods may be used to augment a combined cataract and glaucoma surgical procedure. As a result of its relatively low cost and excellent availability, 5-FU is the most commonly used antimetabolite for glaucoma filtration surgery in Europe,[7] New Zealand, and Australia.[8]

Chen first used MMC intraoperatively in 1981 for patients with refractory glaucoma.[9] Since then its use has grown significantly, from initially being used for high-risk cases to now becoming part of every glaucoma surgeon's armamentarium. In a recent survey of specialist glaucoma physicians practicing in the United States of America, more than two-thirds of cases undergoing primary trabeculectomy had MMC augmented procedures.[10]

In this chapter, the use of antimetabolites in patients undergoing a combined cataract and glaucoma procedure is discussed.

Indications for Surgery

In the past, a trabeculectomy was traditionally performed when patients had uncontrolled intraocular pressure despite maximal medical and/or laser trabeculoplasty treatment. The use of antimetabolites and the establishment of improved surgical techniques have resulted in both increased survival and lower complication rates. A modern trabeculectomy with antimetabolite (either alone or in combination with cataract surgery) may now also be performed in a variety of additional cases, including advanced visual field defect at presentation, rapidly developing field loss, and intolerance to, or non-compliance with, medical treatment.

The choice of whether to use an adjuvant antimetabolite agent or not, which one to use, and at what concentration, is determined by risk stratification. Several schemes have been described. In most of these schemes concurrent intraocular

S. Dhingra (✉)
Department of Ocular Repair and Regeneration Biology, NIHR Biomedical Research Centre, UCL Institute of Ophthalmology and Moorfields Eye Hospital, London EC1V 9EL, UK
e-mail: drsumitdhingra@gmail.com

surgery, including cataract surgery, is a significant risk factor for failure.

We use the Moorfields Florida "More Flow" regime (Table 8.1). This continually evolving regimen is based on both laboratory work and clinical data. In practice, however, as there is significant variation in the surgical technique, the ethnicity of the patients, the personal experience of the surgeon, and the availability of instrumentation and antimetabolites, there is no universally accepted system. The Moorfields Florida More Flow regime places a combined cataract and glaucoma procedure in the intermediate risk category, therefore, recommending that an antimetabolite should be used on every occasion. Indeed, recent or concurrent cataract surgery is a risk factor for failure of a trabeculectomy.[3] Why? A study we carried out looking at anterior chamber flare (which effectively measures blood-

Table 8.1 Moorfields eye hospital (more flow) regimen

Moorfields eye hospital (more flow) intraoperative single-dose anti-scarring regimen v2006 (continuously evolving). Lower target pressures would suggest that a stronger agent was required

Low-risk patients (nothing or intraoperative 5-FU 50 mg/ml[a])[b]
- No risk factors
- Topical medications (beta-blockers/pilocarpine)
- Afro-Caribbean (Elderly)
- Youth <40 with no other risk factors

Intermediate risk patients (intraoperative 5-FU 50 mg/ml[a] or MMC 0.2 mg mg/ml)[b]
- Topical medications (adrenaline)
- Previous cataract surgery without conjunctival incision (capsule intact)
- Several low-risk factors
- Combined glaucoma filtration surgery/cataract extraction with risk factors for hypotony, e.g. high myopes
- Previous conjunctival surgery, e.g., squint surgery/detachment surgery/trabeculotomy

High-risk patients (intraoperative MMC 0.5 mg/ml)[b]
- Neovascular glaucoma
- Chronic persistent uveitis
- Previous failed trabeculectomy/tubes
- Chronic conjunctival inflammation
- Multiple risk factors
- Aphakic glaucoma (a tube may be more appropriate in this case)
- Combined glaucoma filtration surgery/cataract extraction

[a]Intraoperative beta-radiation 1000 cGy can also be used.
[b]Postoperative 5-fluorouracil injections can be given in addition to the intraoperative applications of anti-fibrotic.

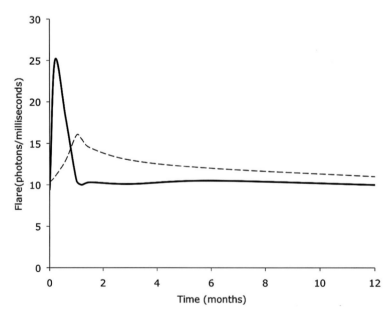

Fig. 8.1 Graph showing anterior chamber flare following trabeculectomy alone (*black line*) and phacoemulsification (*dotted line*). Although there is a higher peak with trabeculectomy, the flare following cataract surgery persists for a much longer period despite the eye being clinically quiet. Adapted from Siriwardena[11]

aqueous barrier breakdown) showed that anterior chamber inflammation is much more prolonged after cataract surgery than after a trabeculectomy, even in clinically quiet eyes (see Fig. 8.1).[11] The aqueous has increased protein, which probably contains a variety of stimulatory cytokines including transforming growth factor beta.[12,13]

Instrumentation

Antimetabolites are cytotoxic agents and therefore must be handled, delivered, and disposed of carefully. Their effect on wound healing is only necessary at the areas of aqueous drainage, i.e., under the flap and the sub-Tenon's drainage area. Contamination to any other area may prevent a normal-healing response, which may result in complications such as wound leaks and thin blebs.

Some hospitals require the use of a separate set of instruments kept on an independent operating trolley that is exclusively used for the application of antimetabolites. This reduces the chance of contamination of any instruments and is in line with general antimetabolite handling policy.

Watertight wound healing is critical at the conjunctival free edge, as otherwise there is a risk of a postoperative wound leak. Therefore, during manipulation it is important that the conjunctiva is not damaged in any way and that any antimetabolites that are used make minimal, if any, contact with the free conjunctival edge. However, there is still a risk during insertion or removal of the antimetabolite-soaked sponges. To accomplish this most safely, we use the non-crushing conjunctival clamps (see Fig. 8.2). These allow the surgeon to safely hold back the conjunctiva, allowing the delivery of the antimetabolite with minimal trauma.

Antimetabolite delivery has been targeted to the wound area by using a sponge or filter paper to administer it. The type of sponge/paper used for this varies and may have an impact on the dosage delivered. Chen et al. originally used a Gelfoam sponge.[9] Now most surgeons use commercially available sponges, which they may cut to size. Attempts have been made to standardize the dose.[14] We prefer medical-grade polyvinyl alcohol (PVA) sponges as they do not fragment easily, unlike methylcellulose sponges.[15] The PVA sponges can be cut into several pieces, which can be placed in a conjunctival pocket to allow them to cover the largest possible area. We now use three PVA whole corneal sponges folded during insertion to minimize any wound edge contact. MMC has primarily been delivered using sponges or paper, and we described the intraoperative 5-FU delivery some years ago using the same technique as MMC.[16]

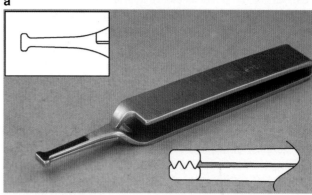

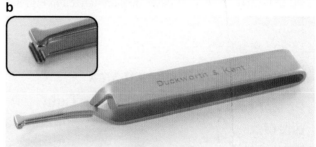

Fig. 8.2 (**a**) T Clamp made by Duckworth-and-Kent. (**b**) T-clamp No 2-686. Courtesy of Duckworth and Kent Ltd., Herts, England

Operative Techniques

There is great variation in the techniques used to deliver intraoperative antimetabolites, and therefore surgeons are best advised to maintain a consistent and safe technique, which they can periodically evaluate. As a complete discussion of the operative technique of a traditional trabeculectomy is beyond the remit of this chapter, the surgical strategies used to allow safe delivery of antimetabolites are discussed here. Further operative tips to reduce specific complications associated with antimetabolite use are discussed in the "Complications" section of this chapter.

For intraoperative use, the antimetabolite should be applied to bare sclera as well as under the conjunctiva as it is in this area that vigorous healing occurs. Although sub-flap treatment has been shown to be safe,[17] it is important to remember the antimetabolite is potentially extremely toxic if it enters the eye, particularly MMC. One drop or less entering the eye is enough to destroy the entire endothelium irreversibly.[18] We now apply the antimetabolites after cutting a scleral flap but before entering the eye. This should reduce the chances of finding scar tissue in the subscleral space, and also allows the surgeon a chance to abandon the use of, or change the type of, antimetabolite used if there are any issues with the flap or scleral integrity, or if there is inadvertent intraocular entry. In combined surgery, we also perform the first part of the trabeculectomy and apply the MMC before we begin the phacoemulsification to reduce the risk of inadvertent anterior chamber entry. Once the application of the antimetabolite has been completed, it is essential to wash the area thoroughly before proceeding and generally at least 20 ml of fluid are used.

Over the years, it has become clear that a focal cystic bleb (especially if an antimetabolite has been used) is prone to leakage, infection, and dysesthesia (Fig. 23.1). Numerous surgical strategies, as well as antimetabolite delivery techniques, can be used to manipulate the healing response, resulting in a diffuse non-cystic bleb with improved appearance and safety.[19] Some of these are summarized in Fig. 8.3.

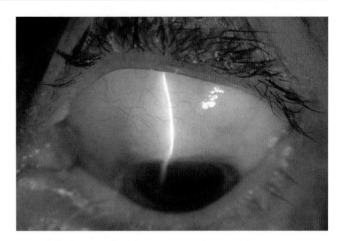

Fig. 8.4 A diffuse bleb that is neither avascular nor focal. Photo courtesy of Bruce E. Prum, MD

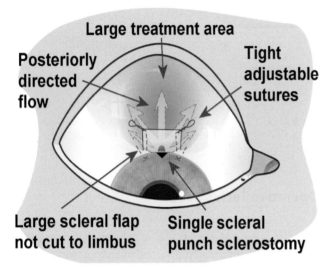

Fig. 8.3 Strategies in antimetabolite delivery and associated surgical techniques that increase safety and improve bleb appearance dramatically. Reproduced from Jones[39] with permission from Lippincott Williams & Wilkins

There are numerous advantages and disadvantages of a limbus-based conjunctival flap versus a fornix-based conjunctival flap. Evidence suggests that with the use of a similar area of MMC treatment, a limbus-based conjunctival flap is more likely to result in a cystic bleb, resulting in increased rates of complications including leakage, blebitis, and endophthalmitis.[19] However, if a large area of MMC treatment is used with a limbus-based flap, it is possible to achieve the same diffuse non-cystic bleb (Fig. 8.4). However, we routinely make a fornix-based conjunctival flap if an antimetabolite is to be used, as this is technically simpler and quicker.

We have shown that treatment of larger areas with antimetabolites resulted in more diffuse bleb.[19] We construct a large sub-Tenon's pocket measuring approximately 15 × 15 mm to allow a large area of antimetabolite treatment.

The antimetabolite must be applied to the subconjunctival tissues; therefore, good dissection of the Tenon's is required. We treat a relatively large area with the use of three PVA corneal sponges delivered with the aid of the non-crushing conjunctival clamp described previously.

Appropriately tensioned sutures are used to reduce the risk of postoperative hypotony. This is especially important in the case of augmented surgery, as the sutures may be the primary regulator for intraocular pressure for many months. A variety of suture techniques such as suture lysis and removable sutures can be used (see Chapter 10). We routinely use at least two "adjustable-type" sutures made of 10-0 nylon suture (10-0 from Alcon Laboratories Inc., Fort Worth, TX) and then assess the need for more (see "Complications" section). These sutures allow gradual titration of the IOP.[20]

Most combined surgery patients receive 3 minutes of MMC at 0.5 mg/ml in our center. In addition, postoperative 5-FU can be given in both non-augmented and augmented trabeculectomy (Table 8.2). In cases of surgery where previous trabeculectomy has been performed with subsequent

Table 8.2 5-FU injection technique

1. Topical anesthesia is given and a speculum is placed to improve access

2. The conjunctiva is blanched with phenylephrine 2.5% or apraclonidine 1%

3. Subconjunctival Healon GV may be injected to act as a "viscoelastic wall," therefore preventing leakage back into the tear film

4. A small-gauge needle (e.g., insulin syringe with 29.5 ga needle) is used to inject 5 mg of 5-FU (0.1 ml of 50 mg/ml) either 90° from the bleb or deep in the superior fornix. The 5-FU is injected slowly under direct visualization so that the injection bleb does not cross into the drainage area. The needle is left in place for a few seconds after injection to facilitate sealing of the entry site and to reduce 5-FU reflux

5. After injection, the eye is irrigated with balanced salt solution (BSS) to remove any residual 5-FU

cataract surgery, we use 5-FU; or sometimes we use an intra-operative exposure of beta irradiation, which reduces the wound-healing response.[21,22]

Postoperative Care

The postoperative care of cataract surgery is very important. The surgeon must be vigilant for any complications that may occur. In the case of a trabeculectomy or combined cataract and trabeculectomy surgery, extra care is necessary as modifications during the postoperative period may be required.

The postoperative regime of combined surgery with antimetabolite includes the use of topical steroids (prednisolone acetate 1%) and topical broad spectrum antibiotics in a similar manner to non-augmented combined surgery. Patients are usually examined at 1 day and 1 week postoperatively, weekly for 4 weeks and then monthly for 6 months. Extra examinations may also become necessary, so it is imperative that the patients are aware of the importance of such an intensive postoperative schedule before having the surgery.

As mentioned previously, in the case of combined cataract and trabeculectomy surgery, antimetabolite use is nearly always indicated; therefore, the scleral flap sutures should be securely tied to decrease the chances of hypotony. As a result of these tight sutures, postoperative massage of the bleb and/or suture manipulation may be subsequently required.

Massage of the bleb to release aqueous early in the postoperative course can be done safely, even if an antimetabolite has been used. However, extra caution is essential as overdrainage carries a high risk of subsequent hypotony. The absence of a wound leak is a prerequisite to any massage.

If the effect of the massage is transient, the sutures can be manipulated to allow increased drainage of aqueous. Interrupted sutures can be lasered (laser suture lysis), and this has been shown to allow serial lowering of IOP. However, this procedure may be associated with significant complications.[23]

An alternative method is to create a releasable suture. The modified technique we use also buries the externalized suture, reducing the risk of infection further.[24] The use of releasable sutures has been shown to reduce the rates of postoperative hypotony and shallow anterior chamber compared to permanent ones.

A recent development is the technique of an adjustable suture, which allows transconjunctival adjustment of tension postoperatively using a specially designed forceps (see Fig. 8.5). This allows a gradual titration of IOP – more gradual than that seen with suture removal or massage.[20,25]

Postoperative 5-FU injections were initially the method of choice; nevertheless, intraoperative use is now becom-

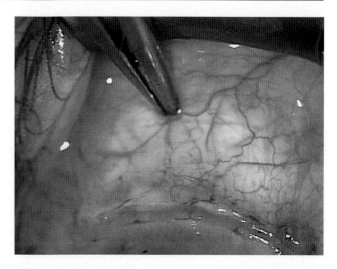

Fig. 8.5 Sutures being adjusted through the conjunctiva with specialized forceps to ensure gradual lowering of intraocular pressure after antimetabolite use

ing more common. However, subsequent postoperative injections of 5-FU can still be given following both augmented and non-augmented surgery if there are any signs of failure, particularly a rising pressure and hypervascularity or a bleb that is going flat (Table 9.4).

Results/Outcomes

As mentioned in Chapter 6, Cohen published one of the first studies of combined ECCE (extracapsular cataract extraction) and trabeculectomy surgery. This was a retrospective study that compared 22 eyes that had received postoperative 5-FU injections following surgery, with patients who had not received the injections. He showed that the 5-FU group had a statistically significant greater improvement of intraocular pressure than the controls.[26] Unfortunately, subsequent studies of combined extracapsular cataract extraction with trabeculectomy surgery have not been able to show any significant benefit from 5-FU.[27,28]

These results are less relevant today, as phacoemulsification surgery is now the preferred method of cataract extraction. Compared to extracapsular technique, there is less trauma and smaller incisions, both of which should result in a reduced stimulus for scarring. The theory, at least, is that in this environment of reduced scarring, the 5-FU may have more chance of having a beneficial effect.

To test this hypothesis, Gandolfi and Vecchi performed a randomized prospective trial, studying the effect of subconjunctival 5-FU injections on patients having combined phacoemulsification cataract extraction with trabeculectomy.

They had 12 eyes in each group and were able to show that, after 1 year, 10 of the 12 eyes in the 5-FU group – compared to only 1 out of 12 in the control group – had pressures less than 15 mmHg. Although the numbers of patients in the trial was small and the follow-up short, the difference was statistically significant.[29]

Unfortunately, the largest randomized control trial of 5-FU for combined phacoemulsification and trabeculectomy surgery did not show similar results. Over an average of 45 months follow-up in 74 patients, there was no improvement in IOP, number of glaucoma medications, visual acuity, or success rates between the two groups.[30]

Overall, the studies of postoperative 5-FU for combined surgery are inconclusive. Intraoperative 5-FU has been shown to be helpful in the laboratory and in clinical practice with trabeculectomy surgery alone. Further studies comparing intraoperative 5-FU with controls for combined surgery need to be done.

Initial studies (although not comparing with controls) of MMC in combined phacoemulsification and trabeculectomy surgery showed it could be used safely with good postoperative outcomes.[31,32]

The first randomized trial looking at MMC in combined cataract extraction and trabeculectomy was unable to show any benefit up to 15 months after surgery.[33] More recently, several randomized control trials (RCT) as reviewed in Chapter 6 have found a benefit.

To review, Cohen showed that in a double-masked RCT evaluating MMC in combined glaucoma and cataract procedures, at 12 months follow-up, the MMC group had a significantly greater reduction in mean intraocular pressure. In addition, through the first 6 months of follow-up, the MMC group required significantly fewer medications. The requirements for additional glaucoma surgery were less in the MMC group than in the placebo, and the filtering blebs were significantly larger at 6 and 12 months.[34]

Carlson had similar results in a double-masked randomized trial. He showed that, throughout the study, the MMC group had IOP 3 mmHg lower than the placebo group. The MMC group also included fewer patients who required pressure lowering medications and less need for laser suture lysis.[35]

After initial results from Shin et al. showing no benefit from MMC, they repeated a large randomized study of MMC for combined cataract and trabeculectomy with subgroup analysis. They found that, although MMC may have no benefit in low-risk cases, in patients who had risk factors for surgical failure, the use of MMC improved the filtration success rates.[36]

When the trials for combined surgery and the use of MMC are combined into a Cochrane systematic review, the results show that MMC has no significant effect on decreasing the failure rate of surgery at 12 months postoperative.

Even after combining three trials, only 167 patients in total were included in the analysis and greater numbers are probably needed to show significance in failure rate. However, the authors did show that MMC resulted in a mean reduction of IOP by 3.34 mmHg (95% CI 2.51–4.16).[37] In their conclusions, the authors argued that the low preoperative pressures in these patient groups made it much more difficult to find a significant outcome effect.

Complications

The use of antimetabolites may increase the likelihood of some of the known complications of cataract and glaucoma surgery (see previous chapter on traditional combined surgery). These specific complications and strategies to prevent them are discussed below.

Hypotony may occur, especially if high-dose MMC has been used. We suggest particular attention is made to flap design, so that the flap is not too small or too thin, otherwise it may not restrict flow. It is crucial to make sure that the flap has been closed adequately. Multiple and extra sutures may be required especially with high-dose MMC. It is helpful for some or all of the sutures to be of the releasable or adjustable (ASC) type, therefore, allowing manipulation at a later stage. Delayed and cautious suture manipulation is crucial as there is a risk of late leakage and hypotony. Extra care must be taken when operating on high-risk patients who may be prone to hypotony, e.g., myopes.

Intraocular pressure titration may be a helpful step in avoiding hypotony and/or too tight sutures. Balanced salt solution is injected through the paracentesis, and based on the opening pressure the sutures can be adjusted.

The antimetabolites increase the risk of wound edge leakage from the conjunctiva. This must be avoided as it may lead to increased fibrosis and failure of the bleb, and it also makes safe and predictable bleb manipulation very difficult. The use of round vascular needles prevents buttonholing the conjunctiva. The suture bites should include both conjunctiva and Tenon's in a single layer for conjunctiva-to-conjunctiva closure. If possible, we avoid a relieving incision in the conjunctiva, as this can be difficult to close. Meticulous conjunctival wound closure is essential, with a final check for a leak at the end of closure. Mattress sutures for a fornix-based flap may also be helpful. To protect the edge of the conjunctiva from trauma and contamination from the antimetabolite during insertion and removal of the sponges, we use a specially designed clamp (see "Instrumentation"). To decrease the chances of wound leak at the limbus, closure with corneal grooves may be helpful. This technique is particularly useful if the conjunctiva is scarred and the tissues are under tension. Although small leaks can be treated conservatively, significant leaks with hypotony and choroidal effusions must be managed by wound re-suturing.

Epithelial erosions may occur as a result of 5-FU in the tear film. The use of intraoperative sponge delivery should reduce the possibility of this. For postoperative injections of 5-FU, we use a long injection track and/or viscoelastic to prevent tear film reflux.

As the antimetabolite is potentially toxic if it enters the eye,[18] applying it before making any scleral incisions can reduce the chances of intraocular penetration. It is then essential to wash the area thoroughly before proceeding.

With the use of antimetabolites there may be an increased risk of bleb breakdown and leakage, which may result in blebitis and endophthalmitis. Having a large surface area for treatment as well as a large scleral flap reduces the chances of a more susceptible cystic bleb. Interpalpebral or inferiorly sited blebs must be avoided if at all possible as the risk of bleb-related problems can rise up to tenfold.[38]

As the antimetabolites are cytotoxic there is a risk of malignancy and tetragenicity. We avoid using these agents if there is any chance of pregnancy.

Acknowledgments The authors' research is supported by the UK National Institute for Health Research (NIHR) Biomedical Research Centre for Ophthalmology, UCL Institute of Ophthalmology and Moorfields Eye Hospital. The views expressed in this publication are those of the authors and not necessarily those of the NIHR. Our work is also supported by Fight for Sight, The Helen Hamlyn Trust (In memory of Paul Hamlyn), Moorfields Trustees, the Medical Research Council, the John Nolan Trust, The Richard Desmond Foundation, and the Michael and Ilse Katz Trust.

References

1. Cairns JE. *Trabeculectomy.* Preliminary report of a new method. *Am J Ophthalmol.* 1968;66:673–679.
2. Watson PG, Barnett F. Effectiveness of trabeculectomy in glaucoma. *Am J Ophthalmol.* 1975;79:831–845.
3. Five-Year Follow-Up of the Fluorouracil Filtering Surgery Study. The fluorouracil filtering surgery study group. *Am J Ophthalmol.* 1996;121:349–366.
4. Blumenkranz M, Hernandez E, Ophir A, Norton EW. 5-fluorouracil: new applications in complicated retinal detachment for an established antimetabolite. *Ophthalmology.* 1984;91:122–130.
5. Heuer DK, Parrish RK 2nd, Gressel MG, Hodapp E, Palmberg PF, Anderson DR. 5-fluorouracil and glaucoma filtering surgery. II. A pilot study. *Ophthalmology.* 1984;91:384–394.
6. Lanigan L, Stürmer J, Baez KA, Hitchings RA, Khaw PT. Single intraoperative applications of 5-fluorouracil during filtration surgery: early results. *Br J Ophthalmol.* 1994;78:33–37.
7. Siriwardena D, Edmunds B, Wormald RP, Khaw PT. National survey of antimetabolite use in glaucoma surgery in the United Kingdom. *Br J Ophthalmol.* 2004;88:873–876.
8. Liu L, Siriwardena D, Khaw PT. Australia and New Zealand survey of antimetabolite and steroid use in trabeculectomy surgery. *J Glaucoma.* 2008;17:423–430.
9. Chen C. Medical Innovation in the effect of fistulizing operation. *Proc Chin Med Assoc.* 1983;30:15.
10. Joshi AB, Parrish RK, Feuer WF. 2002 survey of the American glaucoma society: practice preferences for glaucoma surgery and antifibrotic use. *J Glaucoma.* 2005;14:172–174.
11. Siriwardena D, Kotecha A, Minassian D, Dart JK, Khaw PT. Anterior chamber flare after trabeculectomy and after phacoemulsification. *Br J Ophthalmol.* 2000;84:1056–1057.
12. Cordeiro MF, Gay JA, Khaw PT. Human anti-transforming growth factor-beta2 antibody: a new glaucoma anti-scarring agent. *Invest Ophthalmol Vis Sci.* 1999;40:2225–2234.
13. Cordeiro MF, Bhattacharya SS, Schultz GS, Khaw PT. TGF-beta1, -beta2, and -beta3 in vitro: biphasic effects on Tenon's fibroblast contraction, proliferation, and migration. *Invest Ophthalmol Vis Sci.* 2000;41:756–763.
14. Krommes G, Lieb W, Grehn F. Standardization of the dose of intraoperative mitomycin C in trabeculectomy. *Graefes Arch Clin Exp Ophthalmol.* 2002;240:594–595.
15. Poole TR, Gillespie IH, Knee G, Whitworth J. Microscopic fragmentation of ophthalmic surgical sponge spears used for delivery of antiproliferative agents in glaucoma filtering surgery. *Br J Ophthalmol.* 2002;86:1448–1449.
16. Smith MF, Sherwood MB, Doyle JW, Khaw PT. Results of intraoperative 5-fluorouracil supplementation on trabeculectomy for open-angle glaucoma. *Am J Ophthalmol.* 1992;114:737–741.
17. You YA, Gu YS, Fang CT, Ma XQ. Long-term effects of simultaneous subconjunctival and subscleral mitomycin C application in repeat trabeculectomy. *J Glaucoma.* 2002;11:110–118.
18. Derick RJ, Pasquale L, Quigley HA, Jampel H. Potential toxicity of mitomycin C. *Arch Ophthalmol.* 1991;109:1635.
19. Wells AP, Cordeiro MF, Bunce C, Khaw PT. Cystic bleb formation and related complications in limbus- versus fornix-based conjunctival flaps in pediatric and young adult trabeculectomy with mitomycin C. *Ophthalmology.* 2003;110:2192–2197.
20. Wells AP, Bunce C, Khaw PT. Flap and suture manipulation after trabeculectomy with adjustable sutures: titration of flow and intraocular pressure in guarded filtration surgery. *J Glaucoma.* 2004;13:400–406.
21. Miller MH, Rice NS. Trabeculectomy combined with beta irradiation for congenital glaucoma. *Br J Ophthalmol.* 1991;75:584–590.
22. Kirwan JF, Constable PH, Murdoch IE, Khaw PT. Beta irradiation: new uses for an old treatment: a review. *Eye.* 2003;(London, England)17:207–215.
23. Savage JA, Condon GP, Lytle RA, Simmons RJ. Laser suture lysis after trabeculectomy. *Ophthalmology.* 1988;95:1631–1638.
24. Foster P, Wilkins M, Khaw P. Trabeculectomy with releasable sutures – A modified technique. *Asia Pac J Ophthalmol.* 1996;8:13–16.
25. Ashraff NN, Wells AP. Transconjunctival suture adjustment for initial intraocular pressure control after trabeculectomy. *J Glaucoma.* 2005;14:435–440.
26. Cohen JS. Combined cataract implant and filtering surgery with 5-fluorouracil. *Ophthalmic Surg.* 1990;21:181–186.
27. Hennis HL, Stewart WC. The use of 5-fluorouracil in patients following combined trabeculectomy and cataract extraction. *Ophthalmic Surg.* 1991;22:451–454.
28. Wong PC, Ruderman JM, Krupin T, et al. 5-Fluorouracil after primary combined filtration surgery. *Am J Ophthalmol.* 1994;117:149–154.
29. Gandolfi SA, Vecchi M. 5-fluorouracil in combined trabeculectomy and clear-cornea phacoemulsification with posterior chamber intraocular lens implantation. A one-year randomized, controlled clinical trial. *Ophthalmology.* 1997;104:181–186.
30. Ren J, Shin DH, O'Grady JM, et al. Long-term outcome of primary glaucoma triple procedure with adjunctive 5-fluorouracil. *Graefes Arch Clin Exp Ophthalmol.* 1998;236:501–506.

31. Munden PM, Alward WL. Combined phacoemulsification, posterior chamber intraocular lens implantation, and trabeculectomy with mitomycin C. *Am J Ophthalmol.* 1995;119:20–29.

32. Joos KM, Bueche MJ, Palmberg PF, Feuer WJ, Grajewski AL. One-year follow-up results of combined mitomycin C trabeculectomy and extracapsular cataract extraction. *Ophthalmology.* 1995;102:76–83.

33. Shin DH, Simone PA, Song MS, et al. Adjunctive subconjunctival mitomycin C in glaucoma triple procedure. *Ophthalmology.* 1995;102:1550–1558.

34. Cohen JS, Greff LJ, Novack GD, Wind BE. A placebo-controlled, double-masked evaluation of mitomycin C in combined glaucoma and cataract procedures. *Ophthalmology.* 1996;103:1934–1942.

35. Carlson DW, Alward WL, Barad JP, Zimmerman MB, Carney BL. A randomized study of mitomycin augmentation in combined phacoemulsification and trabeculectomy. *Ophthalmology.* 1997;104:719–724.

36. Shin DH, Kim YY, Sheth N, et al. The role of adjunctive mitomycin C in secondary glaucoma triple procedure as compared to primary glaucoma triple procedure. *Ophthalmology.* 1998;105:740–745.

37. Wilkins M, Indar A, Wormald R. Intra-operative mitomycin C for glaucoma surgery. Cochrane Database Syst Rev. 2005;4:CD002897. DOI: 10.1002/14651858.CD002897.pub2.

38. Wolner B, Liebmann JM, Sassani JW, Ritch R, Speaker M, Marmor M. Late bleb-related endophthalmitis after trabeculectomy with adjunctive 5-fluorouracil. *Ophthalmology.* 1991;98:1053–1060.

39. Jones E, Clarke J, Khaw PT. Recent advances in trabeculectomy technique. *Curr Opin Ophthalmol.* 2005;16:107–113.

Chapter 9

Early Postoperative Bleb Maintenance

Robert T. Chang and Donald L. Budenz

Introduction

After the surgical trabeculectomy, the challenge of maintaining successful filtration begins. Managing blebs in the first 60 days postoperatively frequently involves close follow-up, identification of a leaking or failing bleb, and a systematic approach to deal with these challenges. This chapter focuses on early leaks and bleb encapsulation, while other trabeculectomy-related complications in the posterior segment, including suprachoroidal hemorrhages and choroidals, are discussed in Chapter 12.

It makes sense to review the identification and management of a failing bleb by also covering bleb failure risk factors and bleb failure prevention. Small advances in the trabeculectomy technique will be mentioned; however, specific details on postoperative laser suture lysis and releasables will be included in Chapter 10. It is important to keep in mind that histopathological studies have shown that most early bleb failures have large numbers of inflammatory cells and fibroblasts present.[1] Thus, in addition to careful surgical technique, wound healing plays a significant role in the postoperative success of filtering surgery.

Risk Factors for Bleb Failure

The commonly reported list of risk factors for bleb failure includes previous ocular surgery (failed previous trabeculectomy, cataract extraction, conjunctival incisional procedures), secondary (neovascular or uveitic) glaucoma, black race, long-term therapy with multiple topical anti-glaucoma drugs, and young age.[2] See Table 9.1.

Table 9.1 Risk factors for bleb failure

- Previous conjunctival surgery
- Conjunctival inflammation
- Topical miotics, sympathomimetics
- Uveitis, neovascularization, trauma, ICE
- High preoperative IOP
- High postoperative IOP
- Diabetes
- Race
- Young age

Two large clinical trials, the Fluorouracil Filtering Surgery Study (FFSS) and the Advanced Glaucoma Intervention Study (AGIS), are frequently cited as supporting evidence for the importance of age, ethnicity, and conjunctival status when deciding on the use of antimetabolites during filtering surgery.

The FFSS followed 213 patients with previous cataract or failed filtering surgery randomized to either trabeculectomy alone or trabeculectomy with postoperative subconjunctival 5-fluorouracil (5-FU) injections. Fewer eyes failed in the 5-FU group, and the risk factors for failure included shorter time interval after last conjunctival incisional procedure, increased number of procedures with conjunctival incisions, high intraocular pressure (IOP), and Hispanic ethnicity.[3]

The AGIS produced two major reports demonstrating that trabeculectomy failure was associated with younger age, higher preoperative IOP, diabetes, and one or more postoperative complications, particularly elevated IOP and marked inflammation. AGIS, conducted before the widespread use of antimetabolites in trabeculectomy, consisted of 789 eyes of 591 patients aged 35–80 years with advanced glaucoma randomized to either laser first then subsequent surgery or surgery first then laser followed by surgery. The statistically significant hazard ratios included younger age ($HR = 0.97$, $CI = 0.95$–0.99, $P = 0.005$) and higher preoperative IOP (1.04, 1.01–1.06, $P = 0.002$), though both confidence intervals nearly crossed one. However, the hazard ratios for diabetes (2.86, 1.88–4.36, $P < 0.001$) and postoperative

R.T. Chang (✉)
Department of Ophthalmology, Miller School of Medicine, Bascom Palmer Eye Institute, University of Miami, Miami, FL 33136, USA
e-mail: viroptic@yahoo.com

complications (1.99, 1.35–2.93, $P < 0.001$) were larger, indicating even higher odds of failure.[4] This makes sense for diabetes, since diabetics tend to have poor wound healing, which can cause a trabeculectomy to leak and fail. Complications such as high postoperative IOP or increased inflammation can cause aggressive wound healing with vascularization and fibrosis, leading to subsequent trabeculectomy failure.

An earlier AGIS study looked at bleb encapsulation rates of trabeculectomy in 119 eyes with failed laser compared to 379 eyes without previous laser. Of the multiple factors examined, only male gender and high-school graduation without further formal education were statistically significant. Previous laser was not found to have a statistically significant association with bleb failure.[5]

Smaller, older studies have noted that pseudophakia and aphakia also increase the risk of failure. In a retrospective study of 300 filtering operations, Veldman and Greve[6] reported relatively poor success rates in operations following prior unsuccessful filtering surgery (50.5%) or other surgery (47%), in patients under 50 years of age (61%), and in some types of secondary glaucoma. In aphakia/pseudophakia, the success rate was only 33%. In another retrospective study of 113 patients by Stürmer and colleagues,[7] previous cataract surgery (HR 4.4), argon laser trabeculoplasty (HR 3.4), previous glaucoma filtering surgery (HR 2.5), nonfiltering glaucoma surgery (HR 2.2), and IOP greater than 40 mmHg (HR 2.4) were the major risk factors for glaucoma surgery failure. No direct correlation between success rate and age or racial difference was demonstrated, though the study came out of England, so it would have been more difficult to show a racial difference.

A more recent retrospective cohort study of 73 patients by Fontana and colleagues,[8] however, demonstrated that trabeculectomy with mitomycin C (MMC) in pseudophakia can still have a good outcome of 50 or 67% success at 2 years as defined by an IOP reduction of 30 or 20%, respectively. The majority of cataract wound incisions have now moved from penetrating the conjunctiva via a scleral tunnel to a clear cornea approach.

Prior conjunctival surgery as a risk factor for failure is supported by findings from a prospective study of conjunctival biopsies from 82 patients undergoing filtration surgery, some of whom had prior surgery.[9] Compared with the control tissue after a mean of 5.9 years, conjunctiva from the patients who had undergone previous surgery contained more fibroblasts ($P < 0.001$, $P < 0.05$), macrophages ($P < 0.01$, $P < 0.001$), and lymphocytes ($P = 0.001$, $P < 0.01$) in both superficial and deep substantia propria. Furthermore, it was the trabeculectomy failures that were associated with an increase in number of conjunctival fibroblasts from the intraoperative specimens.[9]

Secondary glaucomas can affect bleb outcome and are listed in Table 9.2.

Table 9.2 Secondary glaucomas

- Neovascular
- Uveitic
- Traumatic
- Iridocorneal endothelial (ICE) syndrome

In neovascular glaucoma, the clinically inflamed eye usually led to an aggressive postoperative wound-healing response and subsequent trabeculectomy failure. In one study by Mietz and colleagues,[10] 534 eyes of 534 patients undergoing trabeculectomy without antimetabolites were evaluated. Failure rates were high in complicated forms of glaucoma such as traumatic (30%), buphthalmos (40%), uveitic (50%), and neovascular (80%). For repeat trabeculectomies, the failure rate was 49% (20 of 41 eyes). In another study of 34 neovascular glaucoma patients undergoing filtering surgery with 5-FU, the 5-year success rate was only 28%, again indicating poor prognosis.[11] Similarly, uveitic inflammation can also cause bleb failure, but it depends largely on the degree and chronicity of active uveitis. This was supported by a study of 20 patients undergoing trabeculectomy without antimetabolites, after maximal intraocular inflammation control 2 months prior to surgery, with resultant adequate outcomes.[12] A case series of 43 patients with uveitis-related glaucoma treated with 5-FU trabeculectomy reported a 5-year success rate of 67%.[13] Both traumatic glaucoma and ICE syndrome are additional risk factors for bleb failure with success rates of filtering surgery with antimetabolites for ICE around 29% at 5 years.[14,15] However, post-traumatic angle recession treated with trabeculectomy with MMC has been shown to achieve a success rate of 66% at 3 years.[16] Interestingly, Jacobi and colleagues have suggested that younger age may not be an independent risk factor, but instead may be correlated with more difficult types of glaucoma at a younger age, but others have disagreed.[17,18] Pediatric glaucoma will not be covered here.

A few small studies have looked at long-term preoperative topical glaucoma therapy. In a retrospective small group analysis, 6 months of additive preoperative treatment with latanoprost did not have a statistically significant effect on the success rate of trabeculectomy.[19] However, a cohort study of 106 patients by Broadway and colleagues[20] noted that the preoperative use of beta blockers and miotics and the addition of sympathomimetics reduced the success rate by 20%. Conversely, cessation of this topical therapy one month before filtering surgery reversed the adverse conjunctival effect of these medications.[21] With beta blockers alone, however, preoperative use of topical medication did not influence the outcome of surgery.[22] With fewer patients on miotics and sympathomimetics currently, it is less relevant, but the key point to remember is that any preoperative inflammatory state can contribute to a higher risk of bleb failure.

Finally, race as a risk factor is more controversial. While AGIS and FFSS appeared to find ethnicity as a statistically significant risk factor, other studies have not. This may be due to population sampling bias. Plus, terms such as "black" race encompass a wide genetic heterogeneity. A study of 90 patients (even groups of white and black) by Broadway and colleagues[23] revealed a tendency for black patients to have more conjunctival fibroblasts from biopsies taken at the time of filtration surgery, but the lower success rate of trabeculectomy in blacks did not reach statistical significance by survival analysis. This finding of increased inflammatory cells in blacks did not agree with a prior study.[24] However, several studies have focused on using 5-FU and MMC to improve filtering surgery outcomes in blacks.[25-27] Today, race is relevant in the decision as to the amount and duration of antimetabolite used in filtering surgery, but there is no definitive standard.

Bleb Failure Prevention

By understanding the risk factors for failure, one can take steps to prevent it. Given that evidence of preoperative inflammation and a tendency toward aggressive wound healing both increase risk, the first step is to take a full medical history and perform a complete ocular exam. Prior surgery, ocular history, and current therapy can all help form an assessment of risk for failure. In addition, the clinician should thoroughly examine the conjunctiva and subconjunctival tissues to assess thickness, scarring and adhesions, blood supply, foreshortening of fornices, and intraocular inflammation. Examination of the fellow eye, particularly if it has undergone previous filtration surgery, may provide valuable bleb information. Any apparent uveitis, blepharitis, or conjunctival inflammation should be treated so that the eye is white and quiet.[2]

Antimetabolites

The next step is to weigh the risk and benefits of antimetabolites, namely 5-FU and MMC. After the surgical decision has already been made, the target IOP needed to preserve vision, the expected lifespan of the patient, the likelihood of scarring, the difficulty of taking the patient to surgery, and the ability to follow-up all start to play a role. Antimetabolite concentration and duration as well as administration intraoperatively or postoperatively need to be determined. In the literature, there are many publications advocating various techniques.

Because definitions of success are different among the various studies and the follow-up timeframe is variable, it is hard to compare them. Most studies support the use of antimetabolites in high-risk filtering surgeries.[28-32] Additionally, many studies indicate that mitomycin offers at least equal or better pressure-lowering effect than 5-FU.[33-36] Though, this point must be balanced against the potential complication rate. A large retrospective chart review of 225 phakic patients by Fontana and colleagues[37] concluded that trabeculectomy with MMC effectively reduces IOP in phakic open-angle glaucoma, but long-term low IOPs are achieved in only half of the cases. To study the dose response relationship of MMC, investigators from Baltimore studied 300 eyes equally divided among therapy with placebo; mitomycin, 0.2 mg/ml, applied for 2 minutes; mitomycin, 0.4 mg/ml, applied for 2 minutes; or mitomycin, 0.4 mg/ml, applied for 4 minutes. After 1 year, length of exposure seemed to be more important than concentration.[38] Other dosing studies indicate that low doses of MMC such as 0.2 or 0.1 mg/ml or less reduce side effects.[39-42] Results are quite variable. A different mitomycin protocol study by Maquet et al.[43] looked at 1-year results from 124 patients divided into four groups: group 1 (without MMC); group 2 (with 0.1 mg/ml MMC); group 3 (with 0.2 mg/ml MMC); and group 4 (with 0.4 mg/ml MMC). Two-minute MMC was used in every case in groups 2, 3, and 4. No significant differences in IOP control and postoperative complications were noticed among the groups. This study included both trabeculectomy alone and combined with phacoemulsification. A prospective trial by Sanders and colleagues[44] of 50 patients compared MMC 0.2 and 0.4 mg/ml in those who have had previous conjunctival incisional surgery. They found treatment failure to be equal after 1 year. Techniques and discussion of combined cataract and glaucoma surgery are covered in Chapters 6 and 7.

Thus, there is no consensus, and depending on the risk factors and patient population, MMC doses range from 0.1 to 0.5 mg/ml with time ranging from seconds to 5 minutes. The 2008 American Glaucoma Society practice preferences survey (unpublished) of 125 respondents reported an average MMC dose of 0.33 mg/ml for an average duration of 2.94 minutes for primary trabeculectomies. For prior failed trabeculectomies, the same data was 0.38 mg/ml and 2.98 minutes, respectively. In the 2002 survey of 100 responses, the average MMC dose for a primary trabeculectomy was 0.36 ± 0.1 mg/ml with an average duration of 2.33 ± 0.77 minutes.[45]

Surgical Techniques

Surgical decisions can also affect blebs, including anesthetic route, flap location, and surgical technique.[2,46] Subconjunctival anesthesia may result in a poorer outcome due to stimulation of fibroblasts.[47] It is prudent to reduce anesthetic volumes of retrobulbar and peribulbar blocks in advanced glaucoma. Topical and intracameral agents with or without mild sedation can work, though the main limitation is lack of akinesia. See Chapter 2. For a traction suture, a 6-0 or 7-0 Vicryl suture placed just anterior to the limbus midway through corneal stroma is ideal, since a superior rectus suture can be associated with bleeding or bleb leaking (Fig. 11.11).

The effectiveness of fornix-based or limbus-based flaps are very similar according to most studies.[48–52] The advantage of fornix-based flaps is a better surgical view and easier creation of diffuse blebs, but there is an increased risk of early wound leakage if not closed properly. Limbus-based flaps do not leak as easily but are more prone to healing with a "ring of steel" or posterior restricting scar. Based on the Moorfield's Safe Surgery trabeculectomy technique, a large half-thickness scleral flap is created but the side cuts are not extended all the way to the limbus. A single scleral punch sclerostomy and tight adjustable sutures are utilized to direct flow posteriorly over a large MMC treatment area.[47] If intraoperative antimetabolites are indicated, they are applied after cutting the flap but before entering the eye. About six 5 × 3 mm sponges are inserted, including under the flap, over a wide area away from the conjunctival edges. For MMC, apply for 3 minutes at either 0.2 or 0.5 mg/ml, since pharmacokinetic studies indicate this is the time frame for a consistent dose to be delivered.[53]

Postoperative Regimen

During the postoperative course, topical steroids are usually prescribed every 1–2 h to decrease inflammation and prevent initial fibroblast proliferation. This approach is supported by the literature.[54–56] To minimize the chance of bleb failure, a typical examination after surgery includes an IOP check and bleb assessment looking for early leaks, signs of infection, and level of inflammation. In the first postoperative month after trabeculectomy surgery, the Collaborative Initial Glaucoma Treatment study (CIGTS) reported the shallow chamber rate as 13% and the bleb encapsulation rate as 12%.[57] The results of a landmark clinical trial, known as the Tube vs. Trab (TVT) study, were published in January 2007. This prospective, randomized, multicenter clinical trial reported the overall complication rate of trabeculectomy surgery during the first year as 57% and most complications were self-limited.[58] See Table 9.3.

Postoperative interventions of the trabeculectomy group included 22% who underwent 5-FU injections, 8% underwent bleb needling, and 1% required suturing of a wound leak. Most patients received limbus-based flaps and MMC

Table 9.3 The most common complications for trabeculectomy in the TVT

- Choroidals effusion
- Shallow or flat anterior chamber
- Wound leak
- Hyphema
- Persistent corneal edema

0.4 mg/ml for 4 minutes. The study notes the current shift toward fornix-based flaps with more diffuse application of MMC at lower doses, which may decrease the rate of bleb leaks.

Identifying a Failing Bleb

The goal of filtering surgery is to create a functioning filtering bleb. Signs of early bleb failure consist of a rise in IOP and an alteration in bleb appearance. A failing bleb includes changes in vascularity, area, height, thickness, and transparency (Fig. 9.1).

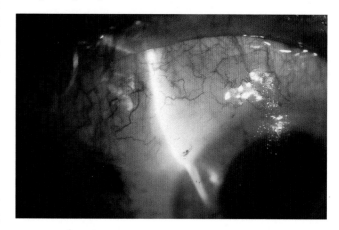

Fig. 9.1 Slit-lamp photo of a failing bleb with increased vascularity

A typical ideal functioning bleb is diffuse and mildly elevated with normal vascularity and conjunctiva thickness (Fig. 9.2). Cystic blebs with large, thin white avascular zones are at high risk for late failure due to leaks. Encysted blebs are walled off by Tenon's and appear elevated and tense (Fig. 9.3). The term "ring of steel" comes from scarring due to a ring of stimulated fibroblasts at the edge of an avascular area.[47] Flat, thickened blebs with increased vascularization are also at high risk for failure due to episcleral fibrosis – the most common cause of long-term failure. Usually, microcysts are mentioned as positive whereas corkscrew vessels are negative, since these vessels are associated with the presence of fibroblasts leading to encapsulation. Numerous small microcysts indicate transconjunctival aqueous flow. Functioning blebs postmortem have been found to have loose connective tissue with tiny clear spaces corresponding to

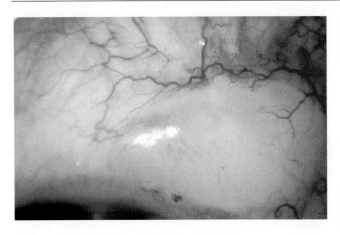

Fig. 9.2 Slit-lamp photo of a normal healthy bleb

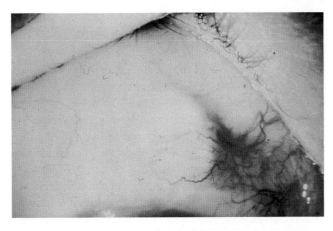

Fig. 9.3 Slit-lamp photo of an encysted bleb. Note the tense surface

microcysts.[47,59] Additionally, a prospective study by Sacu and colleagues[60] looked at 49 patients correlating the morphologic appearance of filtering blebs in the early postoperative period with the outcome of trabeculectomy with mitomycin C (MMC) during the first year. They showed that eyes with conjunctival subepithelial microcysts in the first and second postoperative week had significantly lower IOP than eyes without. Eyes with corkscrew vessels in the first and second postoperative week had significantly higher IOP at 1 year. The only problem with the study is that the use of MMC may have confounded vascularity assessment, since MMC blebs tend to appear more inflamed early on.[60]

Assessing bleb function can be difficult because low IOP in the early postoperative period does not mean the bleb is functioning, particularly if the eye is not producing much aqueous. Thus, subjective evaluation of the healing process has been the standard method. Table 9.4 lists clinical signs that suggest impending bleb failure.

Bleb area is related to outflow and bleb height is related to pressure. Previous papers in the literature have all supported varied assessment of these morphologic features.[61–64]

Table 9.4 Clinical signs suggesting a high likelihood of bleb failure[59]

- Increased bleb vascularity
- High IOP
- Reduced bleb area
- High bleb height
- Presence of Tenon's cyst
- Bleb leak
- Presence of hemorrhage

More recently, two bleb-grading scales have been proposed by Indiana and Moorfields, but neither has become an established method within the glaucoma community. The Indiana Bleb Appearance Grading Scale is a slit-lamp evaluation of bleb height, horizontal extent, vascularity, and leakiness by Seidel testing as compared to standard photographs. The interobserver agreement for vascularity was highest.[63] The Moorfields Bleb Grading System is more detailed with six criteria to assess: two describing area, one describing height, and three describing vascularity.[64] More details about the Moorfields' system and standardized photographs can be found at http://www.blebs.net. Both methods are clinically reproducible, though Moorfields had slightly higher average intraclass correlation coefficient (ICC) values – a measure of reproducibility.[65]

Sometimes bleb failure can be secondary to sclerostomy obstruction. Obstruction can be caused by the entities listed in Table 9.5.

Table 9.5 Causes of sclerostomy obstruction

- Viscoelastic
- Blood or fibrin clot
- Iris
- Vitreous
- Forward rotation of ciliary body
- Lens capsule

The most common cause of obstruction, particularly if the entry point is not anterior enough into the cornea is iris or posterior corneal tissue from an incomplete sclerostomy.[59]

Wound Problems

Finally, early bleb failure due to bleb leakage can be related to poor wound construction or closure technique. Buttonholes in the conjunctiva can lead to leaks in the bleb as seen in Fig. 9.4. Traditionally, fornix conjunctival closure from limbus-based surgery is easier to appose and works best with vascular needles, but the incision must be very posterior to achieve a diffuse bleb. Fornix-based surgery may involve multiple types of closures, but commonly is done with vertical mattress sutures and buried corneal anchor sutures

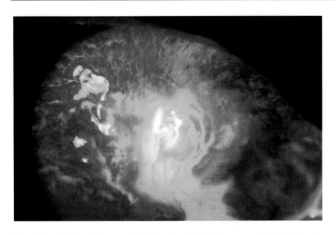

Fig. 9.4 Slit-lamp photo of a bleb painted with fluorescein (Siedel test), which demonstrates an area of aqueous dilution corresponding with a bleb leak

on either side. Leaks occur if two cut ends are not apposed evenly, there is a large amount of wound contraction, or if there are conjunctival defects such as button holes.[47] It is also possible that brisk filtration can lead to a leak if the fluid lifts the conjunctiva off the healing limbal wound, particularly if wound closure is not tight enough. The FFSS determined that if a leak occurred within the first 2 weeks postoperative, the risk for long-term bleb failure increased.[66] This may be due to the fact that early bleb leaks result in flat blebs in which the conjunctiva adheres to the sclera, creating scarring early on.

The reported incidence of bleb leaks within the first year ranges from 0 to 30%.[67] At Moorfields, a prospective, observational case series of 286 sequential trabeculectomies performed over 1 year were analyzed. The rate of moderate and severe leaks was 27%, but 59% did show some leakage at some stage postoperatively, as tested by applying pressure to the conjunctiva, which induced leakage. Two-thirds of those were from fornix-based flaps. The median time to leak was 3.5 days with a median duration of 14 days. More than 75% of leaks occur within the first week. In terms of trabeculectomy success rates as defined by the study, 20% without leaks partially or completely failed compared to 18% with leaks. Therefore, there was no adverse effect of early postoperative leak on outcome.[67] This study cannot be compared directly with FFSS, since it covered a different bleb leak time span, it included both fornix and limbus based flaps, and it did not account for previous conjunctival incisions.

Managing a Failing Bleb

A typical postoperative course for trabeculectomy likely includes an exam on day 1 and 2, twice weekly during weeks 2–4, and once weekly during weeks 5–7. Depending on IOP, anterior chamber (AC) depth, and bleb characteristics, the visit interval can increase. Aqueous suppressants are usually not used postoperatively in order to have normal aqueous flow to establish a filtering bleb. Postoperative 5-FU injections are considered during days 2–14. As a review, Table 9.6 covers the typical scenarios in early trabeculectomy management.[68]

This section will cover the management of two specific bleb-related complications: *postoperative leaks* and *encapsulation*.

Bleb Leaks

Larger bleb leaks often present with low IOP, shallow anterior chamber, and flat blebs. Early bleb leaks are usually caused by surgical trauma to the conjunctiva, so careful operating technique is essential to minimize preventable tears or holes. Spontaneous leaks usually happen in cases following adjunctive use of antimetabolites. Leaks at the limbus occur more often than at the fornix, but increased age and friability of the conjunctiva also predispose to leaks. Seidel testing is used to check for leaks and to estimate the flow rate. Management of leaks can generally be divided into conservative therapy, reformation of the anterior chamber, and surgical repair.[69] Sometimes observation is all that is needed, along with medical control of IOP and use of aqueous suppressants. This is typical if it is a small leak around a suture. Definite streaming usually requires further intervention. Although conservative measures are generally tried first if the leak is small, more aggressive management is started if the leak is complicated by visual loss, hypotony, loss of bleb height, or flattening of the anterior chamber. Patching for the first 24–48 h can work. Several devices, such as shell tamponade[70,71] or a bandage contact lens[72,73] (16–18 mm) can be used to help reform the anterior chamber and to encourage spontaneous closure. Cyanoacrylate and fibrin glue have been tried with some success, but brisk flow prevents the glue from adhering.[74–76] Some have experimented with autologous blood injection to clot late bleb leaks, but this procedure has a risk of causing a hyphema should the blood track into the anterior chamber.[77,78] A blood patch can be combined with a compression suture, which is an X stitch from the posterior aspect of the bleb to the cornea.[79] Others have tested argon or YAG laser to seal the leaky bleb, but at the risk of causing an iatrogenic perforation.[80–83] Persistent leaks generally require surgical revision, though there is some risk of causing scarring and subsequent bleb failure.[84]

Surgical bleb leak revision depends on the dimensions of the bleb and quality of surrounding conjunctiva. This typically involves re-suturing the bleb at the leak site. This

Table 9.6 Bleb evaluation in the immediate postoperative period

IOP (mmHg)	AC depth	Bleb appearance	Clinical diagnosis	Action
<15	Normal	Diffuse	Ideal	Observe medical
>20	Normal	Flat	Tight flap or closed fistula	Massage
>20 2 days after massage	Normal	Flat	Tight flap or closed fistula	Repeat massage Consider LSL
>20	Normal	Elevated, vascular	Encapsulated bleb	Needling Surgical repair
>15	Shallow	Flat	Blocked Sclerostomy Annular choroidals	B-scan? Medical Drainage
<5	Shallow	Flat	Leak Cyclodialysis Serous choroidals	Contact lens Surgical repair Cycloplegia
<5, no leak	Shallow	Elevated, not vascular	Overfiltration	Autologous blood patch Surgical repair
>25	Flat	Flat	Pupillary block Suprachoroidal hemorrhage	Iridectomy Observation then drainage
>25	Flat, PI	Flat	Aqueous misdirection	Medical Laser Surgical

can be done at the slit lamp, and works well for simple limbal leaks from a limbal-based trabeculectomy. One article pending publication, from a group in Japan, mentions the use of transconjunctival scleral flap re-suturing with 10-0 nylon for hypotony, which also has been reported by another group in Germany.[85] There are many other methods in the literature covering such methods as a pedicle flap, a partial excision, and advancement or free conjunctival autologous graft techniques, though most apply to late bleb leaks.[86–94] Re-opening the flap and applying MMC has a high rate of complications. Instead, bleb excision with conjunctival advancement is preferred. Success rates have been reported up to 86%.[90] Oftentimes, scarred cystic conjunctiva and Tenon's fascia surrounding the leaking bleb need to be removed, and relatively uninvolved conjunctiva and Tenon's fascia are mobilized with a large relaxing incision. If no healthy conjunctiva is available, alternatives such as amniotic membrane or donor scleral patch grafts are possibilities.[95–97]

Blocked Aqueous Flow

If the IOP is elevated with a normal to shallow anterior chamber, and a flat bleb, then early bleb failure is due to blockage of aqueous flow. If the iris is occluding the sclerostomy, then pilocarpine drops along with argon laser iridoplasty (200 μm, 200 mW, 200 ms) can be used to shrink the iris away to relieve the blockage. If vitreous is obstructing, attempts can be made to free it with Nd:YAG laser or a vitrectomy may be needed. Sometimes fibrin can be holding the sclerostomy closed, in which case YAG laser through a

gonioprism may also be helpful. Pigment debris collecting at the sclerostomy internal lip over time can also lead to a failing bleb. These cases may benefit from YAG laser, up to 6 mJ, to improve flow.[98,99] Intracameral tissue plasminogen activator (TPA) has been reported to lyse clots blocking filtration. One report looked at reviving previously functional blebs after failure due to other anterior segment surgery.[100] TPA 12.5 μg was injected into the anterior chamber and decreased the IOP back to baseline. Several other studies have looked at TPA 6–12.5 mg for intraocular fibrin after glaucoma surgery.[101–103] See Table 16.1.

If there is no obstruction, the tightness of the flap may be restricting flow.[68] If flow is stopped for too long, scarring of Tenon's may occur. External ocular massage through a closed lid has been used to transiently elevate IOP acutely to force aqueous through the filtering site. This is usually done by pressing the index finger against the inferior sclera through the lower lid for 15 seconds. Patients can be taught to perform this at home, and it can begin as early as postoperative day one. See Fig. 9.5. A later study of 15 patients revealed that digital ocular pressure caused at least a 50% decrease of IOP from baseline in eyes with a well-functioning bleb 3 months to 6 years after filtering surgery. The duration of bleb elevation exceeded 90 minutes in more than 50% of the eyes tested and 180 minutes in more than 30% of the eyes tested.[104] A method proposed by Traverso and colleagues,[105] sometimes referred to by its namesake, promoted aqueous flow by using pressure from an anesthetic-moistened cotton tip applicator applied through the conjunctiva directly adjacent to the flap near a tight suture. This technique separated the flap a little to allow flow and to create an elevated bleb; if unsuccessful, then an excessively tight scle-

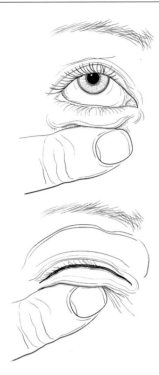

Fig. 9.5 Digital massage throughout the lower lid to push aqueous up through a scarring scleral flap

ral flap was the likely cause of aqueous flow resistance.[105] See Fig. 9.6. If the suture is too tight, laser suture lysis may be performed, though often avoided in the first week and preferably avoided in the second week. This technique is discussed in Chapter 10. It is also helpful for re-establishing flow if the flap is stuck to its base due to blood or fibrin.

Fibrosis/Encapsulation

If the IOP is high with an elevated, vascular bleb, then the concern is early fibrosis and encapsulation. This is a less common complication but has a reported incidence range of 2.5–29%.[106] An encapsulated bleb refers to a high-bleb phase between the second and eighth week postoperatively. It is characterized by a tense, dome-shaped, thick-walled bleb with vascular engorgement of the overlying conjunctiva and coexisting elevated IOP. The aqueous appears walled off beneath a thickened Tenon's but the conjunctiva moves freely over it. A prior Tenon's cyst or previous topical medication or laser are reported risk factors.[107] In a study by Richter and colleagues of 409 surgeries, 14% develop Tenon's cysts over 40 months recognized on average at about 20.4 ± 12.7 days, and 28% required surgical revision.[108] However, this rate may or may not be affected by antimetabolites.[109,110] Yarangümeli et al.[106] reviewed 183 patients and reported a 7.6% cyst formation with a median time to diagnosis of 26 days. The overall prognosis is good even with

conservative management alone, varying from 70% and above. Some cysts may respond to topical steroids, massage, and pressure-lowering drops.[111,112] This means frequent use of anti-inflammatories such as prednisolone acetate. Medical management can be enough until bleb function improves, though a larger portion of patients may need to stay on therapy to achieve adequate pressures. Resistant cases require needling or revision. In a study of 222 eyes by Pederson and colleagues,[113] the overall success rate of needling or bleb revision was 96% after an average follow-up of 20 months (see Fig. 9.3).

Bleb needling is typically performed with a 25- or 30-ga needle at the slit lamp.

- Either 2% lidocaine jelly can be applied or 0.2 ml of 1% lidocaine without epinephrine is used to elevate the conjunctiva from the bleb wall.
- Then, the needle tip is advanced carefully from the side, usually temporally, bevel up.
- Under direct observation through the conjunctiva, the needle enters the thickened bleb cavity for a few millimeters and makes multiple slit openings in the bleb wall.[68]
- With a scarred down scleral flap, it may be necessary to lift the flap. A successful needling may show bleb elevation with lower pressure immediately afterward.
- Additionally, 0.1 ml of 50 mg/ml 5-FU can be administered subconjunctivally, usually away from the bleb site. Others may inject 0.1 ml of MMC 0.04 mg/ml prior to needling (Table 17.1).

If needling does not work the first time, it may take several tries in an attempt to avoid returning to the operating room. See Fig. 16.4 and Table 9.7.

Table 9.7 Bleb needling

Procedure
• Lid speculum
• 25- to 30-ga needle
• Topical fluoroquinolone
• 2% lidocaine jelly or cotton-tipped applicator with topical anesthetic
• Temporal approach, bevel up, few mm from edge of bleb
• Posterior direction, lysis of adhesions with to and fro motion
• May need to lift scleral flap
• ± injection of 0.1 ml of 5-FU or MMC 0.04 mg/ml away from bleb
• Check for bleb elevation, lower IOP afterward
• Look for leaks that may require treatment

Many papers have been published on bleb needling, with more recent methods adding adjunctive antimetabolites.[114–121] Two of the studies using postoperative 5-FU injections after needling reported a mean number of 1.6 and

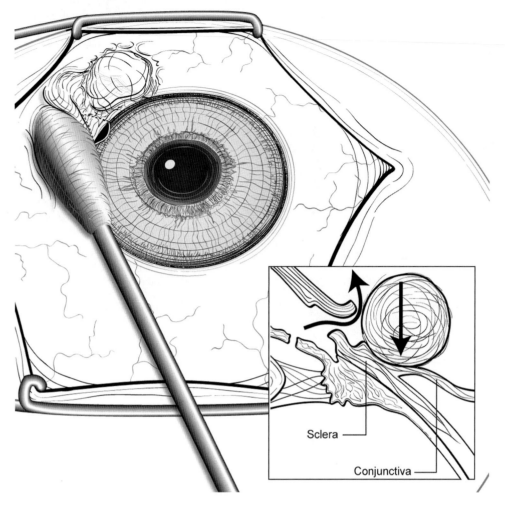

Fig. 9.6 Carlos Traverso Maneuver. The cotton tip applicator soaked in topical anesthetic is used to depress the edge of the scleral flap to encourage flow. This is done with topical anesthetic drops administered beforehand

2.4 injections, respectively.[117,120] A prospective study from Gutierrez-Ortiz et al.[115] showed that MMC needling was more successful if performed within 4 months of trabeculectomy. From the Cochrane reviews, only one small randomized trial of 25 eyes comparing needling versus medical treatment suggested that needling did not significantly reduce IOP and those managed conservatively remained successful.[122] This was a small study by Costa et al.[123] that looked at approximately 3-year pressure control against matched control eyes. In fact, the nonencapsulated control eyes achieved success (pressures less than 21 mmHg with or without medications) better than the needling or the medical treatment group. Risk factors for failure of bleb needling are pre-needling IOP > 30 mmHg, lack of MMC use during the previous filtration surgery, IOP > 10 mmHg immediately afterward, and fornix-based trabeculectomies.[124,125] In those situations, surgical revision is more likely. A Tenon's cyst can be completely excised after the conjunctiva is dissected from the cyst wall and freed from the sclera. A simpler approach is to make a small slit in the side wall of the cyst. In either case, surgical intervention can increase the risk of fibrosis.[126]

Summary

The key to managing early postoperative blebs is to know the potential risk factors, to identify signs of early bleb failure, to focus on bleb failure prevention, and to take a stepwise approach to the medical and surgical management of failing blebs. King an coauthors reviewed 119 consecutive trabeculectomies and noted that 78% underwent postoperative bleb manipulation.[127] Manipulations included massage, releasable suture removal, 5-fluorouracil injections, and needling. This illustrates the intensive care a postoperative trabeculectomy patient can require. Managing the bleb is critical to the success of trabeculectomy.

References

1. Hitchings RA, Grierson I. Clinico pathological correlation in eyes with failed fistulizing surgery. *Trans Ophthalmol Soc UK*. 1983;103(Pt 1):84–88.

2. Broadway DC, Chang LP. Trabeculectomy, risk factors for failure and the preoperative state of the conjunctiva. *J Glaucoma*. 2001 June;10(3):237–249. Review.

3. Five-year follow-up of the fluorouracil filtering surgery study. The fluorouracil filtering surgery study group. *Am J Ophthalmol*. 1996 April;121(4):349–366.

4. AGIS Investigators. The Advanced Glaucoma Intervention Study (AGIS): 11. Risk factors for failure of trabeculectomy and argon laser trabeculoplasty. *Am J Ophthalmol*. 2002 October;134(4):481–498.

5. Schwartz AL, Van Veldhuisen PC, Gaasterland DE, et al. The Advanced Glaucoma Intervention Study (AGIS): 5. Encapsulated bleb after initial trabeculectomy. *Am J Ophthalmol*. 1999 January;127(1):8–19.

6. Veldman E, Greve EL. Glaucoma filtering surgery, a retrospective study of 300 operations. *Doc Ophthalmol*. 1987 September–October;67(1–2):151–170.

7. Stürmer J, Broadway DC, Hitchings RA. Young patient trabeculectomy. Assessment of risk factors for failure. *Ophthalmology*. 1993 June;100(6):928–939.

8. Fontana H, Nouri-Mahdavi K, Caprioli J. Trabeculectomy with mitomycin C in pseudophakic patients with open-angle glaucoma: outcomes and risk factors for failure. *Am J Ophthalmol*. 2006 April;141(4):652–659.

9. Broadway DC, Grierson I, Hitchings RA. Local effects of previous conjunctival incisional surgery and the subsequent outcome of filtration surgery. *Am J Ophthalmol*. 1998 June;125(6):805–818.

10. Mietz H, Raschka B, Krieglstein GK. Risk factors for failures of trabeculectomies performed without antimetabolites. *Br J Ophthalmol*. 1999 July;83(7):814–821.

11. Tsai JC, Feuer WJ, Parrish RK, 2nd, Grajewski AL. 5-Fluorouracil filtering surgery and neovascular glaucoma. Long-term follow-up of the original pilot study. *Ophthalmology*. 1995 June;102(6):887–892; discussion 892–893.

12. Stavrou P, Murray PI. Long-term follow-up of trabeculectomy without antimetabolites in patients with uveitis. *Am J Ophthalmol*. 1999 October;128(4):434–439.

13. Towler HM, McCluskey P, Shaer B, Lightman S. Long-term follow-up of trabeculectomy with intraoperative 5-fluorouracil for uveitis-related glaucoma. *Ophthalmology*. 2000 October;107(10):1822–1828.

14. Mermoud A, Salmon JF, Straker C, Murray AD. Post-traumatic angle recession glaucoma: a risk factor for bleb failure after trabeculectomy. *Br J Ophthalmol*. 1993 October;77(10):631–634.

15. Doe EA, Budenz DL, Gedde SJ, Imami NR. Long-term surgical outcomes of patients with glaucoma secondary to the iridocorneal endothelial syndrome. *Ophthalmology*. 2001 October;108(10):1789–1795.

16. Manners T, Salmon JF, Barron A, et al. Trabeculectomy with mitomycin C in the treatment of post-traumatic angle recession glaucoma. *Br J Ophthalmol*. 2001 February;85(2):159–163.

17. Jacobi PC, Dietlein TS, Krieglstein GK. Primary trabeculectomy in young adults: long-term clinical results and factors influencing the outcome. *Ophthalmic Surg Lasers*. 1999 September–October;30(8):637–646.

18. Gressel MG, Heuer DK, Parrish RK, 2nd. Trabeculectomy in young patients. *Ophthalmology*. 1984 October;91(10):1242–1246.

19. Berthold S, Pfeiffer N. Effect of additive preoperative latanoprost treatment on the outcome of filtration surgery. *Graefes Arch Clin Exp Ophthalmol*. 2006 August;244(8):1029–1034. Epub 2005 December 8.

20. Broadway DC, Grierson I, O'Brien C, Hitchings RA. Adverse effects of topical antiglaucoma medication. II. The outcome of filtration surgery. *Arch Ophthalmol*. 1994 November;112(11):1446–1454.

21. Broadway DC, Grierson I, Stürmer J, Hitchings RA. Reversal of topical antiglaucoma medication effects on the conjunctiva. *Arch Ophthalmol*. 1996 March;114(3):262–267.

22. Johnson DH, Yoshikawa K, Brubaker RF, Hodge DO. The effect of long-term medical therapy on the outcome of filtration surgery. *Am J Ophthalmol*. 1994 February 15;117(2):139–148.

23. Broadway D, Grierson I, Hitchings R. Racial differences in the results of glaucoma filtration surgery: are racial differences in the conjunctival cell profile important? *Br J Ophthalmol*. 1994 June;78(6):466–475.

24. McMillan TA, Stewart WC, Hennis HL, et al. Histologic differences in the conjunctiva of black and white glaucoma patients. *Ophthalmic Surg*. 1992 November;23(11):762–765.

25. Egbert PR, Williams AS, Singh K, et al. A prospective trial of intraoperative fluorouracil during trabeculectomy in a black population. *Am J Ophthalmol*. 1993 November 15;116(5):612–616.

26. Mermoud A, Salmon JF, Murray AD. Trabeculectomy with mitomycin C for refractory glaucoma in blacks. *Am J Ophthalmol*. 1993 July 15;116(1):72–78.

27. Mwanza JC, Kabasele PM. Trabeculectomy with and without mitomycin-C in a black African population. *Eur J Ophthalmol*. 2001 July–September;11(3):261–263.

28. Beckers HJ, Kinders KC, Webers CA. Five-year results of trabeculectomy with mitomycin C. *Graefes Arch Clin Exp Ophthalmol*. 2003 February;241(2):106–110. Epub 2003 January 25.

29. Jacobi PC, Dietlein TS, Krieglstein GK. Adjunctive mitomycin C in primary trabeculectomy in young adults: a long-term study of case-matched young patients. *Graefes Arch Clin Exp Ophthalmol*. 1998 September;236(9):652–657.

30. Perkins TW, Gangnon R, Ladd W, et al. Trabeculectomy with mitomycin C: intermediate-term results. *J Glaucoma*. 1998 August;7(4):230–236.

31. Scott IU, Greenfield DS, Schiffman J, et al. Outcomes of primary trabeculectomy with the use of adjunctive mitomycin. *Arch Ophthalmol*. 1998 March;116(3):286–291.

32. Stone RT, Herndon LW, Allingham RR, Shields MB. Results of trabeculectomy with 0.3 mg/ml mitomycin C titrating exposure times based on risk factors for failure. *J Glaucoma*. 1998 February;7(1):39–44.

33. Akarsu C, Onol M, Hasanreisoglu B. Postoperative 5-fluorouracil versus intraoperative mitomycin C in high-risk glaucoma filtering surgery: extended follow up. *Clin Experiment Ophthalmol*. 2003 June;31(3):199–205.

34. Singh K, Mehta K, Shaikh NM, et al. Trabeculectomy with intraoperative mitomycin C versus 5-fluorouracil. Prospective randomized clinical trial. *Ophthalmology*. 2000 December;107(12):2305–2309.

35. Vijaya L, Mukhesh BN, Shantha B, et al. Comparison of low-dose intraoperative mitomycin-C vs 5-fluorouracil in primary glaucoma surgery: a pilot study. *Ophthalmic Surg Lasers*. 2000 January–February;31(1):24–30.

36. Singh K, Egbert PR, Byrd S, et al. Trabeculectomy with intraoperative 5-fluorouracil vs mitomycin C. *Am J Ophthalmol*. 1997 January;123(1):48–53.

37. Fontana H, Nouri-Mahdavi K, Lumba J, et al. Trabeculectomy with mitomycin C: outcomes and risk factors for failure in phakic open-angle glaucoma. *Ophthalmology*. 2006 June;113(6):930–936. Epub 2006 April 27.

38. Robin AL, Ramakrishnan R, Krishnadas R, et al. A long-term dose-response study of mitomycin in glaucoma filtration surgery. *Arch Ophthalmol.* 1997 August;115(8):969–974.

39. Casson R, Rahman R, Salmon JF. Long term results and complications of trabeculectomy augmented with low dose mitomycin C in patients at risk for filtration failure. *Br J Ophthalmol.* 2001 June;85(6):686–688.

40. Martini E, Laffi GL, Sprovieri C, Scorolli L. Low-dosage mitomycin C as an adjunct to trabeculectomy. A prospective controlled study. *Eur J Ophthalmol.* 1997 January–March;7(1):40–48.

41. Costa VP, Comegno PE, Vasconcelos JP, et al. Low-dose mitomycin C trabeculectomy in patients with advanced glaucoma. *J Glaucoma.* 1996 June;5(3):193–199.

42. Smith MF, Doyle JW, Nguyen QH, Sherwood MB. Results of intraoperative 5-fluorouracil or lower dose mitomycin-C administration on initial trabeculectomy surgery. *J Glaucoma.* 1997 April;6(2):104–110.

43. Maquet JA, Dios E, Aragón J, et al. Protocol for mitomycin C use in glaucoma surgery. *Acta Ophthalmol Scand.* 2005 April;83(2):196–200.

44. Sanders SP, Cantor LB, Dobler AA, Hoop JS. Mitomycin C in higher risk trabeculectomy: a prospective comparison of 0.2- to 0.4-mg/cc doses. *J Glaucoma.* 1999 June;8(3):193–198.

45. Joshi AB, Parrish RK 2nd, Feuer WF. 2002 survey of the American Glaucoma Society: practice preferences for glaucoma surgery and antifibrotic use. *J Glaucoma.* 2005 April;14(2):172–174.

46. Edmunds B, Bunce CV, Thompson JR, et al. Factors associated with success in first-time trabeculectomy for patients at low risk of failure with chronic open-angle glaucoma. *Ophthalmology.* 2004 January;111(1):97–103.

47. Jones E, Clarke J, Khaw PT. Recent advances in trabeculectomy technique. *Curr Opin Ophthalmol.* 2005 April;16(2):107–113.

48. el Sayyad F, el-Rashood A, Helal M, et al. Fornix-based versus limbal-based conjunctival flaps in initial trabeculectomy with postoperative 5-fluorouracil: four-year follow-up findings. *J Glaucoma.* 1999 April;8(2):124–128.

49. Lemon LC, Shin DH, Kim C, et al. Limbus-based vs fornix-based conjunctival flap in combined glaucoma and cataract surgery with adjunctive mitomycin C. *Am J Ophthalmol.* 1998 March;125(3):340–345.

50. Berestka JS, Brown SV. Limbus- versus fornix-based conjunctival flaps in combined phacoemulsification and mitomycin C trabeculectomy surgery. *Ophthalmology.* 1997 February;104(2):187–196.

51. Tezel G, Kolker AE, Kass MA, Wax MB. Comparative results of combined procedures for glaucoma and cataract: II. Limbus-based versus fornix-based conjunctival flaps. *Ophthalmic Surg Lasers.* 1997 July;28(7):551–557.

52. Shuster JN, Krupin T, Kolker AE, Becker B. Limbus- v fornix-based conjunctival flap in trabeculectomy. A long-term randomized study. *Arch Ophthalmol.* 1984 March;102(3):361–362.

53. Khaw PT, Dahlmann A, Mireskandari K. Trabeculectomy technique. *Glaucoma Today.* 2005;3(2):22–29.

54. Fuller JR, Bevin TH, Molteno AC, et al. Anti-inflammatory fibrosis suppression in threatened trabeculectomy bleb failure produces good long term control of intraocular pressure without risk of sight threatening complications. *Br J Ophthalmol.* 2002 December;86(12):1352–1354.

55. Araujo SV, Spaeth GL, Roth SM, Starita RJ. A ten-year follow-up on a prospective, randomized trial of postoperative corticosteroids after trabeculectomy. *Ophthalmology.* 1995 December;102(12):1753–1759.

56. Roth SM, Spaeth GL, Starita RJ, et al. The effects of postoperative corticosteroids on trabeculectomy and the clinical course of glaucoma: five-year follow-up study. *Ophthalmic Surg.* 1991 December;22(12):724–729.

57. Jampel HD, Musch DC, Gillespie BW, et al. Perioperative complications of trabeculectomy in the collaborative initial glaucoma treatment study (CIGTS). *Am J Ophthalmol.* 2005 July;140(1):16–22.

58. Gedde SJ, Herndon LW, Brandt JD, et al. Surgical complications in the tube versus trabeculectomy study during the first year of follow-up. *Am J Ophthalmol.* 2007 January;143(1):23–31. Epub 2006 September 1.

59. Healy PR, Trope GE. The failing bleb: risk factors and diagnosis. In: Trope G, ed. *Glaucoma Surgery.* Boca Raton: Taylor and Francis; 2005:161–162.

60. Sacu S, Rainer G, Findl O, et al. Correlation between the early morphological appearance of filtering blebs and outcome of trabeculectomy with mitomycin C. *J Glaucoma.* 2003 October;12(5):430–435.

61. Picht G, Grehn F. Classification of filtering blebs in trabeculectomy: biomicroscopy and functionality. *Curr Opin Ophthalmol.* 1998 April;9(2):2–8. Review.

62. Crowston JG, Kirwan JF, Wells A, et al. Evaluating clinical signs in trabeculectomized eyes. *Eye.* 2004 March;18(3):299–303.

63. Cantor LB, Mantravadi A, WudDunn D, et al. Morphological classification of filtering blebs after glaucoma filtration surgery: the Indiana bleb appearance grading scale. *J Glaucoma.* 2003;12:266–271.

64. Wells AP, Crowston JG, Marks J, et al. A pilot study of a system for grading of drainage blebs after glaucoma surgery. *J Glaucoma.* 2004 December;13(6):454–460.

65. Wells AP, Ashraff NN, Hall RC, Purdie G. Comparison of two clinical bleb grading systems. *Ophthalmology.* 2006 January;113(1):77–83.

66. Parrish RK, 2nd, Schiffman JC, Feuer WJ, Heuer DK, Fluorouracil filtering surgery study group. Prognosis and risk factors for early postoperative wound leaks after trabeculectomy with and without 5-fluorouracil. *Am J Ophthalmol.* 2001 November;132(5):633–640.

67. Henderson HW, Ezra E, Murdoch IE. Early postoperative trabeculectomy leakage: incidence, time course, severity, and impact on surgical outcome. *Br J Ophthalmol.* 2004 May;88(5):626–629.

68. Lerner SB, Parrish RK. Early postoperative trabeculectomy management. Glaucoma Surgery. Philadelphia, PA: Lippincott Williams & Wilkins, 2003:63–70.

69. Tomlinson CP, Belcher CD, 3rd, Smith PD, Simmons RJ. Management of leaking filtration blebs. *Ann Ophthalmol.* 1987 November;19(11):405–408, 411.

70. Melamed S, Hersh P, Kersten D, et al. The use of glaucoma shell tamponade in leaking filtration blebs. *Ophthalmology.* 1986 June;93(6):839–842.

71. Ruderman JM, Allen RC. Simmons' tamponade shell for leaking filtration blebs. *Arch Ophthalmol.* 1985 November;103(11):1708–1710.

72. Smith MF, Doyle JW. Use of oversized bandage soft contact lenses in the management of early hypotony following filtration surgery. *Ophthalmic Surg Lasers.* 1996 June;27(6):417–421.

73. Blok MD, Kok JH, van Mil C, Greve EL, Kijlstra A. Use of the megasoft bandage lens for treatment of complications after trabeculectomy. *Am J Ophthalmol.* 1990 September 15;110(3):264–268.

74. Asrani SG, Wilensky JT. Management of bleb leaks after glaucoma filtering surgery. Use of autologous fibrin tissue glue as an alternative. *Ophthalmology.* 1996 February;103(2):294–298.

75. Zalta AH, Wieder RH. Closure of leaking filtering blebs with cyanoacrylate tissue adhesive. *Br J Ophthalmol.* 1991 March;75(3):170–173.

76. Kajiwara K. Repair of a leaking bleb with fibrin glue. *Am J Ophthalmol.* 1990 May 15;109(5):599–601. No abstract available.

77. Leen MM, Moster MR, Katz LJ, et al. Management of overfiltering and leaking blebs with autologous blood injection. *Arch Ophthalmol.* 1995 August;113(8):1050–1055.

78. Smith MF, Magauran RG, 3rd, Betchkal J, Doyle JW. Treatment of postfiltration bleb leaks with autologous blood. *Ophthalmology.* 1995 June;102(6):868–871.

79. Palmberg P. Late complications after glaucoma filtering surgery: peril to the nerve. In: Leader BJ, Calkwood JC, eds. Glaucoma and clinical neuro-opthalmology Proceedings of the 45th annual symposium of the new orleans academy of ophthalmology, New Orleans, April 25–28, 1996. The Hague: Kugler Publications; 1998:183–193.

80. Harris LD, Yang G, Feldman RM, et al. Autologous conjunctival resurfacing of leaking filtering blebs. *Ophthalmology.* 2000 September;107(9):1675–1680.

81. Geyer O. Management of large, leaking and inadvertent filtering blebs with the neodymium: YAG laser. *Ophthalmology.* 1998;105:983–987.

82. Baum M, Weiss HS. Argon laser closure of conjunctival bleb leak. *Arch Ophthalmol.* 1993 April;111(4):438. No abstract available.

83. Hennis HL, Stewart WC. Use of the argon laser to close filtering bleb leaks. *Graefes Arch Clin Exp Ophthalmol.* 1992;230:53–541.

84. Loane ME, Galanopoulos A. The surgical management of leaking filtering blebs. *Curr Opin Ophthalmol.* 1999 April;10(2):121–125. Review.

85. Eha J, Hoffmann EM, Wahl J, Pieffer N. Flap suture-a simple technique for the revision of hypotony maculopathy following trabeculectomy with mitomycin C. *Graefe's Arch Clin Exp Ophthalmol.* 2008;246:869–874.

86. Anand N, Arora S. Surgical revision of failed filtration surgery with mitomycin C augmentation. *J Glaucoma.* 2007 August;16(5):456–461.

87. Tannenbaum DP, Hoffman D, Greaney MJ, Caprioli J. Outcomes of bleb excision and conjunctival advancement for leaking or hypotonous eyes after glaucoma filtering surgery. *Br J Ophthalmol.* 2004 January;88(1):99–103.

88. Desai K, Krishna R. Surgical management of a dysfunctional filtering bleb. *Ophthalmic Surg Lasers.* 2002 November–December;33(6):501–503.

89. Schnyder CC, Shaarawy T, Ravinet E, Achache F, Uffer S, Mermoud A. Free conjunctival autologous graft for bleb repair and bleb reduction after trabeculectomy and nonpenetrating filtering surgery. *J Glaucoma.* 2002 February;11(1):10–16.

90. Van de Geijn EJ, Lemij HG, de Vries J, et al. Surgical revision of filtration blebs: a follow-up study. *J Glaucoma.* 2002 August;11(4):300–305.

91. La Borwit SE, Quigley HA, Jampel HD. Bleb reduction and bleb repair after trabeculectomy. *Ophthalmology.* 2000 April;107(4):712–718.

92. Wadhwani RA, Bellows AR, Hutchinson BT. Surgical repair of leaking filtering blebs. *Ophthalmology.* 2000 September;107(9):1681–1687.

93. Myers JS, Yang CB, Herndon LW, et al. Excisional bleb revision to correct overfiltration or leakage. *J Glaucoma.* 2000 April;9(2):169–173.

94. O'Connor DJ, Tressler CS, Caprioli J. A surgical method to repair leaking filtering blebs. *Ophthalmic Surg.* 1992 May;23(5):336–338.

95. Rauscher FM, Barton K, Budenz DL, et al. Long-term outcomes of amniotic membrane transplantation for repair of leaking glaucoma filtering blebs. *Am J Ophthalmol.* 2007 June;143(6):1052–1054.

96. Melamed S, Ashkenazi I, Belcher DC, 3rd, Blumenthal M. Donor scleral graft patching for persistent filtration bleb leak. *Ophthalmic Surg.* 1991 March;22(3):164–165.

97. Harizman N, Ben-Cnaan R, Goldenfeld M, et al. Donor scleral patch for treating hypotony due to leaking and/or overfiltering blebs. *J Glaucoma.* 2005 December;14(6):492–496.

98. Cohn HC, Whalen WR, Aron-Rosa D. YAG laser treatment in a series of failed trabeculectomies. *Am J Ophthalmol.* 1989 October 15;108(4):395–403.

99. Oh Y, Katz LJ. Indications and technique for reopening closed filtering blebs using the Nd:YAG laser – a review and case series. *Ophthalmic Surg.* 1993 September;24(9):617–622.

100. Smith MF, Doyle JW. Use of tissue plasminogen activator to revive blebs following intraocular surgery. *Arch Ophthalmol.* 2001 June;119(6):809–812.

101. Burnstein Y, Higginbotham EJ. Report of tissue plasminogen activator (tPA) injection in a very low dose for the treatment of posttrabeculectomy fibrin. *J Glaucoma.* 1998 October;7(5):361.

102. Foo K, Workman D. TPA for sclerostomy occlusion. *Aust N Z J Ophthalmol.* 1996 November;24(4):391–392.

103. Lundy DC, Sidoti P, Winarko T, et al. Intracameral tissue plasminogen activator after glaucoma surgery. Indications, effectiveness, and complications. *Ophthalmology.* 1996 February;103(2):274–282.

104. Kane H, Gaasterland DE, Monsour M. Response of filtered eyes to digital ocular pressure. *Ophthalmology.* 1997 February;104(2):202–206.

105. Traverso CE, Greenidge KC, Spaeth GL, Wilson RP. Focal pressure: a new method to encourage filtration after trabeculectomy. *Ophthalmic Surg.* 1984 January;15(1):62–65.

106. Yarangümeli A, Köz OG, Kural G. Encapsulated blebs following primary standard trabeculectomy: course and treatment. *J Glaucoma.* 2004 June;13(3):251–255.

107. Feldman RM, Gross RL, Spaeth GL, et al. Risk factors for the development of Tenon's capsule cysts after trabeculectomy. *Ophthalmology.* 1989 March;96(3):336–341.

108. Richter CU, Shingleton BJ, Bellows AR, et al. The development of encapsulated filtering blebs. *Ophthalmology.* 1988 September;95(9):1163–1168.

109. Azuara-Blanco A, Bond JB, Wilson RP, et al. Encapsulated filtering blebs after trabeculectomy with mitomycin-C. *Ophthalmic Surg Lasers.* 1997 October;28(10):805–809.

110. Campagna JA, Munden PM, Alward WL. Tenon's cyst formation after trabeculectomy with mitomycin C. *Ophthalmic Surg.* 1995 January–February;26(1):57–60.

111. Scott DR, Quigley HA. Medical management of a high bleb phase after trabeculectomies. *Ophthalmology.* 1988 September;95(9):1169–1173.

112. Sherwood MB, Spaeth GL, Simmons ST, et al. Cysts of Tenon's capsule following filtration surgery. Medical management. *Arch Ophthalmol.* 1987 November;105(11):1517–1521.

113. Pederson JE, Smith SG. Surgical management of encapsulated filtering blebs. *Ophthalmology.* 1985 July;92(7):955–958.

114. Ares C, Kasner OP. Bleb needle redirection for the treatment of early postoperative trabeculectomy leaks: a novel approach. *Can J Ophthalmol.* 2008 April;43(2):225–228.

115. Gutierrez-Ortiz C, Cabarga C, Teus MA. Prospective evaluation of preoperative factors associated with successful mitomycin C needling of failed filtration blebs. *J Glaucoma.* 2006;15:98–102.

116. Shetty RK, Wartluft L, Moster MR. Slit-lamp needle revision of failed filtering blebs using high-dose mitomycin C. *J Glaucoma.* 2005 February;14(1):52–56.

117. Broadway DC, Bloom PA, Bunce C, et al. Needle revision of failing and failed trabeculectomy blebs with adjunctive 5-fluorouracil: survival analysis. *Ophthalmology.* 2004 April;111(4):665–673. Erratum in: Ophthalmology. 2005 January;112(1):66.

118. Pasternack JJ, Wand M, Shields MB, Abraham D. Needle revision of failed filtering blebs using 5-Fluorouracil and a combined ab-externo and ab-interno approach. *J Glaucoma.* 2005 February;14(1):47–51.

119. Iwach AG, Delgado MF, Novack GD, et al. Transconjunctival mitomycin-C in needle revisions of failing filtering blebs. *Ophthalmology.* 2003 April;110(4):734–742.

120. Durak I, Ozbek Z, Yaman A, et al. The role of needle revision and 5-fluorouracil application over the filtration site in the management of bleb failure after trabeculectomy: a prospective study. *Doc Ophthalmol.* 2003 March;106(2):189–193.

121. Ophir A, Wasserman D. 5-Fluorouracil-needling and paracentesis through the failing filtering bleb. *Ophthalmic Surg Lasers.* 2002 March–April;33(2):109–116.

122. Feyi-Waboso A, Ejere HO. Needling for encapsulated trabeculectomy filtering blebs. *Cochrane Database Syst Rev.* 2004;(2):CD003658. Review.

123. Costa VP, Arcieri ES, Freitas TG. Long-term intraocular pressure control of eyes that developed encapsulated blebs following trabeculectomy. *Eye.* 2006 March;20(3):304–308.

124. Shin DH, Kim YY, Ginde SY, et al. Risk factors for failure of 5-fluorouracil needling revision for failed conjunctival filtration blebs. *Am J Ophthalmol.* 2001 December;132(6):875–880.

125. Hawkins AS, Flanagan JK, Brown SV. Predictors for success of needle revision of failing filtration blebs. *Ophthalmology.* 2002 April;109(4):781–785.

126. Sherwood MB. Tenon's cysts. In: Mark Sherwood M, Spaeth G, eds. *Complications of Glaucoma Therapy,* New Jersey: SLACK, 1990:293–299.

127. King AJ, Rotchford AP, Alwitry A, Moodie J. Frequency of bleb maipulations after trabeculectomy surgery. *Br J Ophthalmol.* 2007;91:873–877.

Chapter 10

Laser Suture Lysis and Releasable Sutures

Anastasios Costarides and Prathima Neerukonda

Introduction

Since first being described by Cairns in 1968, trabeculectomy, with guarded filtration, has become the preferred surgical method of reducing intraocular pressure.[1] The goal of trabeculectomy is to create a balance between aqueous humor inside the eye and the filtering conjunctival bleb. To establish this balance, a scleral flap must be created that is loose enough to allow outflow, but tight enough to prevent postoperative hypotony.[2,3] A number of adverse events may occur with overfiltration from loose sutures, including shallow chambers, choroidals, suprachoroidal hemorrhages, maculopathy, and progressive cataract formation.[2–8] Tight closure of the flap can avoid these complications but at the peril of achieving the desired intraocular pressure. To manage these dueling forces, laser suture lysis and the use of releasable suture are commonly employed.[9]

Laser Suture Lysis

Laser suture lysis (LSL) has become an accepted procedure to manage postoperative filtering blebs.[2,9] It was first described in 1983 by Lieberman using a Goldman goniolens.[3] Since its initial description, many lenses have been used to perform laser suture lysis (see Table 10.1, Figs. 10.1 and 10.2).[10]

Procedure Technique

If LSL is to be done, it is best not to massage the eye and elevate the bleb as this will make viewing sutures more

Table 10.1 Lenses for laser suture lysis

- Flat edge of a Zeiss four mirror lens
- Goldmann three mirror lens
- Hoskins lens
- Ritch suture lysis lens
- Blumenthal lens

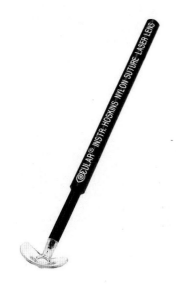

Fig. 10.1 Hoskins lens. Photo courtesy of Ocular Instruments Inc., Bellevue, WA

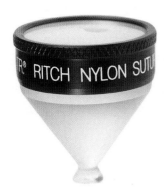

Fig. 10.2 Ritch lens. Photo courtesy of Ocular Instruments Inc., Bellevue, WA

A. Costarides (✉)
Emory Eye Center, Emory University School of Medicine, Atlanta, GA, 30033, USA
e-mail: acostar@emory.edu

difficult. After placing a drop of topical anesthetic in the eye, a suture lysis lens is placed on the conjunctiva overlying the scleral flap. A vasoconstrictor, such as 2.5% phenylephrine, can also be placed to help blanch the conjunctiva for easier suture visualization. If using the Hoskins lens, the flange assists by elevating the upper lid. With light pressure of the lens over the surgical site, the superficial conjunctival vessels blanch and the bleb flattens, revealing the underlying sutures (Fig. 10.3). The standard argon laser parameters are as follows: 50–100 μm size, 0.07–0.1 s, and 400–600 mW. Krypton red wave length can be used if there is subconjunctival hemorrhage overlying the area for laser suture lysis. Ideally, a suture is chosen for lysis to increase flow toward the 12 o'clock limbus. Rarely, LSL is used to direct flow away from a small bleb leak.

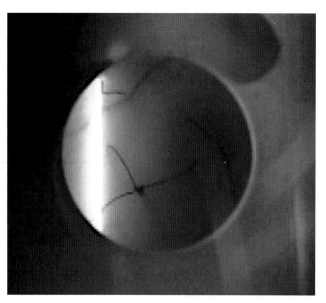

Fig. 10.3 The view of a 10-0 nylon suture after placement of a Hoskins lens

Intraocular pressure and the size of the bleb are noted after the procedure. Ideally, the bleb will rise, signifying reduced resistance to aqueous outflow, and the intraocular pressure will be lower. The Carlos Traverso maneuver of light focal pressure at the edge of the flap may be needed to elevate the bleb following LSL (Fig. 9.6).[11] Some ophthalmologists give 5 mg in 0.1 ml 5-fluorouracil (5-FU) subconjunctival injections following LSL.

Outcomes/Complications

With the addition of the antimetabolite mitomycin-C (MMC), the duration of efficacy of laser suture lysis, after surgery, is prolonged. Originally, the maximum reduction in IOP after laser suture lysis in eyes undergoing trabeculectomy without mitomycin-C was within 2 weeks.[2] With the introduction of mitomycin-C, sutures may be cut 6 weeks after surgery and it has even been reported to help after 21 weeks from the surgery date.[4] Larger responses to suture lysis are typically obtained closer to the time of surgery.[12]

Laser suture lysis is associated with a low incidence of long-term complications.[5] The most common complication after laser suture lysis is overfiltration causing hypotony and its associated sequelae, including hypotony maculopathy, choroidals, flat chambers, and progressive lens opacity.[6] Also, hyphema, wound leaks, and malignant glaucoma have been reported to occur.[7,8] Most complications can be handled medically for the majority of cases. With the use of adjunctive MMC, to avoid early postoperative hypotony, laser suture lysis may be delayed.[13]

Releasable Sutures

The releasable suture technique is an alternative to laser suture lysis and is founded on the same premise of controlling postoperative intraocular pressure. The method most commonly used was described by Cohen and Osher in 1988; since then many modifications of the original technique have been reported.[14] It offers the advantage of possible postoperative titration of the flow under the trabeculectomy flap, without the need for laser technology.[15]

Operative Technique

Several techniques for placement have been developed and have been reviewed by de Barros et al.[16] The authors' preferred technique is as follows:

- A 10-0 nylon suture is first passed through the sclera posterior to the scleral flap and brought through the scleral flap itself (Fig. 10.4).
- The suture is tied with a quadruple throw slipknot and tightened until adequate outflow is achieved (Fig. 10.5).
- The suture is then passed through the base of the scleral flap, under the conjunctival insertion, and through partial thickness cornea (Fig. 10.6).
- Two to three remaining sutures are placed depending on the type of scleral flap. The suture passed through the cornea is cut flush against the epithelium to avoid an exposed surface (Fig. 10.7a–c).

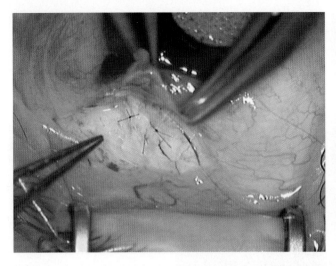

Fig. 10.4 A 10-0 nylon suture is passed through the sclera posterior to the scleral flap

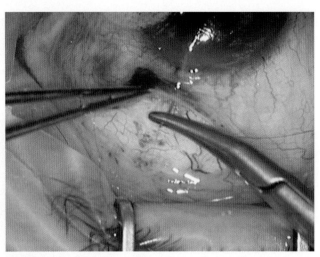

Fig. 10.6 The suture is passed through the base of the scleral flap, under the conjunctival insertion, and through partial thickness cornea

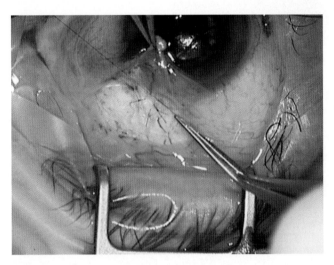

Fig. 10.5 The suture is tied with a quadruple throw slipknot

Postoperatively, the sutures are released at the slit lamp, with the patient under topical anesthetic and topical antibiotic drops, by pulling the suture with a jeweler's forceps. Ideally, the bleb will rise and the intraocular pressure will be lower. Again, some focal pressure near the flap may be required to increase the flow of aqueous and 5-FU injection is an option.

Results/Outcomes/Complications

Typically, sutures are removed within 2 weeks if no adjunctive metabolites are used. In trabeculectomies with antimetabolites, there is a longer grace period for removal just as in laser suture lysis.[12,17] If a releasable does not release, laser suture lysis may be employed if available. Both techniques have similar mechanisms of action with similar complications. The main complication is hypotony and its sequelae, including flat anterior chamber, choroidal detachment, progressive cataract formation, suprachoroidal hemorrhage, hypotony maculopathy, and decreased vision.[18] Unlike laser suture lysis, the use of releasable sutures can be associated with additional complications such as suture tract leaks and corneal abrasions from exposed sutures. The exposed suture may also serve as a conduit for infection.[19] To avoid a conduit for infection, techniques in which the suture is buried in the cornea are preferred.

Summary

Intraocular pressure reduction can effectively be achieved with laser suture lysis and releasable sutures in both the early postoperative period and later in the postoperative period if antimetabolites are used.

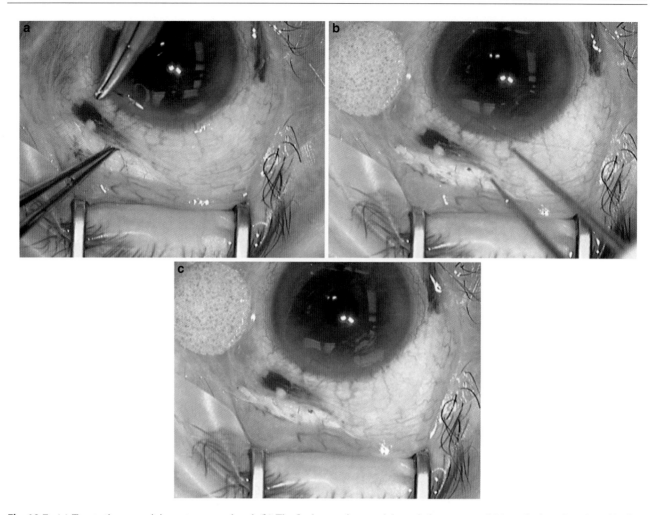

Fig. 10.7 (**a**) Two to three remaining sutures are placed. (**b**) The final suture is passed through the cornea and (**c**) cut flush against the epithelium to avoid an exposed surface

References

1. Cairns JE. Trabeculectomy. Preliminary report of a new method. *Am J Ophthalmol*. 1968;66:673–679.
2. Savage JA, Condon GP, Lytle RA, Simmons RJ. Laser suture lysis after trabeculectomy. *Ophthalmology*. 1988;95:1631–1637.
3. Lieberman MF. Suture Lysis by laser and goniolens. *Am J Ophthalmol*.1983;95:257–258.
4. Pappa KS, Derick RJ, Weber PA. Late argon laser suture lysis after MMC trabeculectomy. *Ophthalmology*. 1993;100:1268–1274.
5. Macken P, Buys Y, Trope GE. Glaucoma laser suture lysis. *Br J Ophthalmol*. 1996;80:398–401.
6. Jampel HD, Pasquale LR, Dibernardo C. Hypotony maculopathy following trabeculectomy with mitomycin C. *Arch Ophthalmol*. 1992;110:1049–1050.
7. Schwartz AL, Weiss HS. Bleb leak with hypotony after laser suture lysis and trabeculectomy with mitomycin C. *Arch Ophthalmol*. 1992;110:1049.
8. DiSclafani M, Lieberman JM, Ritch R. Malignant glaucoma following argon laser release of scleral flap sutures after trabeculectomy. *Am J Opthalmol*. 1989;108:597–598.
9. Hoskins HD, Migliazzo C. Management of failing filtering blebs with the argon laser. *Opthalmic Surg*. 1984;15:731–733.
10. Ritch R, Potash SD, Liebmann JM. A new lens for argon laser suture lysis. *Ophthalmic Surg*. 1994;25:126–127.
11. Kapetansky FM. Laser suture lysis after trabeculectomy. *J Glaucoma*. 2003;12:316–320.
12. Aykan U, Bilge AH, Akin T, Certetl I, Bayer A. Laser suture lysis or releasable sutures after trabeculectomy. *J Glaucoma*. 2007;16:240–244.
13. Morinelli EN, Sidoti PA, Heuer DK, et al. Laser suture lysis after mitomycin C trabeculectomy. *Ophthamology*.1996;03:306–314.
14. Cohen JS, Osher RH. Releasable scleral flap suture. *Ophthalmol Clin North Am*. 1988;1:187–197.
15. Raina UK, Tuli D. Trabeculectomy with releasable sutures: a prospective, randomized pilot study. *Arch Ophthalmol*. 1998;116:1288–1293.
16. de Barros M, Daniela S, Gheith ME, Ghada A, Katz JL. Releasable suture technique. *J Glaucoma*. 2008;17:414–421.
17. Tezel G, Lolker AE, Kass MA, Wax MB. Late removal of releasable sutures after trabeculectomy or combined trabeculectomy with cataract extraction supplemented with antifibrotics. *J Glaucoma*. 1998;7:75–81.
18. Sathyan P, Singh G, Au Eong K, et al. Suprachoroidal hemorrhage following removal of releasable suture after combined phacoemulsification-trabeculectomy. *J Cataract Refract Surg*. 2007;33:1104–1105.
19. Kolker AE, Kass MA, Rait JL. Trabeculectomy with releasable sutures. *Trans Am Ophthakmol Soc*. 1993;91:131–145.

Chapter 11

Cataract Surgery Combined with Glaucoma Drainage Devices

Ramesh S. Ayyala and Brian J. Mikulla

Introduction

Frequently, patients may develop both glaucoma and a cataract, and the treatment of one possibly aids in the development of the other as a number of studies have observed an increase in cataracts among patients using anti-glaucoma medications.[1–4] When medical management fails to adequately control a patient's intraocular pressure (IOP) and the patient's cataract becomes visually significant, the question arises as to how best to treat the patient surgically. A lack of consensus regarding the preferred surgical sequence for treating a patient with cataract and glaucoma led the American Academy of Ophthalmology to request a systematic literature review, which exhibited strong evidence for better intraocular pressure control after combined glaucoma and cataract surgery versus cataract surgery alone and weak evidence for better intraocular pressure control with trabeculectomy alone verses combined surgery.[5] Another systematic literature review found insufficient data to determine if combined surgery versus sequentially staged surgeries resulted in better outcomes.[6]

Glaucoma drainage devices (GDD) have been utilized for years and have frequently been alternatives in patients who have a high risk of failing a traditional trabeculectomy, either because of past surgeries or the presence of secondary glaucomas. Cataract surgery combined with a glaucoma drainage device tube implant can be an effective course of treatment in patients with refractory glaucoma.

Indications for Surgery

Combined cataract and glaucoma surgery is indicated for patients with a visually significant cataract and glaucoma

Table 11.1 Indications for glaucoma tube implant

1. Prior failed trabeculectomy
2. History of blebitis
3. Hypotony from chronic or recurrent bleb leak
4. Superior subconjunctival scar tissue of any etiology
5. History of scleral buckle surgery
6. Prior penetrating keratoplasty
7. Uveitic glaucoma
8. Traumatic glaucoma
9. Chronic angle-closure glaucoma
10. Neovascular glaucoma (NVG)
11. Iridocorneal endothelial (ICE) syndrome
12. Anirida

that is uncontrolled under 2 or more anti-glaucoma medications.[7] Trabeculectomy is frequently the glaucoma procedure of choice, but for patients with conjunctival scarring secondary to prior surgeries and those with secondary glaucomas, trabeculectomy has a lower success rate. In these patients, tube implantation can provide an alternative means of successfully reducing intraocular pressure.[8] Combined GDD surgery and phacoemulsification with posterior chamber intraocular lens (IOL) implantation is indicated in patients with visually significant cataract in the setting of a variety of complicated glaucomas as listed in Table 11.1 and Figs. 11.1 and 11.2.

Operative Techniques

Glaucoma drainage devices (GDD) consist of a tube attached to a plate. The three main ones in current use include the Ahmed glaucoma valve (AGV) (New World Medical, Rancho Cucamonga, CA) the Baerveldt glaucoma implant (BGI) (American Medical Optics, Santa Ana, CA), and the Molteno implant (IOP Inc., Costa Mesa, CA). There are no known advantages of one over the other in terms of long-term surgical success rate. The choice of which GDD to use is dependent upon the individual surgeon's preference. Each GDD has its own protocol and best practices for

R.S. Ayyala (✉)
Department of Ophthalmology, Tulane University School of Medicine, New Orleans, LA 70112, USA
e-mail: rayyala@tulane.edu

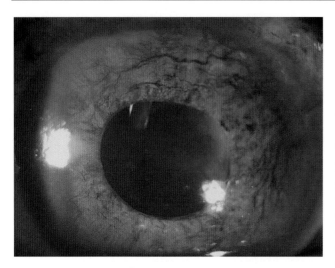

Fig. 11.1 A slit lamp photograph of an eye 1 day following a combined AGV and a cataract surgery with PC IOL. Note the well-formed anterior chamber with no bleeding due to retained viscoelastic. The AGV tube is behind the iris and over the PC IOL

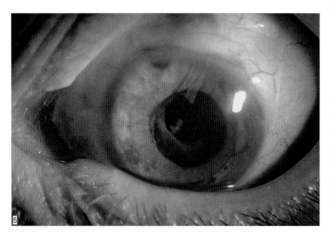

Fig. 11.2 Slit lamp photo of a patient with uveitis who underwent implantation of an AGV, lysis of posterior synechiae, superior scleral tunnel cataract extraction by phacoemulsification with implantation of PC IOL, and peripheral iridectomy due to the granulomatous nature of her disease. A capsulotomy was done several months postoperatively. Photograph courtesy of Tom Monego, Dartmouth Hitchcock Medical Center (DHMC), Lebanon, NH

implementation, the exhaustive details of which are beyond the scope of this chapter. Instead, it is important to discuss considerations for approach and alterations in technique when combining cataract surgery with tube implantation.

Anesthesia

Retrobulbar anesthesia is preferred to peribulbar so as to prevent an increase in intraocular pressure when injecting the solution.[7] Topical anesthesia with sub-Tenon's injection in the area of the surgery is another technique that is effective. See Chapter 2.

Surgical Sites

The area of the eye chosen for tube implantation depends largely on previous surgeries performed on the eye and the impact they have had on tissue health, such as conjunctival scarring and scleral thinning. Additionally, the approach for the cataract surgery needs to be taken into account, since the tube of the GDD is introduced into the anterior chamber through a needle track to obtain a tight fit, to avoid hypotony. This precludes using a single opening into the anterior chamber to perform both procedures, as could be done with a phacotrabeculectomy. With other factors being equal, a superonasal or superotemporal placement of a drainage device and temporal approach for cataract extraction will provide easier surgical access.

Which One First?

At the time of surgery, some surgeons prefer to implant the GDD into the sub-Tenon's pocket and secure it to the sclera, before performing the cataract surgery through an adjacent scleral tunnel technique or via a temporal scleral or clear cornea approach. The authors' personal preference is to perform the cataract surgery through a clear cornea temporal incision followed by the GDD implantation.

Cataract Surgery – Surgical Pearls

1. Temporal limbal/corneal incision is the preferred incision.
2. Pupil: Small pupil/synechial attachments to the lens capsule are often present in these patients with glaucoma either because of the drops (pilocarpine) or because of the underlying conditions (uveitis or neovascular glaucoma or trauma). A floppy-iris-like syndrome is very frequently seen in these situations. The authors prefer to inject 0.1 cc of preservative-free lidocaine 1% mixed with 1 in 10,000 preservative-free epinephrine (mixed 50:50) via the paracentesis site.[9,10]

    This mixture provides the required anesthesia for pupil manipulation and will help dilate the pupil and stabilize the iris in case of floppy iris syndrome. This is followed by the injection of 0.1 cc of viscoelastic (avoid high molecular weight viscoelastics). Pupil stretching and/or synechiolysis in patients with underlying diseases such uveitis

Fig. 11.3 Collar button manipulator, which is useful for lysis of posterior synechiae and pupil stretching. Photo courtesy of Storz Instruments, Bausch & Lomb, Rochester, NY

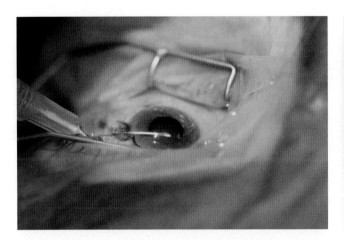

Fig. 11.4 Cataract extraction from a clear cornea incision in the superior-temporal quadrant. Note the formation of continuous capsulorexhis with the cystotome to measure about 6 mm

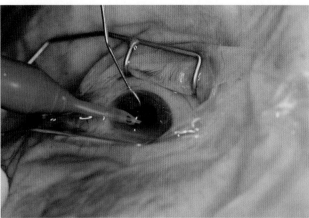

Fig. 11.5 Phacoemulsification using the down sculpting technique followed by chopping with the second instrument

or neovascular glaucoma should be done in an atraumatic fashion. The authors prefer to use the collar button to stretch the pupil and dilate the pupil to approximately 7 mm (Fig. 11.3). Re-injection of viscoelastic will stabilize the iris and maintain the dilated pupil size. See also Chapter 3.

3. A 6-mm capsulorhexis is preferred. This will allow for proper positioning of the IOL inside the capsular bag and also prevent the IOL from forward displacement and pupillary capture, in the event the patient develops hypotony and/or choroidal effusions following glaucoma surgery (Fig. 11.4).

4. Following the implantation of the IOL, after cataract extraction, leave the viscoelastic in the anterior chamber (AC) to maintain the IOP for the GDD surgery. Also, the retained viscoelastic will help prevent immediate postoperative hypotony (Figs. 11.5 and 11.6).

5. Always close the cataract incision site with a 10-0 nylon suture at the end of the surgery and make the wound water tight (Figs. 11.7 and 11.8). Intracameral injection of Decadron (dexamethasone sodium phosphate, APP pharmaceuticals, Schaumburg, IL) 0.4 mg in 0.1 cc, used by the author, at the end of the case helps in preventing postoperative inflammation, especially in African-American patients.

6. In patients with uveitis with glaucoma and cataracts, a GDD with smaller surface area (such as the pediatric Ahmed valve, FP8 or S3, New World Medical, Rancho Cucamonga, CA) is advisable, to prevent postoperative hypotony.

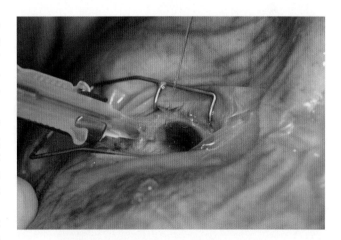

Fig. 11.6 Foldable intraocular lens implantation, then no irrigation-aspiration after the IOL implantation to prepare the eye for glaucoma surgery. The viscoelastic material is retained in the eye to prevent bleeding from the rubeotic blood vessels, while maintaining the IOP

In patients with uveitis with glaucoma and cataract, intravitreal injection through the pars plana of 4 mg triamcinolone acetonide (Triesence, Alcon, Fort Worth, TX) or Kenalog (Bristol Meyer, New York, NY) in 0.1 cc of 40 mg/ml suspension is advisable to prevent postoperative inflammation.[11,12] In patients with NVG and cataract, intravitreal injection of bevacizumab (Avastin, Genetech, South San Francisco, CA) through the pars plana is helpful if the patient has a tendency to bleed from the iris vessels or has proliferative diabetic retinopathy. See the retinal surgeon's advice[13,14] (Fig. 11.9).

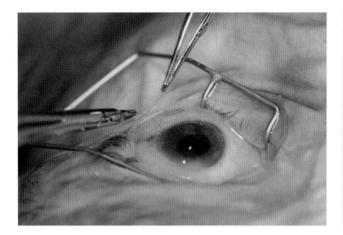

Fig. 11.7 Closure of the clear cornea wound with 10-0 nylon suture

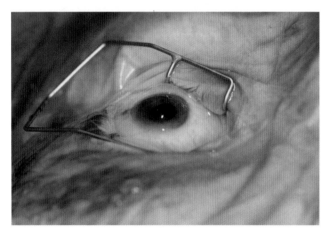

Fig. 11.8 The final appearance of the eye after cataract surgery and before implantation of a GDD

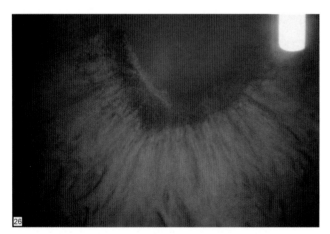

Fig. 11.9 Slit lamp photograph of an eye with neovascular glaucoma and dense nuclear cataract. At the time of GDD implantation, CE/IOL may be considered to improve the view for retinal laser and intravitreal bevacizumab to help control the neovascularization in the short term. Photo courtesy of Tom Monego at DHMC, Lebanon, NH

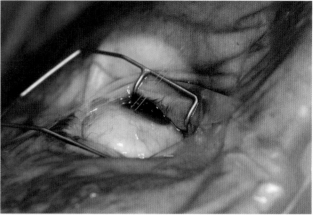

Fig. 11.10 A 7-0 Vicryl suture is placed through the 12 o'clock limbus to help position the eye inferiorly and obtain adequate exposure of the superior conjunctiva

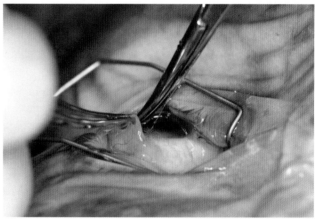

Fig. 11.11 Limbal peritomy at 12 o'clock position

Ahmed Glaucoma Valve Implantation

1. 7-0 Vicryl stay suture is placed through 12 o'clock limbus to help rotate the eye inferiorly and expose the superior conjunctiva adequately (Fig. 11.10).
2. Limbal peritomy at 12 o'clock with Westcott scissors (Fig. 11.11).
3. Sub-Tenon's injection of lidocaine-epinephrine into the quadrant of surgery. Injection of this mixture achieves multiple objectives: anesthesia, dissection of the sub-Tenon's tissue in an atraumatic fashion, and vasoconstriction for prevention/control of bleeding. The mixture can be injected posterior into the muscle cone to achieve more anesthesia.
4. Further dissection with Westcott scissors followed by underwater cautery.
5. The Ahmed valve is then primed with balanced salt solution (BSS) (Fig. 11.12).

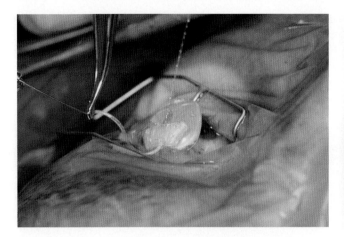

Fig. 11.12 Ahmed glaucoma valve is primed with balanced salt solution (BSS) with a 27-gauge cannula

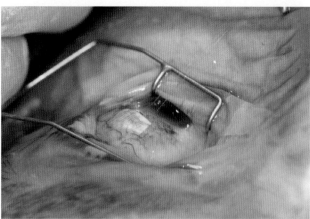

Fig. 11.14 Scleral patch graft is placed on the tube and secured to the surrounding episcleral with 10-nylon sutures

6. The end-plate is inserted into the sub-Tenon's pocket and secured to the sclera 8–10 mm posterior to the limbus (Fig. 11.13a, b).
7. A 23-ga butterfly needle is used to make an entry into the anterior chamber (AC). Make sure that the entry into the AC is through the trabecular meshwork so as to position the tube on the surface of the iris and away from the cornea.
8. This is followed by the placement of the scleral patch graft over the tube and closure of the conjunctiva[15] (Fig. 11.14).

Alternative Techniques

Some surgeons prefer to secure the GDD first to the sclera followed by cataract surgery. Then they will insert the tube into the anterior chamber and complete the GDD surgery. Here is a brief description of this technique.

Baerveldt Implant with Cataract Surgery

First, a fornix-based flap of Tenon's tissue and conjunctiva is raised in the superotemporal quadrant. Next, muscle hooks are used to isolate the superior and lateral rectus muscles, which allows for a wing of the Baerveldt implant to be positioned under the belly of each muscle (Fig. 11.15a, b). After suturing the implant to the sclera, the drainage tube is occluded near the implant using a polyglactin suture. Optionally, one to three fenestrations can be made in the drainage tube proximal to the occluding suture to allow for minor aqueous outflow over the average 5-week period it

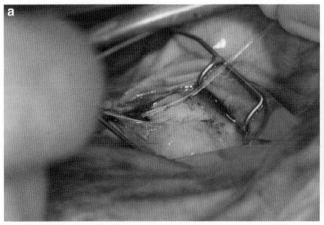
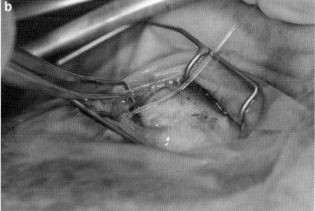

Fig. 11.13 (a) The end-plate of the valve is tucked into the sub-Tenon's pocket in the quadrant, usually superior temporal and (b) secured with two interrupted 10-nylon sutures

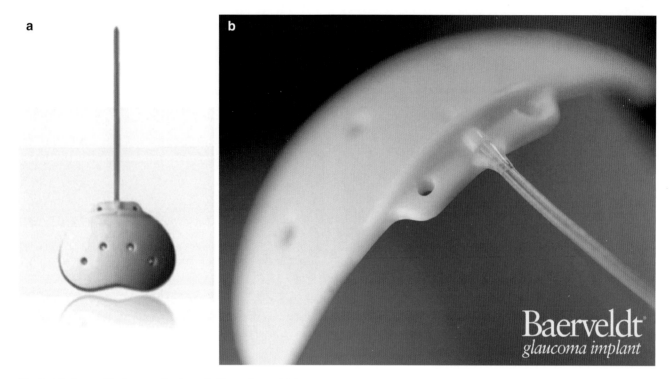

Fig. 11.15 Baerveldt glaucoma implants (BGI). (**a**) Baerveldt 250 and (**b**) Baerveldt 350. Figures courtesy of American Medical Optics (AMO), Santa Ana, CA

takes for the implant to begin full functionality. At this point phacoemulsification can be performed. Once the eye is closed, the drainage tube is trimmed to the required length with a forward-facing bevel and inserted into the anterior chamber through a track formed by a 23-ga needle (Figs. 11.16 and 11.17). As with the AGV technique, the drainage tube is covered with a piece of donor cornea, sclera, or dura mater, and the conjunctival flap is replaced.[15] Finally, subconjunctival injections of steroids and antibiotics are given.[8]

Postoperative Care

Postoperative care consists of topical application of antibiotics, cyclopentolate 1%, and non-steroidal anti-inflammatory such as ketorolac tromethamine ophthalmic solution (Acular, Allergan, Irvine, CA) drops four times/day for 1 week and topical steroids eight times a day with gradual tapering over a 4–8 week period with regular follow-up visits.[7]

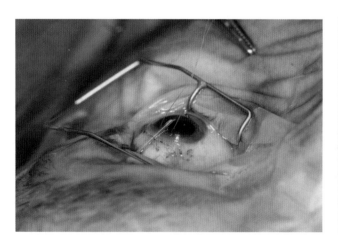

Fig. 11.16 The silicone tube is cut with the bevel facing up 0.5 mm beyond the pupillary margin

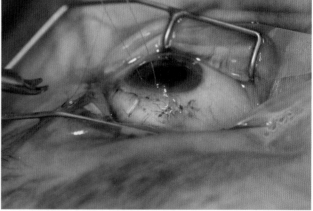

Fig. 11.17 Tube inserted into the AC and the tube is secured to the episcleral with 10-nylon suture

With the Molteno and Baerveldt implants, patients should be seen every 2 weeks until the drainage tube has opened, as evidenced by a drop in intraocular pressure and the presence of a distended bleb over the drainage plate. Before the tube opens, patients should continue to take their hypotensive medications to control their intraocular pressure. As the tube opens, the hypotensive medications should be readjusted based on the intraocular pressure.[16]

Complications and the Intraoperative Period

Complications during cataract surgery that can have an impact on the combination surgery are as follows:

a. Capsular rupture with loss of nuclear pieces into the vitreous cavity. Should this happen, the following points can be helpful:

   1. Inject small quantities of viscoelastic into the anterior chamber and reassess the situation. If the capsular bag contains nuclear pieces and/or cortex, then every attempt must be made to remove them successfully. Judicious use of viscoelastic using the cannula as a support mechanism, similar to a conventional second instrument, along with careful phaco technique will help in removing the rest of the nuclear pieces. The challenge is in removing the cortical material in the presence of vitreous. One method is to use the anterior vitrector to perform anterior vitrectomy followed by cortical aspiration, using the same instrument but just switching from vitrectomy mode to irrigation–aspiration (IA) mode. By switching between the anterior vitrectomy and the IA mode, one can successfully remove all the cortical material and the vitreous from the anterior chamber. Another method is to use a manual technique as with a Simcoe type cannula. Vitreous can be stained with Kenalog for easier visualization, as described in Chapter 16.
   2. Once this is achieved, one should reassess the remaining capsular bag and make a decision regarding the placement of the intraocular lens. If there is only a small rent in the posterior capsule and the bag itself is intact and stable, then careful insertion of the posterior chamber foldable IOL is feasible. If the rent is big, the bag is found to be unstable, or if the surgeon is unsure, it is better to insert a 3-piece IOL into the sulcus. Should there be no capsular support at all, then the choice is to suture the 3-piece IOL to the iris or place an anterior chamber IOL.
   3. In all these situations, 0.1 cc of triamcinolone acetonide should be injected into the vitreous cavity

through the cataract wound site and the rent in the posterior capsule. This will help in preventing postoperative complications such as cystoid macular edema and inflammation and may aid in vitreous visualization. See Table 16.2.[13,14]

   4. Once the IOL is inserted, then the rest of the viscoelastic is retained in the anterior chamber and the cataract wound site is secured with interrupted 10-0 nylon sutures. This is followed by the GDD implantation.
   5. The patient should be referred to the retina surgeon for pars plana vitrectomy and lens removal in cases with retained nuclear pieces.

b. Capsular rupture with vitreous prolapse into the anterior chamber: Complete and careful anterior vitrectomy should be performed prior to tube implantation. Presence of vitreous in the anterior chamber can potentially obstruct the tube opening by plugging it which leads to sudden increase in the IOP and GDD surgery failure. More importantly, the resulting vitreous traction can induce retinal tear/detachment in the opposite direction.

   As mentioned previously, complete and careful vitrectromy during the surgery is the best prevention. Should this complication be seen in the postoperative period, YAG vitreolysis can be tried in the clinic.[17] If that does not succeed and/or there is too much vitreous in the anterior chamber, the patient should be taken back to the operating room and a complete core vitrectomy should be performed, preferably from a pars plana approach with a retina specialist.

Complications in the Immediate Postoperative Period

1. Watch for choroidal effusions and shallowing of the anterior chamber. Should this happen, use cycloplegics to deepen the anterior chamber and topical and oral steroids to help reduce the choroidal effusion. Anterior chamber reformation should be considered in cases with flat chambers from over filtration or those with very shallow chambers with significant choroidal effusions. Choroidal effusion drainage should be considered in cases with kissing choroidal effusions. See Chapter 12.

2. Suprachoroidal hemorrhage should be suspected in patients with severe ocular pain, shallow anterior chamber, moderate to elevated IOP, and choroidal effusion with a dark appearance. B-scan will help in making the diagnosis. Small- to moderate-size hemorrhages can be treated conservatively with oral steroids, pain

medications, and topical steroids and cycloplegic agents. Moderate to severe suprachoroidal hemorrhages need to be drained. See Chapter 12.

3. Hyphema can be seen in some patients, especially in patients with NVG. Most times, hyphema will resolve without any additional measures. Anterior chamber washout should be considered in patients with total hyphema with tube blockage and elevated IOP. Intracameral injection of tissue plasminogen activator (TPA) (12.5 μg) can also be considered in cases with tube obstruction with hyphema or fibrin.[18] See Chapter 16.

4. Anterior dislocation of the intraocular lens with pupillary capture: This is usually seen in patients with hypotony, shallow chambers, and choroidal effusion. The IOL can be repositioned into the bag by injecting viscoelastic into the anterior chamber and using gentle manipulation of the IOL with viscoelastic cannula. This can be performed either at the slit lamp, using sterile technique or in the main operating room depending on the patient's and the surgeon's preferences.

5. Endophthalmitis should be suspected in patients with pain, conjunctival injection, cells and flare in the anterior chamber, and vitritis. As in any patient postoperative an intraocular surgery, this should be recognized immediately and treated promptly with the help of a retina surgeon.

Complications in the Late Postoperative Period

Failure of the GDD in the early and late postoperative period[19]: Failure of the GDD appears to be of multifactorial etiology. Excessive fibrous reaction around the bleb appears to be the major cause of long-term glaucoma drainage device failure. Failure appears to be more common in the first postoperative year than subsequent years.

Other factors that can contribute to the failure include biomaterial of the GDD, end-plate design, and possible inflammatory factors in the aqueous in these complicated eyes.

Corneal Decompensation and Glaucoma Drainage Devices

Corneal decompensation appears to be one of the main complications following glaucoma drainage device surgery. It has been reported in up to 30% of the patients with long-term follow-up.[19] Graft failure from decompensation or rejection in patients with penetrating keratoplasty and glaucoma following glaucoma drainage device surgery has been reported in the range of 10–51% (an average of 36.2%).[19]

The etiology of corneal decompensation and graft failure is probably multifactorial.

Results/Outcomes

Surgical outcomes following combined phaco/GDD surgery in published literature supports the concept that in select cases this approach achieves excellent results, both in terms of vision recovery and IOP control.

A report from Singapore reviewed 32 eyes with either an Ahmed or a Baerveldt implant placement, 16 cases each, combined with phacoemulsification in Asian eyes. Follow-up was only 6–22 months, but the results were promising with the mean IOP reduced from 28 mmHg to a mean of 15.2 mmHg for the group. Four eyes failed to achieve IOP control, one eye lost more than one line of vision, and six eyes experienced a period of hypotony.[20]

Nassiri et al.[21] studied the efficacy and safety of combined phacoemulsification and Ahmed valve glaucoma drainage implant with respect to visual acuity improvement, intraocular pressure (IOP) control, and requirement for anti-glaucoma medications. They reported a cumulative success of 87.8% at 1 year for 41 eyes. The mean visual acuity improved from 0.73 ± 0.5 to 0.16 ± 0.16 ($P = 0.000$). The mean IOP decreased from 28.2 ± 3.1 to 16.8 ± 2.1 ($P = 0.000$, 40.4%), while the number of anti-glaucoma medications decreased from 2.6 ± 0.66 to 1.2 ± 1.4 ($P = 0.000$). The absolute and relative success rates were 56.1 and 31.7%, respectively; five eyes (12.2%) were considered failures. There were no intraoperative complications; postoperative complications occurred in eight eyes (19.5%). A hypertensive phase was detected in 12 (29.3%) eyes.

A longer term study of 42 eyes, which utilized intraoperative and postoperative antimetabolites, reported 100% success at 1 year and 84% success at 6 years, with a mean intraocular pressure of 12.9 mmHg and a mean number of medications of 1.2.[22]

Hoffman et al.[8] studied cataract surgery combined with Baerveldt implant. They reported cumulative survival of 89% at 18 months for the 33 eyes in their study with a mean intraocular pressure and number of medications needed to control intraocular pressure of 13.1 mmHg and 0.4, respectively, at 18 months. The results of patients' visual acuity in that study were not as good as past phacotrabeculectomy studies, but the authors note that preexisting conditions, such as advanced glaucoma, limited the ability to improve visual acuity after cataract removal.

A long-term study of the Molteno implant showed that all of the patients were able to maintain intraocular pressure below 21 mmHg, with or without hypotensive medication. Interestingly, the same study noted that, with time, the intraocular pressure control of the patients with the Molteno implant improved, resulting in less hypotensive medications and lower pressures.[23]

Summary

Combined cataract and glaucoma drainage device implantation offers an effective option for surgically managing patients with refractory glaucoma and visually significant glaucoma. The combined procedure provides the benefits of a single trip to the operating room, versus performing the operations sequentially, and has not been shown to increase the chances of failure of the drainage device.[21]

References

1. Heijl A, Leske MC, Bengtsson B, et al. Reduction of intraocular pressure and glaucoma progression: results from the early manifest glaucoma trial. *Arch Ophthalmol.* 2002;120(10):1268–79.

2. Kass MA, Heuer DK, Higginbotham EJ, et al. The ocular hypertension treatment study: a randomized trial determines that topical ocular hypotensive medication delays or prevents the onset of primary open-angle glaucoma. *Arch Ophthalmol.* 2002;120(6):701–13; discussion 829–30.

3. Leske MC, Wu S, Nemesure B, Hennis A. Risk factors for incident nuclear opacities. *Ophthalmology.* 2002;109(7):1303–8.

4. Chandrasekaran S, Cumming RG, Rochtchina E, Mitchell P. Associations between elevated intraocular pressure and glaucoma, use of glaucoma medications, and 5-year incident cataract: the blue mountains eye study. *Ophthalmology.* 2006;113(3):417–24.

5. Friedman DS, Jampel HD, Lubomski LH, et al. Surgical strategies for coexisting glaucoma and cataract: an evidence-based update. *Ophthalmology.* 2002;109(10):1902–13.

6. Jampel HD, Friedman DS, Lubomski LH, et al. Effect of technique on intraocular pressure after combined cataract and glaucoma surgery: An evidence-based review. *Ophthalmology.* 2002;109(12):2215–24; quiz 2225, 2231.

7. Rivier D, Roy S, Mermoud A. Ex-PRESS R-50 miniature glaucoma implant insertion under the conjunctiva combined with cataract extraction. *J Cataract Refract Surg.* 2007;33(11):1946–52.

8. Hoffman KB, Feldman RM, Budenz DL, et al. Combined cataract extraction and Baerveldt glaucoma drainage implant: indications and outcomes. *Ophthalmology.* 2002;109(10):1916–20.

9. Backstrom G, Behndig A. Redilation with intracameral mydriatics in phacoemulsification surgery. *Acta Ophthamol Scan.* 2006;84:100–4.

10. Nikeghbali A, Falavarjani KG, Kheirkhah A, et al. Pupil dilation with intracameral lidocaine during phacoemulsification. *J Cataract Refract Surg.* 2007;33:101–3.

11. Park CH, Jaffe GJ, Fekrat S. Intravitreal triamcinolone acetonide in eyes with cystoid macular edeam associated with central retinal vein occlusion. *Am J Ophthalmol.* 2003;136:419–25.

12. Martidis A, Duker JS, Greenberg PB, et al. Intravitreal triamcinolone for refractory diabetic macular edema. *Ophthalmology.* 2002;109:920–7.

13. Wakabayashi T, Oshima Y, Sakaguchi H, et al. Intravitreal bevacizumab to treat iris neovascularization and neovascular glaucoma secondary to ischemic retinal diseases in 41 consecutive cases. *Ophthalmology.* 2008;115:1571–80.

14. Sothornwit N. Intravitreal bevacizumab for Ahmed glaucoma valve implantation in neovascular glaucoma: a case report. *J Med Assoc Thai.* 2008;91S:S162–5.

15. Smith MF, Doyle WD, Ticrney JW. A comparison of glaucoma drainage implant tube coverage. *J Glaucoma.* 2002;11:143–7.

16. Molteno AC, Bevin TH, Herbison P, Houliston MJ. Otago glaucoma surgery outcome study: long-term follow-up of cases of primary glaucoma with additional risk factors drained by Molteno implants. *Ophthalmology.* 2001;108(12):2193–200.

17. Fankhauser F, Kwanseiwska S. Laser vitreolysis. A review. *Ophthalmologica.* 2002;216:73–84.

18. Lundy DC, Sidoti P, Winarko T, Minckler D, Heuer DK. Intracameral tissue plasminogen activator after glaucoma surgery. Indications, effectiveness and complications. *Ophthalmology.* 1996;103:274–82.

19. Hong CH, Arosemena A, Zurakowski D, Ayyala RS. Glaucoma drainage devices: A systematic literature review and current controversies. *Surv Ophthalmol.* 2005;50:48–60.

20. Chung AN, Aung T, Wang JC, Chew PTK. Surgical outcomes of combined phacoemulsification and glaucoma drainage implant surgery for Asian patients with refractory glaucoma with cataract. *Am J Ophthalmol.* 2004;137:294–300.

21. Nassiri N, Nassiri N, Sadeghi Yarandi S, Mohammadi B, Rahmani L. Combined phacoemulsification and Ahmed valve glaucoma drainage implant: a retrospective case series. *Eur J Ophthalmol.* 2008;18(2):191–8.

22. Alvarado JA, Hollander DA, Juster RP, Lee LC. Ahmed valve implantation with adjunctive mitomycin c and 5-fluorouracil: long-term outcomes. *Am J Ophthalmol.* 2008;146:276–84.

23. Molteno ACB, Whittaker KW, Bevin TH, Herbison P. Otago glaucoma surgery outcome study: long term results of cataract extraction combined with Molteno implant insertion or trabeculectomy in primary glaucoma. *Br J Ophthalmol.* 2004;88(1):32–5.

Chapter 12

Choroidal Detachment Following Glaucoma Surgery

Diego G. Espinosa-Heidmann

Introduction

The presence of serous or hemorrhagic fluid accumulation in the suprachoroidal space is defined as a choroidal detachment.[1] The pathophysiology of this fluid collection is not clearly understood, but it occurs as a result of multiple mechanisms such as ocular hypotony, surgical trauma, altered integrity of the ocular vasculature, as well as inflammation. A choroidal detachment can be seen after several clinical settings such as a combined cataract and glaucoma surgery, a cataract extraction, or a retinal detachment, as a result of ocular inflammation or due to spontaneous development.[2] It usually occurs at any time in the postsurgical period more frequently during the first week. There is also an idiopathic form, in nanophthalmos and in association with increased episcleral venous pressure presenting as an intraoperative choroidal effusion during glaucoma or cataract surgery (see Table 12.1).

Serous Choroidal Detachment

Choroidal detachments were first noted in the 1860s, but it was not until 1900 that Fuchs reported that they were a frequent complication of surgery such as cataract surgery.[3,4]

The frequency and degree of postoperative hypotony have decreased due to improved microscopic surgical techniques. The use of fine suture material and more exact wound closure techniques have resulted in a decrease in overfiltration and wound leaks. At the same time, the recent introduction of antimetabolite drug therapy during or following filtration surgery has again increased the incidence rate of hypotony-associated choroidal detachments.

D.G. Espinosa-Heidmann (✉)
Duke University Eye Center, Durham, NC 27710, USA
e-mail: diego.espinosa-heidmann@duke.edu

Table 12.1 Clinical Settings in which choroidal detachment may occur

- Cataract surgery
- Filtration surgery
- Retinal reattachment surgery
- Intraocular surgery in eyes with enlarged episcleral vessels
- Before or after intraocular surgery in nanophthalmos
- Non-surgical ocular trauma
- Inflammatory disorders affecting the eye (i.e., choroiditis, scleritis)
- Ocular tumors (primary or metastatic)

The suprachoroidal space is a potential space situated between the choroid and the sclera.[5] When filled with blood or fluid it becomes a true space, of which the boundaries are the scleral spur anteriorly and the optic disc posteriorly. The choroid is firmly attached to the sclera at the ampullae of the vortex veins. These attachments are responsible for the typical lobular appearance of a large choroidal detachment. The suprachoroidal space normally contains approximately $10 \mu l$ of fluid.[6] A choroidal detachment is defined as a separation of the uvea from the sclera; therefore, a choroidal effusion is serous fluid within the suprachoroidal space. As mentioned previously, hypotony and inflammation appear to be causative factors responsible for this accumulation of fluid in the suprachoroidal space.[7]

Chandler made important initial observations about the nature of this condition. He noted that if the eye was soft and there was no obvious choroidal detachment, a sclerectomy would demonstrate fluid in the suprachoroidal space, that suprachoroidal fluid had to extend to the scleral spur for aqueous production to be reduced, and that it was essential to maintain re-formation of the anterior chamber if repeated drainage of fluid was required.[8,9] The validity of these observations is now established.

Choroidal serous detachments are usually asymptomatic. They can be associated with a positive scotoma. The clinical features of serous choroidal detachment include low intraocular pressure (IOP), shallow to flat anterior chamber, overfiltration of a filtering bleb, and the possibility of a wound leak. It may occur anywhere in the fundus, but it is usually found anterior to the equator on either side of the midline in the inferonasal or inferotemporal quadrants of the globe. Upon clinical examination it appears as a brown, balloon-like choroidal elevation, most efficiently examined by indirect ophthalmoscopy, but it can also be viewed by direct ophthalmoscopy, biomicroscopy, and can be imaged frequently by ultrasonography.

There can be idiopathic conditions associated with ciliochoroidal serous effusion, which can lead to forward rotation of the lens-iris diaphragm and angle-closure glaucoma. The first condition is nanophthalmos, which is an ocular anomaly characterized by a small eye with a small cornea, shallow anterior chamber, narrow angle, and high lens/eye volume ratio.[10] The eyes are highly hyperopic due to the short axial length (<20 mm). Uveal effusion and non-rhegmatogenous retinal detachment may follow intraocular surgery in these cases. Histopathologic studies reveal an unusually thick sclera with irregular interlacing collagen bundles, fraying of collagen fibrils, reduced glycosaminoglycans, and elevated fibronectin.[10] It has been proposed that the uveal effusion may be due to reduced scleral permeability to proteins by the thickened sclera or compression of venous drainage channels by the dense collagen around the vortex veins. See also Chapter 19. The second condition, uveal effusion syndrome, has similarities to nanophthalmos with the exception that the eye is of normal size. It is characterized by dilated episcleral vessels, thickened or detached choroid and ciliary body, and rhegmatogenous retinal detachment. The sclera may be thickened and impermeable due to structural abnormalities such as impaired deposits of glycosaminoglycans, dilated endoplasmic reticulum, and large glycogen-like granules in scleral cells.[10] Other conditions with elevated episcleral venous pressure and prominent episcleral veins must also be ruled out as causes for choroidal detachments such as idiopathic episcleral venous pressure glaucoma, dural shunt, carotid-cavernous sinus fistula, and Sturge-Weber syndrome. Eyes with these abnormalities often develop an intraoperative choroidal effusion that may mimic an intraoperative expulsive hemorrhage. Often, it is recommended that a prophylactic posterior sclerostomy may reduce the complications associated with intraoperative choroidal effusion in these eyes.

Suprachoroidal Hemorrhage

Suprachoroidal hemorrhage (SCH) is defined as blood, as opposed to serous fluid, within the suprachoroidal space. Suprachoroidal hemorrhage can be classified with respect to size and extent of hemorrhage, by their relation to intraocular surgery, or by the precipitating event. When categorized with respect to size, it can vary from a small area of

involvement to massive involvement. This massive involvement can be sufficiently large to force the inner surfaces into direct apposition, usually within the center of the posterior chamber. This extensive type of hemorrhage is commonly defined as a "kissing suprachoroidal hemorrhage" or massive suprachoroidal hemorrhage with central retinal apposition. The timing of development of suprachoroidal hemorrhage with relation to intraocular surgery is another method of classifying the condition. Here it may develop at the time of the intraocular surgery, representing intraoperative suprachoroidal hemorrhage, which in many cases is associated with the expulsion of intraocular contents through the surgical wound (i.e., expulsive suprachoroidal hemorrhage). Suprachoroidal hemorrhage that develops in the postoperative period is termed "postoperative suprachoroidal hemorrhage" or "delayed suprachoroidal hemorrhage." This type occurs in a closed system and is not typically associated with expulsion of intraocular contents. Finally, suprachoroidal hemorrhage can be categorized by the precipitating events such as penetrating or blunt trauma. This type of suprachoroidal hemorrhage is considered a distinct entity by itself and will not be considered here.[7]

Several theories have been postulated to explain suprachoroidal hemorrhage. Hypotony appears to be the major precipitating factor resulting in rupture of a long or short ciliary artery.[11] Another theory is that hypotony causes a choroidal effusion that stretches and ruptures a long or a short posterior ciliary artery.[12-15] Obstruction of venous outflow from the vortex veins may also be a precipitating factor that may lead to a suprachoroidal hemorrhage.[16] Suprachoroidal hemorrhage is a relatively rare event that has been reported to occur in the setting of all types of intraocular procedures including cataract extraction, penetrating keratoplasty, glaucoma filtering surgery, and vitreoretinal surgery.[17-25] The occurrence of this complication during the advent of modern techniques of intraocular surgery has even made this complication almost non-existent. The incidence of expulsive suprachoroidal hemorrhage during glaucoma surgery has been reported to be approximately 0.15%.[26] On the other hand, the incidence of delayed suprachoroidal hemorrhage is higher, as reported by various authors, when compared to the former.[21,27,28] This type of delayed suprachoroidal hemorrhage is believed to be precipitated by prolonged postoperative hypotony and inflammation.

Multiple studies have indicated that multiple risk factors are associated with the development of both intraocular and delayed suprachoroidal hemorrhage (SCH). These systemic, ocular, intraoperative, and postoperative risk factors are summarized in Table 12.2.[29-31]

Before surgery, certain preventive measures should be employed in patients at high risk for the development of suprachoroidal hemorrhage. These measurements should be

Table 12.2 Risk factors for SCH

1. Systemic
    Advanced age
    Arteriosclerosis
    HTN
    Blood dyscrasia/Coagulation defects
    Diabetes
2. Ocular
    Glaucoma
    Myopia
    Aphakia/pseudophakia
    Choroidal inflammation
    Recent intraocular procedures
    SCH in the fellow eye
3. Perioperative risk factors
    Retrobulbar anesthesia without epinephrine
    Precipitous drop of IOP
    Valsalva maneuvers
    Vitreous loss
4. Postoperative risk factors
    Postoperative trauma
    Ocular hypotony
    Valsalva maneuvers
    TPA administration

Table 12.3 Prophylactic measures to avoid choroidal effusions

1. Preoperative
    Perform complete ophthalmic evaluation to rule out ocular risk
        factors
    Perform complete medical evaluation to rule out systemic risk
        factors
    Avoid aspirin and other anticoagulants to prevent coagulation
        problems
2. Operative
    Use minimal preoperative phenylephrine to avoid systemic
        hypertension
    Use epinephrine in lid blocks to produce vasoconstriction of
        vessels
    Lower IOP before incision by the use of intravenous
        hyperosmotic agents
    Or carbonic anhydrase inhibitor (CAI)
    Avoid rapid decompression of the globe
    Avoid Valsalva maneuvers
    Recognize suprachoroidal hemorrhage early if it occurs
3. Postoperative
    Avoid eye trauma or eye pressure
    Avoid hypotony
    Avoid Valsalva maneuvers

followed before, during, and after surgery. Please refer to Table 12.3.

A favorable outcome after intraoperative or delayed suprachoroidal hemorrhage requires early recognition. Early signs of an intraoperative suprachoroidal hemorrhage include a sudden increase in IOP with firming of the globe, loss of the red reflex, and shallowing of the anterior chamber with forward displacement of the iris and lens or lens implant,

with or without vitreous prolapse. Immediate tamponade of the globe is required by either direct digital pressure or rapid suturing of all surgical incisions. If intraocular contents are expelled, they should be reposited as quickly as possible. Sometimes, acutely, posterior sclerotomies need to be performed in order to successfully accomplish reduction of intraocular content, but this still remains debatable. Delayed suprachoroidal hemorrhage behaves differently from intraoperative suprachoroidal hemorrhage. This usually presents with the sudden onset of severe ocular pain with subsequent loss of vision. Headache, nausea, or vomiting may accompany the ocular pain. On clinical examination, there is shallowing of the anterior chamber, vitreous prolapse into the anterior chamber in aphakic or pseudophakic eyes, and loss of the red reflex. On fundoscopic examination, dark elevated dome-shaped lesions are seen occupying the equatorial fundus and on occasions there is an extension to the posterior pole. Intraocular pressure may be low, normal, or elevated.

Role of Ultrasound in SCH

Ultrasound can be extremely useful in the diagnosis of serous choroidal detachment as well as suprachoroidal hemorrhage. It can help in the diagnosis and management of these conditions. Ultrasound can determine the location and extent of suprachoroidal hemorrhage, as well as determine the status of the retina and vitreous. Also, differentiation between hemorrhagic choroidal detachment and serous choroidal effusion can be used with the combination of A- and B-scans. In suprachoroidal hemorrhage, the suprachoroidal space is typically filled with opacities denoting the presence of clotted blood evident in the B-scans as opposed to the absence of these images in serous choroidal detachments. These clots are seen as highly reflective, solid-appearing masses with irregular internal structures and irregular shapes. In subsequent follow-ups, liquefaction of these blood clots occurs, which, on average, has been reported to take from 7 to 14 days.[7,32,33] See Fig. 12.1. The A-scans show a steeply rising double-peaked wide spike characteristic of a choroidal detachment with lower reflective spikes in the suprachoroidal space, indicating clotted blood. Ultrasound can be a useful adjunct in determining the optimal time for drainage by delaying drainage until there is echographic evidence indicating liquefaction of the suprachoroidal hemorrhage.[32–34] This can minimize probing of the suprachoroidal space for residual clots, a maneuver that may cause further bleeding or retinal damage. Computed tomography and the use of magnetic resonance can also aid in the differentiation of serous and hemorrhagic choroidal detachments as well, but are not as cost-effective.

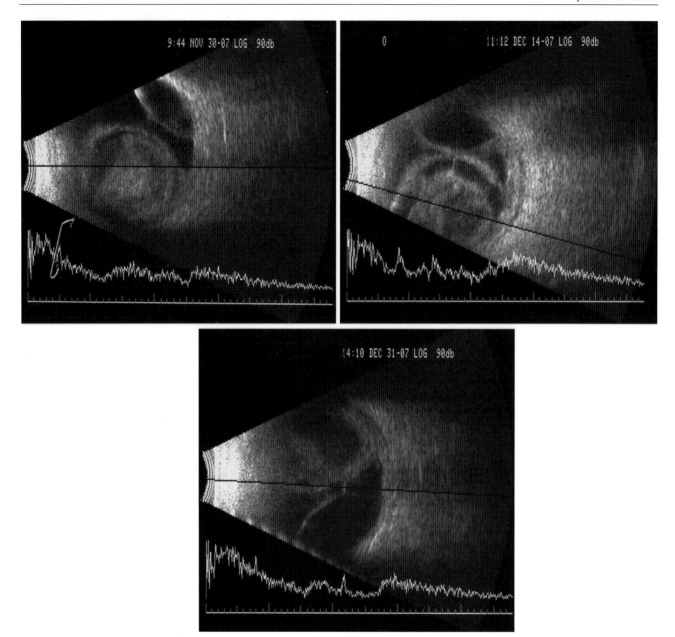

Fig. 12.1 B-scan ultrasound image that illustrates suprachoroidal hemorrhage with clot contraction and liquefaction

Medical Management

Choroidal detachments are usually not a clinically significant concern if there is just serous fluid as opposed to blood. As indicated previously, in the context of glaucoma surgery, there can be a flat chamber associated with serous choroidal detachment, which would require reformation. Here it is important to differentiate between the former and other complications, such as an overfiltration due to failure to adjust the scleral flap resistance enough during filtration surgery, a wound leak, an aqueous hyposecretion from inflammation, or a forward displacement of the lens-iris diaphragm by aqueous misdirection.[35] For most cases when there is just diversion of fluid into the uveal-scleral tract, as in serous choroidal detachment, it resolves spontaneously or with conservative medical treatment without sequelae[36] (Figs. 12.2 and 12.3a, b). Even suprachoroidal hemorrhages may resolve with medical management (Fig. 12.4).

The goal of medical management is achieving decreased inflammation and increased IOP.[1] Topical prednisolone acetate or dexamethasone every 1–2 h, as well as dexamethasone ointment at bedtime, are used to minimize intraocular

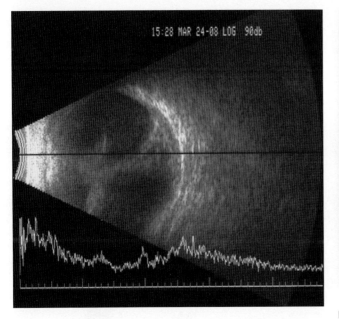

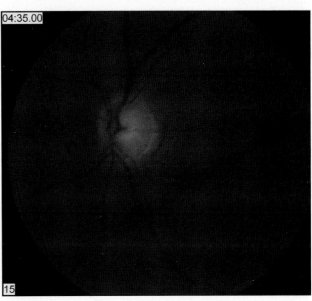

Fig. 12.2 This B-scan ultrasound shows large serous choroidal detachment, which resolved completely with conservative treatment, despite "kissing" for several days

Fig. 12.3 (**a, b**) These fundus photographs illustrate the near resolution of a low-lying serous choroidal effusion. Photographs courtesy of Tom Monego at Dartmouth Hitchcock Medical Center (DHMC), Lebanon, NH

inflammation. The use of mydriatic and cycloplegic agents, such as atropine 1% or shorter acting agents, results in diminished ciliary body tone and posterior displacement of the lens-iris diaphragm as well as controls ocular pain if present. If the anterior chamber is very shallow, a dilating course of neo-synephrine 2.5% and tropicamide 1% administered every 5 minutes, four times, twice a day can be helpful in promoting deepening of the anterior chamber. The use of prednisone (80 mg/daily), a systemic steroid, is controversial but can be effective in some refractory cases. A polymethyl methacrylate (PMMA) glaucoma shell can also be used to manage an early choroidal detachment by promoting deepening of the anterior chamber if excessive filtration is the factor contributing to the serous effusion.

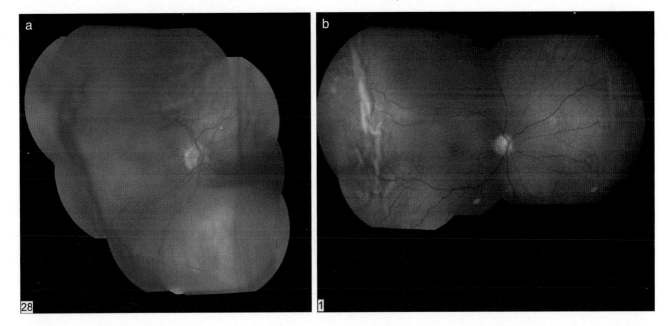

Fig. 12.4 This fundus photograph shows resolving hemorrhagic choroidal detachment. Note the wrinkling of the retina on the domed surface. Courtesy of CRP at DHMC, Lebanon, NH

Surgical Management

When the choroidal detachment persists despite medical therapy and there is anterior chamber shallowing, there can be consequences that might indicate a more aggressive course of action. The consequences of prolonged absence of the anterior chamber are summarized in Table 12.4.

Table 12.4 Consequences of prolonged absence of the anterior chamber

- Closure of a previously open angle by peripheral anterior synechiae
- Failure of filtration bleb in filtration procedures for glaucoma
- Anterior capsular and/or subcapsular cataracts
- Hastening of nuclear sclerotic cataractous changes
- Damaged corneal endothelium with bullous keratopathy
- Formation of posterior synechiae
- Hypotony maculopathy if associated low IOP

In these cases, it may be indicated to do surgical drainage of the suprachoroidal fluid. The procedure is known as a choroidal tap (Table 12.5). Here the anterior chamber reformation is combined with posterior sclerotomies that allow drainage of the suprachoroidal space (see Fig. 12.5).

Table 12.5 Performing a choroidal tap

1. Peribulbar block with a mixture of 2% lidocaine with epinephrine plus 0.75% bupivacaine without epinephrine and hyaluronidase applied in four quadrants (1–2 cc per quadrant) is preferred over a retrobulbar block, especially if the eye is extremely soft. This lessens the risk of intraocular needle perforation and diminishes the possibility of a retrobulbar hemorrhage, which would prove difficult for re-formation of the anterior chamber. Neither Honan's balloon nor digital pressure compression is used
2. Sterile preparation of the eye and drapes are applied in the usual fashion for eye surgery
3. Bridle sutures may be used in the superior and inferior rectus muscle only if there is not a bleb that can be compromised with this maneuver. If a bleb is present, then a bridle suture is not indicated and clear cornea Vicryl or silk sutures are placed anterior to the limbus to control the globe position
4. A paracentesis should be made with a very sharp blade very slowly to avoid a rapid entry in the anterior chamber, which can result in damage to the iris or lens. Then using a 27-gauge cannula, the anterior chamber is reformed with balanced salt solution. If the anterior chamber is resistant to reformation, an air bubble or viscoelastic material can be used
5. A horizontal conjunctival incision is made 3–6 mm from the limbus in the quadrants where the drainage is going to be made. If a bleb is present, then the drainage should be away from the quadrant where the filtering bleb is located. Unipolar diathermy is applied to visible episcleral vessels to minimize bleeding
6. The sclera is penetrated by a scratch-down technique to enter the suprachoroidal space with a diamond blade, or a duller blade such as a Beaver no. 67 or a Bard-Parker no. 15 blade. The incision is 2–3 mm in length and is placed perpendicular to the limbus in a radial configuration. It is recommended that two sclerostomies be created to completely evacuate the suprachoroidal space. See Fig. 12.5.

Table 12.5 (continued)

7. Clear to yellowish-tinged fluid often drains spontaneously once the incision is carried into the suprachoroidal space. Once the fluid stops, the tip of a cyclodialysis spatula can be inserted into the suprachoroidal space in a circumferential fashion (parallel to the limbus). This maneuver can be performed in both directions
8. The anterior chamber is reformed periodically with balanced salt solution when the eye softens. This cycle of anterior chamber reformation and fluid drainage is repeated until no further fluid drains from the sclerostomy. Using two fine-tipped forceps to elevate one edge of the sclerostomy wound while alternately depressing the opposite edge with a cotton-tipped applicator permits more effective fluid release
9. Once the anterior chamber has been reformed and the choroidal effusions have been drained, the sclerostomy openings are left open and the conjunctiva is closed with 10-0 absorbable suture
10. The eye is then gently patched and an eye shield placed after subconjunctival steroid injection and atropine plus antibiotic ointment are applied to the conjunctival sac

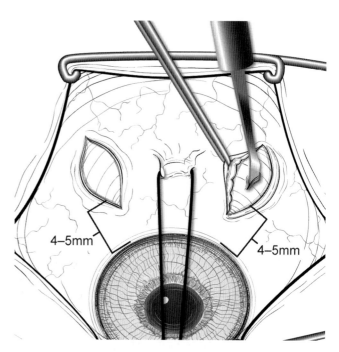

Fig. 12.5 Illustration of a choroidal tap. The conjunctiva has been opened 5 mm from the limbus in the quadrant. A blade is being used to scratch down through the sclera to the level of the suprachoroidal space to allow exit of the fluid

The indications for early surgical drainage, in the presence of suprachoroidal hemorrhage, may be in part similar to the ones observed in serous choroidal detachments such as lens-cornea touch, progressive corneal edema, progressive cataract formation, failing filtering bleb with shallow anterior chamber in an inflamed eye, wound leak and flat anterior chamber, and development of angle-closure glaucoma associated with anterior rotation of the ciliary body.[5,7] More specifically, the indications for drainage and intraocular surgery for suprachoroidal hemorrhage include the presence of a retinal detachment, central retina apposition that may cause retinal adhesions, vitreous incarceration into a surgical wound, a breakthrough vitreous hemorrhage, retained lens material during cataract surgery, and intractable eye pain[7] (Fig. 12.6). With these later complications, suprachoroidal hemorrhage drainage may require sclerotomies 12–14 mm posterior to the limbus to evacuate blood that has accumulated in the posterior pole area. Consultation with a retinal specialist is indicated when there is any indication that the structures of the posterior segment are jeopardized from the hemorrhage. Vitrectomy techniques to manage the vitreoretinal complications and the use of intraocular expandable gases that can effectively decrease the incidence of re-bleeding and tamponade the choroid and retina in their anatomic positions, so that reoperation is less likely, may be needed as well.[7,37]

It is important that when retinal detachments are associated with choroidal detachment, a distinction be made between retinal detachment of serous origin and retinal detachments of a tractional or rhegmatogenous cause. Serous detachments are typically dome shaped, low lying, and situated over areas of choroidal hemorrhage. Traction retinal detachments are taut areas of retinal separation, with apparent areas of vitreoretinal traction. Rhegmatogenous retinal detachments are usually more elevated and bullous, and may not be overlying an area of choroidal hemorrhage. The importance relies in the fact that serous retinal detachments can be observed closely with a high rate of spontaneous resolution. On the other hand, rhegmatogenous and tractional retinal detachments remain a common indication for surgical intervention.[38–41]

Central retinal apposition, or kissing choroidals, has traditionally been considered to be an absolute indication for surgical drainage. It has been reported that the retinal surfaces in apposition become fixed. The duration of central retinal apposition in suprachoroidal ranges from 10 to 25 days with decrease in elevation after the third week. Despite this prolonged apposition, no evidence of persistent retinal

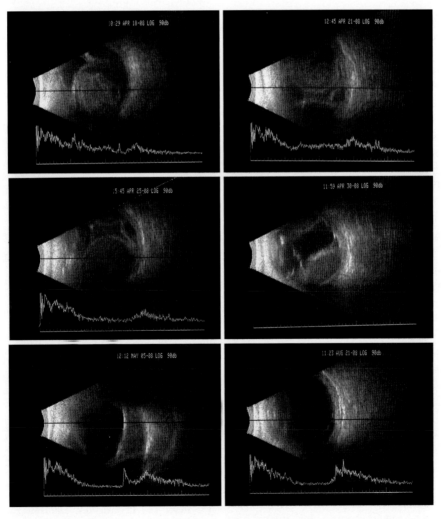

Fig. 12.6 B-scan ultrasound that illustrates the clearing of a large postoperative suprachoroidal hemorrhage that required pars plana vitrectomy to relieve retinal traction

adherence, either clinically or echographically, has been noted in many cases. Therefore, central retinal apposition may be a relative rather than an absolute indication for early surgical intervention.[34,41–43]

Surgical Approach

In a patient with suprachoroidal hemorrhages, the surgical approach may be one of two choices:

1. Drainage procedure to remove the suprachoroidal hemorrhage or
2. vitreoretinal surgery in combination with a drainage procedure to remove not only the hemorrhage in the suprachoroidal space but also to remove vitreous hemorrhage, to remove retained lens material, to relieve vitreoretinal traction, and to re-establish the normal anatomic configuration of the posterior segment.[7]

When a drainage procedure is contemplated, the optimal time for intervention can be critical for success. Mean clot lysis time for a suprachoroidal hemorrhage has been reported to be between 7 and 14 days.[24] See Fig. 12.1. Attempts to drain before clot lysis has occurred are usually unsuccessful. It is therefore recommended that drainage in patients with suprachoroidal hemorrhage be deferred for 1–2 weeks, preferably with clot lysis confirmed by ultrasound. Some authors recommend an infusion system or an anterior chamber maintainer to form the anterior chamber during drainage of the suprachoroidal blood, while maintaining uniform IOP.[44–47] Another alternative is the use of a continuous-infusion air pump through a 25-, 27-, or 30-gauge needle inserted through the limbus.[21,48] The air pump insufflation pressure is preset to 20–30 mmHg. A potential disadvantage of this technique versus the use of balanced salt solution is the loss of detailed visualization of the posterior segment because of the air-fluid interface reflections, which will make identification of peripheral retinal tears or areas of vitreoretinal traction more difficult to detect at the time of surgery. When retinal detachment, vitreoretinal traction, vitreous hemorrhage, and/or dislocated lens fragments are present in the setting of a suprachoroidal hemorrhage, vitreoretinal surgery at the time of the drainage procedure is advisable.[7] Vitreoretinal surgery will re-establish the normal anatomic configuration of the globe by controlled removal of vitreous and vitreous debris, relief of vitreoretinal traction, and reattachment of detached retina. In these instances the drainage of suprachoroidal blood should be first with the purpose of restoring the normal anatomic location of the pars plana, anterior retina, and vitreous base before attempting the introduction of an infusion cannula and instruments into the eye for the conventional three-port pars plana vitrectomy. Internal tamponade with a long-acting gas as mentioned earlier or silicone oil may also be required to successfully restitute the normal anatomy of the posterior pole.

Outcomes

Cantor and coauthors reviewed the outcomes of drainage of serous choroidals in 63 eyes following glaucoma surgery, including combined trabeculectomy with cataract extraction. The patients were initially treated medically. At 1 month, 59% had resolution of the choroidal effusions and 77% at 12 months. In the eyes with flat anterior chambers, this condition resolved with drainage. Likewise, visual improvement occurred in eyes that underwent drainage for loss of vision. Seventy-seven percent of the phakic eyes went on to develop cataract within the year. Some eyes required more than one drainage procedure.[49]

References

1. Bellows AR, Chylack LT, Jr, Hutchinson BT. Choroidal detachment. Clinical manifestation, therapy and mechanism of formation. *Ophthalmology*. 1981;88(11):1107–1115.
2. Berke SJ, Bellows AR, Shingleton BJ, Richter CU, Hutchinson BT. Chronic and recurrent choroidal detachment after glaucoma filtering surgery. *Ophthalmology*. 1987;94(2):154–162.
3. Knapp H. Die intraocularen Geschwülste. Karlsruhe: CF Müller; 1868.
4. Fuchs E. Ablosung der aderhaut nach staroperation. *Arch Ophthalmol*. 1900;51(199).
5. Brubaker RF, Pederson JE. Ciliochoroidal detachment. *Surv Ophthalmol*. 1983;27(5):281–289.
6. Hawkins WR, Schepens CL. Choroidal detachment and retinal surgery. *Am J Ophthalmol*. 1966;62(5):813–819.
7. Chu TG, Green RL. Suprachoroidal hemorrhage. *Surv Ophthalmol*. 1999;43(6):471–486.
8. Chandler PA. Primary glaucoma; complications of surgery; causes of failures and methods of prevention and correction. *Trans Am Acad Ophthalmol Otolaryngol*. 1949;53:224–231.
9. Chandler PA. Complications after cataract extraction: clinical aspects. *Trans Am Acad Ophthalmol Otolaryngol*. 1954; 58(3):382–396.
10. Ward RC, Gragoudas ES, Pon DM, Albert DM. Abnormal scleral findings in uveal effusion syndromes. *Am J Ophthalmol*. 1988;106:139.
11. Manschot WA. The pathology of expulsive hemorrhage. *Am J Ophthalmol*. 1955; 40(1):15–24.
12. Maumenee AE, Schwartz MF. Acute intraoperative choroidal effusion. *Am J Ophthalmol*. 1985;100(1):147–154.
13. Beyer CF, Peyman GA, Hill JM. Expulsive choroidal hemorrhage in rabbits. A histopathologic study. *Arch Ophthalmol*. 1989;107(11):1648–1653.

14. Wolter JR. Expulsive hemorrhage: a study of histopathological details. *Graefes Arch Clin Exp Ophthalmol.* 1982;219(4): 155–158.

15. Wolter JR, Garfinkel RA. Ciliochoroidal effusion as precursor of suprachoroidal hemorrhage: a pathologic study. *Ophthalmic Surg.* 1988;19(5):344–349.

16. Zauberman H. Expulsive choroidal haemorrhage: an experimental study. *Br J Ophthalmol.* 1982;66(1):43–45.

17. Davison JA. Acute intraoperative suprachoroidal hemorrhage in capsular bag phacoemulsification. *J Cataract Refract Surg.* 1993;19(4):534–537.

18. Eriksson A, Koranyi G, Seregard S, Philipson B. Risk of acute suprachoroidal hemorrhage with phacoemulsification. *J Cataract Refract Surg.* 1998;24(6):793–800.

19. Duncker GI, Rochels R. Delayed suprachoroidal hemorrhage after penetrating keratoplasty. *Int Ophthalmol.* 1995;19(3): 173–176.

20. Ingraham HJ, Donnenfeld ED, Perry HD. Massive suprachoroidal hemorrhage in penetrating keratoplasty. Am J Ophthalmol. 1989;108(6):670–675.

21. Givens K, Shields MB. Suprachoroidal hemorrhage after glaucoma filtering surgery. Am J Ophthalmol. 1987;103(5):689–694.

22. Gressel MG, Parrish RK, Heuer DK. Delayed nonexpulsive suprachoroidal hemorrhage. *Arch Ophthalmol.* 1984;102(12): 1757–1760.

23. Fastenberg DM, Perry HD, Donnenfeld ED, Schwartz PL, Shakin JL. Expulsive suprachoroidal hemorrhage with scleral buckling surgery. *Arch Ophthalmol.* 1991;109(3):323.

24. Lakhanpal V. Experimental and clinical observations on massive suprachoroidal hemorrhage. *Trans Am Ophthalmol Soc.* 1993;91:545–652.

25. Piper JG, Han DP, Abrams GW, Mieler WF. Perioperative choroidal hemorrhage at pars plana vitrectomy. A case-control study. *Ophthalmology.* 1993;100(5):699–704.

26. Speaker MG, Guerriero PN, Met JA, Coad CT, Berger A, Marmor M. A case-control study of risk factors for intraoperative suprachoroidal expulsive hemorrhage. *Ophthalmology.* 1991;98(2):202–209.

27. Ruderman JM, Harbin TS Jr, Campbell DG. Postoperative suprachoroidal hemorrhage following filtration procedures. *Arch Ophthalmol.* 1986;104(2):201–205.

28. Paysse E, Lee PP, Lloyd MA, et al. Suprachoroidal hemorrhage after Molteno implantation. *J Glaucoma.* 1996;5(3): 170–175.

29. Jeganathan VSE, Ghosh S, Ruddle JB, et al. Risk factors for delayed suprachoroidal haemorrhage following glaucoma surgery. *Br J Ophthalmol.* 2008;92:1393–1396.

30. Tuli ST, WuDunn D, Ciulla TA, Cantor LB. Delayed suprachoroidal Hemorrhage after glaucoma filtration procedures. *Ophthalmology.* 2001;108:1808–1811.

31. The Fluorouracil Filtering Surgery Study Group. Risk factors for suprachoroidal hemorrhage after filtering surgery. *Am J Ophthalmol.* 1992;113:501–507.

32. Le Quoy O, Girard P. Postoperative choroidal hemorrhage. Surgical indications. J Fr Ophtalmol. 1995;18(2):96–105.

33. Reynolds MG, Haimovici R, Flynn HW Jr, DiBernardo C, Byrne SF, Feuer W. Suprachoroidal hemorrhage. Clinical features and results of secondary surgical management. *Ophthalmology.* 1993;100(4):460–465.

34. Chu TG, Cano MR, Green RL, Liggett PE, Lean JS. Massive suprachoroidal hemorrhage with central retinal apposition. A clinical and echographic study. *Arch Ophthalmol.* 1991;109(11): 1575–1581.

35. Liebmann JM, Ritch R. Complications of glaucoma surgery. The Glaucomas. Philadelphia: Mosby; 2008:1703–1736.

36. Bellows R. Postoperative management following filtration surgery. In: Epstein DL, Allingham RR, Schuman JS, eds. Glaucoma. Baltimore, MD: Williams & Wilkins, 1997:541.

37. Desai UR, Peyman GA, Chen CJ, et al. Use of perfluoroperhydrophenanthrene in the management of suprachoroidal hemorrhages. *Ophthalmology.* 1992;99(10):1542–1547.

38. Brucker AJ, Hopkins TB. Retinal detachment surgery: the latest in current management. *Retina.* 2006;26(6 Suppl): S28–S33.

39. Schwartz SG, Flynn HW. Primary retinal detachment: scleral buckle or pars plana vitrectomy? *Curr Opin Ophthalmol.* 2006;17(3):245–250.

40. Ghazi NG, Green WR. Pathology and pathogenesis of retinal detachment. *Eye.* 2002;16(4):411–421.

41. Berrocal JA. Adhesion of the retina secondary to large choroidal detachment as a cause of failure in retinal detachment surgery. Mod Probl Ophthalmol. 1979;20:51–52.

42. Lakhanpal V, Schocket SS, Elman MJ, Dogra MR. Intraoperative massive suprachoroidal hemorrhage during pars plana vitrectomy. *Ophthalmology.* 1990;97(9):1114–1119.

43. Scott IU, Flynn HW Jr, Schiffman J, Smiddy WE, Murray TG, Ehlies F. Visual acuity outcomes among patients with appositional suprachoroidal hemorrhage. *Ophthalmology.* 1997;104(12): 2039–2046.

44. Baldwin LB, Smith TJ, Hollins JL, Pearson PA. The use of viscoelastic substances in the drainage of postoperative suprachoroidal hemorrhage. *Ophthalmic Surg.* 1989;20(7):504–507.

45. Davison JA. Vitrectomy and fluid infusion in the treatment of delayed suprachoroidal hemorrhage after combined cataract and glaucoma filtration surgery. *Ophthalmic Surg.* 1987;18(5): 334–336.

46. Eller AW, Adams EA, Fanous MM. Anterior chamber maintainer for drainage of suprachoroidal hemorrhage. *Am J Ophthalmol.* 1994;118(2):258–259.

47. Birt CM, Berger AR. Anterior chamber maintenance during drainage of a suprachoroidal hemorrhage in two phakic eyes. *Ophthalmic Surg Lasers.* 1996;27(9):739–745.

48. Abrams GW, Thomas MA, Williams GA, Burton TC. Management of postoperative suprachoroidal hemorrhage with continuous-infusion air pump. *Arch Ophthalmol.* 1986;104(10): 1455–1458.

49. WuDunn D, Ryser D, Cantor LB. Surgical drainage of choroidal effusions following glaucoma surgery. *J Glaucoma.* 2005;14: 103–108.

Chapter 13

Cataract Extraction Combined with Endoscopic Cyclophotocoagulation

Steven D. Vold

Introduction

Some of the earliest work regarding cyclodestruction as a means to treat glaucoma occurred when Heine observed decreases in intraocular pressure with detachments of the ciliary body.[1] Verhoeff followed by surgically excising the ciliary body in 1924.[2] Vogt later popularized the use of a penetrating diathermy technique to destroy the ciliary body in the late 1930s.[3,4] In 1950, Bietti became the first person to correlate cyclocryotherapy with intraocular pressure (IOP) reduction.[5] Purnell advocated a transscleral ultrasound radiation to produce the desired destruction in the early 1960s.[6] Since that time, cyclophotocoagulation through either a transpupillary route or a contact or non-contact transscleral route has been popularized utilizing a multitude of different lasers.[7,8]

These various attempts at decreasing intraocular pressure via cyclodestruction share a common set of disadvantages and associated complications. In each of these procedures, the surgeon is attempting to ablate the tissue surrounding fragile ocular structures in a fashion with limited ability to assess anatomic accuracy or qualitative effect. Complications include prolonged hypotony, pain, uveitis, hemorrhage, choroidal effusion, anterior segment ischemia, scleromalacia, failure and need to retreat, and postoperative visual loss associated with chronic cystoid macular edema. Traditionally, these procedures had been limited to patients with refractory glaucomas after failure of other surgical options in patients that already had poor visual acuity.[7,8] More recently studies have suggested patients can enjoy the effects of adequate glaucoma treatment and retain good vision long-term after transscleral laser cyclodestruction with newer lasers.[9]

Endoscopic cyclophotocoagulation (ECP) is a relatively new, Food and Drug Administration (FDA)-approved procedure developed by Martin Uram to minimize the disadvantages of more traditional cyclodestructive procedures while maximizing the advantage of ablating the ciliary body epithelium to decrease IOP. It employs the use of a laser endoscope containing three fiber groupings: the image guide, the light source, and the semiconductor diode laser. This technology allows direct visualization of the ciliary epithelium so that the highly titratable laser energy can be delivered to the source of aqueous production in a precise manner, limiting damage to the underlying ciliary body and surrounding tissue.[10]

Indications for Surgery

The indications for performing ECP remain somewhat controversial and continue to be debated. In light of the complications potentially associated with this procedure, cautious patient selection for this procedure has been advised. ECP has been utilized in a wide variety of glaucoma types including primary open-angle, angle-closure, pigmentary, neovascular, traumatic, pediatric, and other refractory glaucomas.[11–21]

Cyclodestructive procedures have been classically reserved for cases of glaucoma that are refractory to medical therapy, outflow surgeries, and eyes with poor or no vision potential. This is understandable in light of the relatively crude and poorly titratable technology previously available. In these sick eyes with imprecise and sometimes severe treatments, poor treatment outcomes were common and were to be expected.

With the advent of improved laser technologies, the use of scleral transillumination, and endoscopic techniques, the accuracy of treatment location and precision in energy delivery has dramatically improved.[22] These advancements challenge where cyclophotocoagulation fits into the glaucoma treatment paradigm. Evidence is growing that supports cyclophotocoagulation as a viable

S.D. Vold (✉)
Boozman-Hof Regional Eye Clinic, Rogers, AR 72757, USA
e-mail: svold@cox.net

treatment in patients with less severe glaucomas and good vision potential.[9] Unfortunately, no long-term randomized prospective studies that compare ECP to transscleral cyclophotocoagulation and trabeculectomy are currently available.

In recent years, ECP has been increasingly utilized in conjunction with cataract extraction as an initial glaucoma surgery. Early studies seem to support that ECP is effective in lowering IOP and suggest an excellent safety profile in this setting.[23–26] With extensive ECP experience, Berke suggests performing ECP in combination with small-incision cataract surgery in patients with cataract and moderate glaucoma on two or more medications. He performs phacoemulsification with intraocular lens implantation alone in patients with cataract and mild, well-controlled glaucoma on a single, well-tolerated glaucoma medication (see Chapter 2). In patients with cataract and advanced glaucomatous optic nerve damage on maximum medical therapy, he generally performs phacotrabeculectomy with intraoperative mitomycin C[26] (see Chapter 6). The clinical experience of this author mirrors the findings of Berke and colleagues. Visually significant cataract is commonly the driving force in the decision to proceed with phaco-ECP in patients with both cataract and glaucoma under this treatment paradigm.

Despite extensive positive anecdotal experience, more prospective well-controlled long-term studies are necessary to more accurately determine the actual benefits and indications of ECP. Intraocular pressure spikes, increased postoperative inflammation, intraocular lens dislocation, and long-term efficacy remain concerns potentially associated with combined phaco-ECP.[27] Cautious utilization of this technology is appropriate, especially in patients with pseudoexfoliation syndrome, inflammatory disease, cystoid macular edema, macular degeneration, and diabetic retinopathy. The true benefit of ECP on intraocular pressure reduction has been questioned as well. Cataract surgery is well known to lower intraocular pressure in certain glaucoma patients.[28,29,30] The long-term efficacy and potential implications on concurrent ocular diseases remain largely unknown.

Instrumentation

Ocular endoscopy was first suggested by Thorpe in 1934.[31] Interestingly, no other reports were published until Norris and Cleasby described an endoscope for ophthalmology in 1978.[32] In 1986, Patel and colleagues were the first to report endolaser treatment of the ciliary body for uncontrolled glaucoma.[18] However, this was done using scleral depression through an operating microscope, not with an endoscope. Uram developed an intraocular laser endoscope with both vitreoretinal and anterior segment applications, and reported his initial results treating neovascular glaucoma in 1992.[11]

The unit developed by Uram has two basic sets of instrumentation: the laser endoscope and the equipment console. The laser endoscope has three fiber groupings: the image guide, the light guide, and the semiconductor diode laser guide, which is set to the 810-nm wavelength (Fig. 13.1). These three exist as either an 18- or 20-gauge endoprobe with a 110° field of view and depth of focus from 1 to 30 mm. The light guide employs a 175 W xenon light source. The laser has an up to 2.0 W power output. Both straight and curved endoscopic probes are available. The laser endoscope is connected to the console that contains all of the instrumentation used for endoscopy including the video camera, light source, video monitor, and video recorder (Fig. 13.2). The surgeon controls the progress of surgery by viewing the video monitor, rather than viewing through the operating microscope (Fig. 13.3).

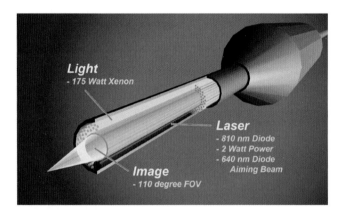

Fig. 13.1 ECP probe. Image courtesy of EndoOptiks Corp., Little Silver, NJ

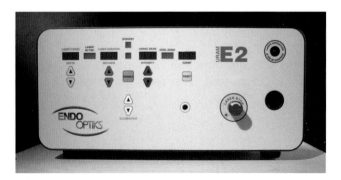

Fig. 13.2 ECP console. Photo courtesy of EndoOptiks Corp., Little Silver, NJ

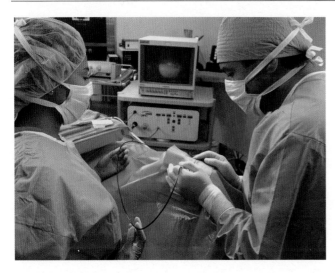

Fig. 13.3 ECP surgical set-up. Photo courtesy of EndoOptiks Corp., Little Silver, NJ

Operative Technique

With endoscopic cyclophotocoagulation, ciliary processes may be accessed from either a limbal or a pars plana approach (Fig. 13.4). Assessment of lens and vitreous status is important in determining an ECP surgical plan. Mechanism of glaucoma, level of intraocular pressure, and previous surgical intervention should also be considered.

Ciliary processes may be accessed from an anterior approach in phakic, pseudophakic, and aphakic eyes. The limbal approach is generally recommended in patients undergoing ECP combined with cataract surgery and intraocular lens implantation. The incision should be at least 1.5–2.0 mm in length. Both clear corneal and the scleral tunnel incisions commonly used in cataract surgery provide adequate access for the endoscope. Topical, extraconal, and intraconal regional block techniques all provide acceptable anesthesia.

In phakic eyes that are not undergoing phaco but ECP only, an "over-the-capsule" approach may be used. Sodium hyaluronate is injected posterior to the iris but anterior to the capsule. Hyaluronate-based viscoelastics are entirely transparent to the diode laser wavelength, allowing laser transmission across the viscoelastic cushion without generating more thermal energy. This maneuver causes anterior displacement of the iris and posterior movement of the lens, creating a wide approach to the ciliary process. High viscosity viscoelastics such as Healon GV or Healon5 (Abbott Medical Optics, Abbott Park, IL) maintain this space well and prevent any potential contact of the laser endoscope with the iris and lens throughout the procedure. Any adhesions between the lens capsule and the iris are severed by viscoelastic or mechanical dissection. Endolaser cyclophotocoagulation may then be performed. Once ECP has been completed, thorough removal of the viscoelastic is vital to preventing early postoperative intraocular pressure rises.

In pseudophakic patients with posterior chamber lenses or in patients undergoing ECP combined with cataract surgery, a similar approach is used. In combined surgery, cataract surgery is typically performed first. Sodium hyaluronate is then injected posterior to the iris but anterior to the lens capsule and lens implant, creating open access to the ciliary processes. Clear corneal incisions may be preferable as it may allow for easier access to a wider treatment area and preservation of the conjunctiva in the event that filtering surgery is required in the future. If capsular rupture occurs during cataract surgery, vitreous should be carefully removed from the anterior chamber prior to proceeding with ECP. This author would likely not proceed with ECP after complicated cataract surgery or in patients with a loose zonular apparatus. ECP performed in these circumstances potentially leads to complications associated with both poor intraocular lens support and increased postoperative inflammation.

In aphakic eyes, vitreous must be removed before any endoscope manipulation occurs in the region of treatment. An anterior chamber maintainer is generally required making viscoelastic use optional. Surgeons must be aware that lens remnants, gliotic capsule, and opacified vitreous may overlie the ciliary processes preventing their visualization and treatment. In these situations, removal of fibrotic material may need to be performed, and a pars plana approach may be useful. With a pars plana surgical approach, the laser endoscope is inserted through the pars plana 3.5–4.0 mm from the limbus. The tip is directed in an anterior direction, and the cil-

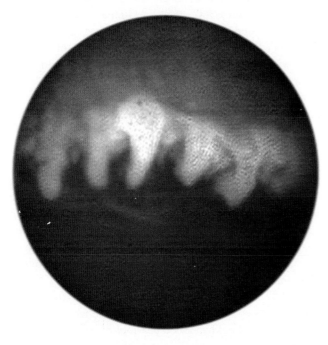

Fig. 13.4 Treated ciliary processes. Photo courtesy of EndoOptiks Corp., Little Silver, NJ

iary processes are easily viewed and photocoagulated. A pars plana approach is discouraged in phakic patients as the crystalline lens will obscure visualization of the ciliary processes with this technique.

One of the great advantages of ECP over transscleral cyclophotocoagulation techniques is the ability to deliver laser energy in a highly titratable fashion to the ciliary processes. The optimum tissue effect is to whiten the ciliary process and effect visible tissue shrinkage (Fig. 13.4). Photocoagulation is applied with the endoscope 1.0–3.0 mm from the ciliary processes with power levels of the 810-nm semiconductor diode laser titrated upward from lower power levels to achieve whitening and shrinkage of the ciliary processes. A slow continuous wave application of the laser treatment allows surgeons to methodically "paint" the entirety of each ciliary process in a smooth, well-controlled fashion.

Treatment of at least 300° is often required to get optimal intraocular pressure reduction with ECP.[33] Using the straight probe, two-site surgery is often required to achieve adequate treatment. The curved endoscope probe enhances a surgeon's ability to expand the ciliary process treatment area through smaller incisions (Table 13.1). Gas bubble formation, pigment dispersion, audible "popping" sounds, photocoagulation of non-ciliary process tissue, and inclusion of prosthetic material in the treatment zone should be avoided.

Table 13.1 Tips for ECP success

Treat at least 270–300°
Go back over treated areas to enhance treatment efficacy
Treat the ridge of the process first so that shrinkage exposes the valley better
Ensure you treat both the anterior and posterior aspect of the process
Slower burns of two seconds that avoid "popping" ciliary processes are preferable

Postoperative Care

The postoperative course following ECP is one of the most attractive features associated with this operation. In most patients, postoperative management of both ECP alone and also combined ECP and cataract surgery is similar to that encountered with cataract surgery alone. The perioperative use of topical broad-spectrum antibiotic, topical prednisolone acetate 1%, and topical non-steroidal anti-inflammatory medication are generally recommended. Postoperative anti-inflammatory medication regimens rarely require more than four times a day dosing with proper patient selection and good surgical technique. In the immediate postoperative period, aggressive use of topical or systemic glaucoma medication may be helpful in preventing early postoperative intraocular pressure spikes. Glaucoma medica-

tions are often slowly tapered down over the first 4–6 weeks after surgery.

With early aggressive management of inflammation, complications such as posterior and anterior synechiae, posterior capsule opacification, and cystoid macular edema mirror those experienced in patients undergoing cataract surgery alone. Patients are commonly examined at 1 day, 1 week, 4 weeks, 3 months, and 6 months postoperatively. This is a significant reduction in postoperative visits when compared to most postoperative care regimens after standard filtration surgery.

Results/Outcomes

Precise tissue localization and ability to potentially titrate laser treatment are major reasons why ECP may be superior to transscleral cyclodestruction in both efficacy and safety. Histopathologic studies have shown that eyes treated with transscleral cyclodestruction had coagulative changes to the ciliary muscle and surrounding tissue with inaccurate and incomplete atrophy of the ciliary body epithelium where the aqueous is produced. This is in contradistinction to those eyes treated with ECP, which showed precise damage to only the ciliary body epithelium in the areas intended by the surgeon with no other involved structures damaged.[34–36] Recent studies performing ciliary body fluorescein angiography on patients who have failed transscleral cyclodestructions showed that less than 120° of ablation was achieved in all of the eyes studied, even when the surgeon had documented attempted 360° ablation. Similar histological evidence suggested that those patients who had received ECP appeared to have accurate and thorough ablation of intended tissues.[37] This study highlights the difficulty in providing a surgical procedure to a delicate area blindly with hopes of adequate treatment without overtreating and suggests the potential solution of ECP.

The first patients treated by ECP were treated for neovascular glaucoma and published as a small retrospective study of ten treated eyes in 1992 by Uram who holds the ECP patent. Uram reported intraocular pressure below 21 mmHg in nine of the ten eyes, with only three eyes requiring postoperative glaucoma medication at a mean follow-up of 8.8 months. Ciliary processes were treated contiguously for 90–180°. Chronic hypotony was the only major complication occurring in two eyes with preexisting chronic retinal detachments.[11]

In 1997, Chen and colleagues reported the retrospective results of 68 eyes from 68 patients with refractory glaucomas, most of whom had failed previous incisional glaucoma surgery or transscleral cyclophotocoagulation. Eyes received between 180° and 360° of ciliary body epithelium treatment.

During the mean follow-up period of 12.9 months, mean intraocular pressure decrease from 27.7 mmHg preoperatively to 17.0 mmHg postoperatively. Sixty-one eyes (90%) achieved an intraocular pressure ≤ 21 mmHg. Best-corrected visual acuity was stable or improved in 64 eyes. No cases of hypotony or phthisis bulbi were observed.[12]

In 2004, Lima and colleagues performed a randomized prospective study of 68 eyes in 68 patients comparing ECP and the Ahmed drainage implant in the treatment of refractory glaucomas. Ciliary processes were treated for 210° in the ECP group. Surgical success was defined as an intraocular pressure greater than 6 mmHg and below 21 mmHg at 24 months of follow-up with or without maximum tolerated therapy. Preoperative intraocular pressures dropped from approximately 41 mmHg preoperatively to between 14 and 15 mmHg postoperatively in both groups. Kaplan–Meier survival curve analysis showed a probability of success of 70.59 and 73.53% for the Ahmed and ECP groups, respectively. Complications of choroidal detachment (Ahmed 17.64%, ECP 2.94%) and shallow anterior chambers (Ahmed 17.64%, ECP 0.0%) were much less frequent in the ECP treatment group.

In their study published in 2004, Wilensky and Kammer challenged the assumption that transscleral cyclophotocoagulation should be reserved for eyes with poor vision potential. In their observational case series of 21 eyes, they found that only 3 of 21 eyes had significantly worse best-corrected visual acuities after a mean follow-up of 40.7 months. Unfortunately, a single treatment provided inadequate long-term intraocular pressure control in 19 of the 21 eyes.[9]

Uram published the initial study evaluating outcomes in patients who underwent combined phacoemulsification and intraocular lens implantation with ECP for the management of glaucoma and cataracts in 1995. In this study, he treated ciliary processes contiguously for 180° in ten eyes. An average decrease in intraocular pressure of 57% from 31.5 mmHg preoperatively to 13.5 mmHg postoperatively occurred over a mean follow-up of 19.2 months using this technique. Five of these eyes maintained favorable IOP without any glaucoma medications.[23]

In 1999, Gayton and colleagues compared outcomes of ECP with phacoemulsification and intraocular lens implantation versus trabeculectomy with phacoemulsification and intraocular lens implantation. In this randomized prospective study of 58 eyes in 58 patients, 240–270° of treatment were performed. Only 14 of the 29 patients undergoing trabeculectomy were given an antifibrotic agent (mitomycin-C). With a mean follow-up of 2 years, 30% of ECP patients achieved intraocular pressure control below 19 mmHg without medication and 65% with medication. Forty percent of trabeculectomy eyes achieved this level of intraocular pressure control without medication and 52% with medication. Four ECP patients (14%) and three trabeculectomy patients (10%) were considered treatment failures and required additional surgical intervention. In this study, ECP produced less inflammation than trabeculectomy as assessed by anterior chamber cell and flare measurements on slit lamp examination.[24]

In the largest prospective study published thus far, Berke compared ECP combined with phacoemulsification and intraocular lens implantation to phacoemulsification with intraocular lens implantation alone in 2006. In his study, the ciliary process epithelium received between 180° and 360° of treatment. In the ECP treatment group of 626 eyes, intraocular pressures dropped from 19.08 mmHg preoperatively to 15.73 mmHg postoperatively with a mean follow-up of 3.2 years. The numbers of glaucoma medications were reduced from 1.53 meds preoperatively to 0.65 meds postoperatively. In the 81 eyes undergoing cataract surgery alone, intraocular pressures slightly increased from 18.16 mmHg preoperatively to 18.93 mmHg postoperatively, with the number of glaucoma medications remaining unchanged at 1.20 meds both before and after surgery. Cystoid macular edema developed in 1% of eyes in each treatment group. No serious complications were reported in either group.[25,26]

Complications

The most common risks for glaucoma patients undergoing cataract surgery with or without ECP include vision loss, excessive pain, hemorrhage, infection, inflammation, retinal detachment, blindness, retained lens material, zonular dehiscence, need for additional surgeries including trabeculectomy, failure of the procedure, posterior capsule opacification, ptosis, diplopia, cystoid macular edema, and risks of anesthesia including death. The additional risks of glaucoma patients undergoing cataract surgery with the ECP procedure include hypotony, ciliary block glaucoma, and phthisis bulbi.[7,22,38–41] Sympathetic ophthalmia has been reported with transscleral cyclophotocoagulation, but never been reported with ECP to the author's knowledge.

Summary

Endoscopic cyclophotocoagulation (ECP) is an effective tool for the treatment of refractory glaucomas and appears to play a role in the management of patients with both cataract and glaucoma. Despite the problems of previous cyclodestructive procedures, initial ECP studies are promising and appear to suggest that this procedure is different from previous transscleral cyclodestructive techniques. ECP appears to be a relatively safe and appealing surgical option in patients with good vision potential and in the setting of cataract surgery.

ECP offers the advantages of precise tissue treatment, short surgical times, rapid postoperative recovery, and reduced complications. Further study is required to better define its long-term efficacy and its role in the management of glaucoma.

References

1. Heine L. Die Cyklodialyse, eine neue glaucomoperation. *Deutsche Med Wochenschr*. 1905;31:824–825.
2. Verhoeff FH. Cyclectomy: a new operation for glaucoma. *Arch Ophthalmol*. 1924;53:228–229.
3. Vogt A. Versche zur intraokularen Druckherabsetzung mittels Diatermiesehadigung des Corpus ciliare (Zyklodiatermiestichelung). *Klin Monatsbl Augenheilkd*. 1936;97:672–677.
4. Vogt A. Cyclodiathermypuncture in cases of glaucoma. *Br J Ophthalmol*. 1940;24:288–297.
5. Bietti G. Surgical intervention on the ciliary body: new trends for the relief of glaucoma. *JAMA*. 1950;142:889–897.
6. Purnell EW, Sokollu A, Torchia R, et al. Focal chorioretinitis produced by ultrasound. *Invest Ophthalmol*. 1964;3:657–664.
7. Mastrobattista JM, Juntz M. Ciliary body ablation: where are we now and how did we get here? Surv Ophthalmol. 1996;41(3):193–213.
8. Pastor SA, Singh K, Lee DA, et al. Cyclophotocoagulation: a report by the American Academy of Ophthalmology. *Ophthalmology*. 2001;108(11):2130–2138.
9. Wilensky JT, Kammer J. Long-term visual outcome of transscleral laser cyclotherapy in eyes with ambulatory vision. *Ophthalmology*. 2004;111:1389–1392.
10. Uram M. Endoscopic cyclophotocoagulation in glaucoma management. *Curr Opin Ophthalmol*. 1995;6(2):19–29.
11. Uram M. Ophthalmic laser microendoscope ciliary process ablation in the management of neovascular glaucoma. *Ophthalmology*. 1992;99(12):1823–1828.
12. Chen J, Cohn RA, Lin SC, et al. Endoscopic photocoagulation of the ciliary body for treatment of refractory glaucomas. *Am J Ophthalmol*. 1997;124(6):787–796.
13. Plager DA, Neely DE. Intermediate-term results of endoscopic diode laser cyclophotocoagulation for pediatric glaucoma. *J AAPOS*. 1999;3(3):131–137.
14. Neely DE, Plager DA. Endocyclophotocoagulation for management of difficult pediatric glaucomas. J AAPOS. 2001;5:221–229.
15. Lima FE, Magacho L, Carvalho DM, et al. A prospective, comparative study between endoscopic cyclophotocoagulation and the Ahmed drainage implant in refractory glaucoma. *J Glaucoma*. 2004;13:43–47.
16. Mora JS, Iwach AG, Gaffney MM, et al.: Endoscopic diode laser cyclophotocoagulation with a limbal approach. *Ophthalmic Surg Lasers*. 1997;28(2):118–123.
17. Barkana Y, Morad Y, Ben-nun J. Endoscopic photocoagulation of the ciliary body after repeated failure of trans-scleral diode-laser cyclophotocoagulation. *Am J Ophthalmol*. 2002;133:405–407.
18. Patel A, Thompson JT, Michels RG, et al. Endolaser treatment of the ciliary body for uncontrolled glaucoma. *Ophthalmology*. 1986;93:825–830.
19. Zarbin MA, Michels RG, deBustros S, et al. Endolaser treatment of the ciliary body for severe glaucoma. *Ophthalmology*. 1988;95:1639–1648.
20. Lai JS, Tham CC, Chan JC, et al. Diode laser transscleral cyclophotocoagulation as primary surgical treatment for medically uncon-

trolled chronic angle closure glaucoma: long-term outcomes. *J Glaucoma*. 2005;14:114–119.
21. Lin SC, Chen J, Hwang DG, et al. Endoscopic cyclophotocoagulation for the treatment of glaucoma in keratoplasty patients. *Invest Ophthalmol Vis Sci*. 1998;39:2157–B14.
22. Lin S. Perspective: endoscopic cyclophotocoagulation. *Br J Ophthalmol*. 2002;86:1434–1438.
23. Uram M. Combined phacoemulsification, endoscopic ciliary process photocoagulation, and intraocular lens implantation in glaucoma management. *Ophthalmic Surg*. 1995;26(4):346–352.
24. Gayton JL, Van Der Karr M, Sanders V. Combined cataract and glaucoma surgery: trabeculectomy versus endoscopic laser cycloablation. *J Cataract Refract Surg*. 1999;25:1214–1219.
25. Berke SJ, Cohen AJ, Sturm RT, et al. Endoscopic cyclophotocoagulation(ECP) and phacoemulsification in the treatment of medically controlled primary open-angle glaucoma. *J Glaucoma*. 2000;9(1):2000. abstract.
26. Berke SJ. Endolaser cyclophotocoagulation in glaucoma management. *Tech Ophthalmol*. 2006;4:74–81.
27. Netland PA, Mansberger SL, Lin S. Uncontrolled intraocular pressure after endoscopic cyclophotocoagulation. J Glaucoma. 2007;16:165–167.
28. Heltzer J, Lieberman M. The effect of clear cornea phacoemulsification on intraocular pressure in normal and glaucomatous patients. *J Glaucoma*. 2000;9(1):103. abstract.
29. Mathalone N, Hyams M, Neiman S, et al. Long-term intraocular pressure control after clear corneal phacoemulsification in glaucoma patients. *J Cataract Refract Surg*. 2005;31:479–483.
30. Poley BJ, Lindstrom RL, Samuelson TW. Long-term effects of phacoemulsification with intraocular lens implantation in normotensive and ocular hypertensive eyes. *J Cataract Refract Surg*. 2008;34:735–742.
31. Thorpe HE. Ocular endoscope. *Trans Am Acad Ophthalmol Otolaryngol*. 1934;39:422–424.
32. Norris JL, Cleasby GW. An endoscope for ophthalmology. *Am J Ophthalmol*. 1978;85:420–427.
33. Kahook MY, Lathrop KL, Noecker RJ. One-site versus two-site endoscopic cyclophotocoagulation. *J Glaucoma*. 2007;16:527–530.
34. Trevisani MG, Allingham RR, Shields MB. Histologic comparison of contact transscleral diode cyclophotocoagulation and endoscopic diode cyclophotocoagulation. *Invest Ophthalmol Vis Sci*. 1995;36(4):S331. abstract.
35. Shields MB, Chandler DB, Hickingbotham D, et al. Intraocular cyclophotocoagulation histopathologic evaluation in primates. *Arch Ophthalmol*. 1985;103:1731–1735.
36. Francis B, Flowers B, Alvarado JA. Endoscopic cyclophotocoagulation (ECP) and other cyclodestructive modalities: a histopathologic comparison. *Medtronics*. Unpublished.
37. Uram M. Endoscopic fluorescein angiography of the ciliary body in glaucoma management. *Ophthalmic Surg Lasers*. 1997;27:174–178.
38. Edward DP, Brown SVL, Higginbotham E, et al. Sympathetic ophthalmia following neodymium:YAG cyclotherapy. *Ophthalmic Surg*. 1989;20:544–546.
39. Lam S, Tessler HH, Lam BL, et al. High incidence of sympathetic ophthalmia after contact and noncontact neodymium:YAG cyclotherapy. *Ophthalmology*. 1992;99:1818–1822.
40. Bechrakis NE, Muller-Stolzenurg NW, Helbig H, et al. Sympathetic ophthalmia following laser cyclophotocoagulation. *Arch Ophthalmol*. 1994;112:80–84.
41 Azuara-Blanco A, Dua HS. Malignant glaucoma after diode laser cyclophotocoagulation. *Am J Ophthalmol*. 1999;127:467–469.

Chapter 14

Approach to Cataract Extraction Combined with New Glaucoma Devices

Diamond Y. Tam and Iqbal Ike K. Ahmed

Introduction

Both the incidence of glaucoma and cataract increases in the aging population, and the surgical treatment of glaucoma increases the rate of progression of cataractous lens opacity. So, it follows that the simultaneous surgical treatment of both pathologies with cataract extraction, intraocular lens implantation, and intraocular pressure (IOP) lowering surgery benefits the patient with fewer procedures. This thereby decreases cumulative recovery time, time for visual rehabilitation, and intraoperative risk. Furthermore, a cataractous lens, which may sometimes be large in size, occupying a large antero-posterior space, or a forward positioned crystalline lens as with weakened zonules or microspherophakia, may cause narrowing of the anterior chamber angle, and even precipitate angle closure with a pupillary block mechanism or via a mass effect. In these circumstances, removal of the crystalline lens may not only improve visual function in patients but also aid in the management of the glaucoma, or assist in opening the angle to facilitate the performance of glaucoma surgery.

In the 1960s, concurrent surgical treatment of cataract and glaucoma was first described with combining cataract extraction and thermal sclerostomy,[1,2] which was followed in the late 1960s and early 1970s by cataract extraction in conjunction with trabeculectomy.[3,4] While trabeculectomy, first described by Cairns,[5] has a well-documented IOP-lowering effect,[6] and has been enhanced by the use of adjunctive antimetabolites,[7–9] a significant short- and long-term risk profile exists for the patient with traditional penetrating trabeculectomy. In a recent study, the rate of long-term hypotony related to trabeculectomy was 42%.[6] This is an unacceptable and unsafe high rate of a potentially visually

Table 14.1 Short- and long-term risks of traditional filtration surgery

- Blebitis, endophthalmitis
- Hypotony, overfiltration
- Thin-walled avascular blebs, bleb leaks, dysesthesia, overhang, encapsulation
- Corneal dellen, endothelial cell loss
- Episcleral fibrosis
- Aqueous misdirection

devastating complication. Other short- and long-term risks of traditional penetrating surgery are listed in Table 14.1 among others, the vast majority of which are lifetime risks in patients who undergo penetrating trabeculectomy.[10]

Likewise, tube shunts, valved devices, and seton implants, while effective also in IOP lowering, have a significant risk of hypotony and suprachoroidal hemorrhage. They also share some common risks and postoperative challenges with trabeculectomy such as encapsulation of the filtering bleb as well as bleb fibrosis. While filtration of aqueous humor into the post-equatorial conjunctival space, further from the metabolically active limbal zone, may be less likely to cause these problems, tube shunt devices present their own unique set of possible postoperative complications as listed in Table 14.2 .

Table 14.2 Possible complications unique to tube shunts

- Such as tube or plate exposure
- Tube lumen occlusion
- Corneal endothelial loss even with proper tube positioning
- Tube migration
- Ptosis
- Diplopia

Some recent reports have suggested that cataract extraction and IOL implantation alone decrease IOP and glaucoma medication dependence, with the patients having higher preoperative IOPs receiving the greatest benefit.[11,12] See Chapter 4. However, it is worth noting that as a cataractous lens increases in size with time, a concurrent shallowing of the anterior chamber and narrowing of the angle and even

D.Y. Tam (✉)

Department of Ophthalmology, University of Toronto, Toronto, ONT, Canada

e-mail: diamondtam@gmail.com

intermittent or chronic angle closure may result. It is these patients who may benefit the most from cataract extraction and IOL implantation, in terms of IOP reduction as well as lessened progression of glaucomatous optic neuropathy. The studies reporting the beneficial effect of phacoemulsification on IOP do not stratify patients according to preoperative gonioscopic findings, which may potentially be an important predictor of those patients who may most benefit from cataract extraction used as a method of lowering IOP.

In the authors' experience, patients with high preoperative IOPs and glaucomatous disease in the presence of an open angle typically require concurrent glaucoma surgical therapy and cataract extraction for adequate control of the disease. While traditionally patients were only able to receive penetrating trabeculectomy along with its significant short- and long-term risks, new glaucoma surgical devices are emerging that provide surgeons and patients with potentially safer alternatives. With the aim of increasing safety while maintaining a high degree of efficacy for glaucoma patients both intra- and postoperatively, new devices and procedures for the surgical treatment of glaucoma will be reviewed in this chapter. These new procedures and devices provide surgeons with the option to lower the risk profile associated with subconjunctival filtration surgery by augmenting the conventional outflow pathway or the uveoscleral suprachoroidal outflow pathway.

In this chapter, we will discuss cataract extraction and intraocular lens implantation in combination with the following:

- Ex-PRESS shunt subconjunctival filtration device (Optonol Ltd., Neve Ilan, Israel)

- *Ab externo* Schlemm's canal surgery in non-penetrating canaloplasty (iScience Interventional Inc., Menlo Park, CA)
- *Ab interno* approaches to Schlemm's canal in the trabecular microbypass iStent® (Glaukos Corp., Laguna Hills, CA) and the Trabectome micro-electrocautery device (NeoMedix Corp., San Juan Capistrano, CA)
- Suprachoroidal filtration devices such as the gold microshunt (SOLX Inc., Waltham, MA)

Indications for surgery, instrumentation, operative technique, postoperative considerations, complications, the best available data, and a discussion on each device will follow, as well as comparison to traditional trabeculectomy and tube shunt procedures.

The Ex-PRESS Shunt

Indications for Surgery

The Ex-PRESS mini glaucoma shunt was originally designed for implantation directly under the conjunctiva allowing aqueous humor to travel through the shunt unimpeded into the subconjunctival space (Fig. 14.1). This allowed for decreased surgical time compared with traditional subconjunctival filtration trabeculectomy. However, unacceptably high rates of hypotony, conjunctival erosion, and shunt migration led to the placement of the shunt under a trabeculectomy-style scleral flap.[13-15] Different models/designs of the shunt are available varying in ostium size

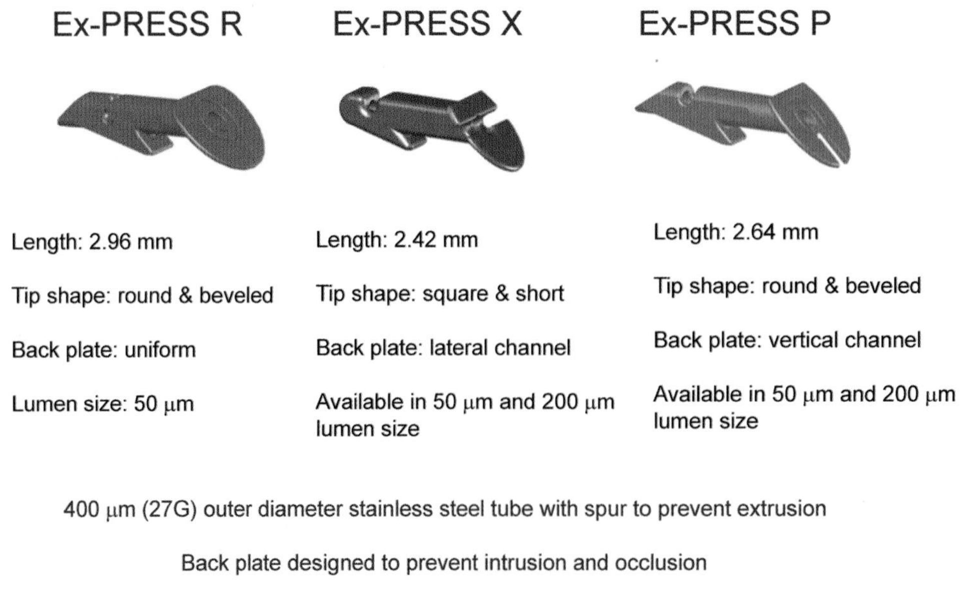

Ex-PRESS R

Length: 2.96 mm

Tip shape: round & beveled

Back plate: uniform

Lumen size: 50 μm

Ex-PRESS X

Length: 2.42 mm

Tip shape: square & short

Back plate: lateral channel

Available in 50 μm and 200 μm lumen size

Ex-PRESS P

Length: 2.64 mm

Tip shape: round & beveled

Back plate: vertical channel

Available in 50 μm and 200 μm lumen size

400 μm (27G) outer diameter stainless steel tube with spur to prevent extrusion

Back plate designed to prevent intrusion and occlusion

Fig. 14.1 Schematic diagram of the Ex-PRESS shunt models and their specifications

as well as ostium placement and footplate design. No data currently exists comparing the different shunt models.

The rate of egress of aqueous humor from the anterior chamber to the subconjunctival space in trabeculectomy varies primarily via two surgical variables: ostium size and scleral flap tension. As a result, significant variability from case to case, even with the same surgeon, may be encountered with a lack of predictability in IOP postoperatively. Furthermore, although its IOP lowering effect is well established, the long-term hypotony rate of 42%[6] reveals the lack of control that surgeons have over the amount of filtration in trabeculectomy.

The Ex-PRESS shunt, with the fixed constant lumen size of 50 μm, aims to improve the safety and control of aqueous outflow in penetrating subconjunctival filtration surgery. Not only is the lumen size fixed, aiding in consistency and reproducibility between cases and patients, but the entry incision into the anterior chamber is smaller than in trabeculectomy and no surgical iridectomy is required. The surgeon need only be concerned about scleral flap suture tension and not the size of a trabeculectomy ostium. In addition, although the labeled use of the device is only open-angle glaucoma surgery, it has been the authors' experience that the device is equally as effective with similar outcomes in open- and closed-angle glaucomas. Therefore, when a patient is considered for conventional trabeculectomy, the use of an Ex-PRESS device under the scleral flap should be given consideration to potentially improve safety and reliability both intraoperatively and postoperatively. One study comparing the Ex-PRESS shunt to trabeculectomy revealed less hypotony and hypotony-related complications in the early postoperative period for patients receiving the Ex-PRESS shunt.[13–15] As the Ex-PRESS shunt is a subconjunctival bleb forming procedure, the shunt must be placed superiorly for the same reasons that trabeculectomy is performed superiorly.

Instrumentation and Operative Technique

As in combined cataract extraction with trabeculectomy, the lensectomy and intraocular lens (IOL) implantation should be performed first to ensure anterior chamber stability, to deepen the anterior chamber, and to prevent excessive irrigation of fluid into a subconjunctival bleb. Prior to beginning surgery, inspection of the conjunctiva superiorly should be undertaken and the surgeon should plan the location of the future bleb. The placement of the paracentesis or side port incision should be away from the area of anticipated filtering surgery, and may need to be placed slightly more centrally into clear cornea to ensure that the conjunctiva is not disturbed. This is especially true superiorly where the conjunc-

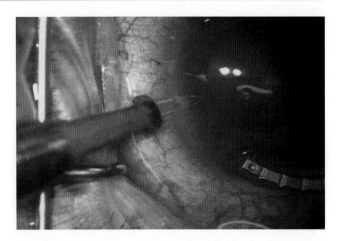

Fig. 14.2 The paracentesis location for phacoemulsification. Note that the entry is made anterior to the conjunctival insertion at the limbus and slightly away from the anticipated superior area of intended glaucoma surgery

tival insertion may be more anterior. This resultant side port incision may be somewhat closer to the main incision and more central than the surgeon is accustomed to (Fig. 14.2). The authors advise the use of a temporal clear corneal or limbal incision for the cataract extraction, to minimize manipulation, to optimize handling of conjunctival tissues, and to avoid any potential disturbance to tissues superiorly where the bleb will reside. Should a superior incision be chosen, it must be in clear cornea to avoid trauma to the conjunctival insertion. After completion of successful lensectomy and insertion of the IOL, viscoelastic should be left in the anterior chamber without being evacuated to assist in anterior chamber stabilization. A suture should be placed into the main incision to ensure watertight closure in cases combined with glaucoma surgery, as a low IOP postoperatively may result in wound incompetence and gape leading to a risk of endophthalmitis. The intraocular pressure should remain reasonably high when attention is turned to the glaucoma procedure to ensure adequate globe and scleral rigidity for ease of maintaining tissue planes during scleral dissection. This may be achieved with the residual viscoelastic and injection of balanced saline solution (BSS) with a blunt cannula through the paracentesis incision. Injection of BSS or viscoelastic may be repeated during the scleral dissection as required to maintain tension in the globe.

To proceed to the insertion of the Ex-PRESS shunt, the surgeon must move to sit superiorly with appropriate adjustments to the microscope and foot pedal controls. A conjunctival peritomy is performed as per the surgeon's usual trabeculectomy technique. It is the authors' preference to begin the peritomy approximately 1 mm posterior to the limbus, leaving a skirt of limbal conjunctiva remaining (Fig. 14.3). Light cautery is then applied to the scleral surface if necessary. Similarly, the dissection of the partial thickness scleral

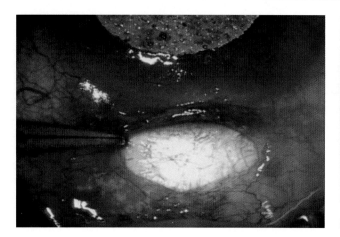

Fig. 14.3 The conjunctival peritomy. Note the anterior tag of conjunctiva at the limbus left behind to facilitate closure at the conclusion of the case

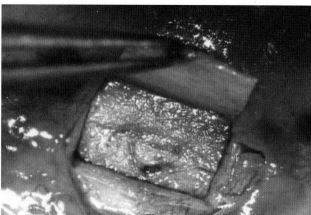

Fig. 14.5 Under the scleral flap, the white hue of the scleral spur is visible in between corneal tissue anteriorly and the sclera posteriorly

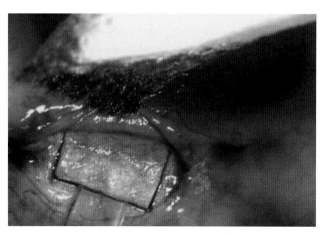

Fig. 14.4 The scleral flap dissection for the Ex-PRESS shunt

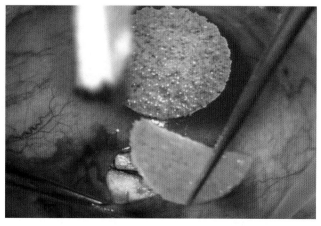

Fig. 14.6 Mitomycin C is soaked onto a half surgical sponge. In this case, a hemi-corneal light shield that is to be placed into the subconjunctival space for local treatment

flap is performed with a crescent blade, in the same manner as in conventional trabeculectomy (Fig. 14.4). The shape of the flap may be of the surgeon's choice, but the overall dimensions of the scleral flap may need to be slightly larger to provide full scleral coverage of the footplate of the Ex-PRESS shunt. Adequate exposure of the scleral spur must be attained during dissection of the scleral flap. It is recommended that the flap dissection be carried forward into clear cornea to allow for full visualization of the spur where the Ex-PRESS shunt will be inserted into the anterior chamber (Fig. 14.5). At this time, as per the surgeon's choice, antimetabolites such as mitomycin-C (MMC) may be applied subconjunctivally and under the scleral flap with a similar technique that would be used for traditional trabeculectomy (Fig. 14.6). After copious irrigation of the antimetabolite from the surgical field, the scleral flap is lifted to visualize and properly identify anatomical landmarks. A sapphire blade manufactured by Optonol, designed for the insertion of

the Ex-PRESS shunt, is then used to make an entry into the anterior chamber at the level of the scleral spur (Fig. 14.7). Of paramount importance, during this step, is the angle of entry of the shunt into the anterior chamber. A posteriorly directed shunt may contact iris and result in iris occlusion of the ostia present on the shunt. A shunt angled excessively anteriorly may result in contact with the cornea resulting in endothelial trauma. The entry of the sapphire blade is angled parallel to the iris plane for proper shunt placement. If the sapphire blade is unavailable, a 25-gauge needle may be used to enter the anterior chamber. The shunt is manufactured preloaded on an injector system. In this system, the surgeon's index finger depresses a portion of the shaft of the injector, which in turn indents a thin malleable central metal fixation rod holding the device at the tip. Once the rod has been crimped, the device is released at the tip of the injector (Fig. 14.8).[16] Due to the design of the small horizontal slit entry into the anterior chamber, the shunt may need to be inserted into the

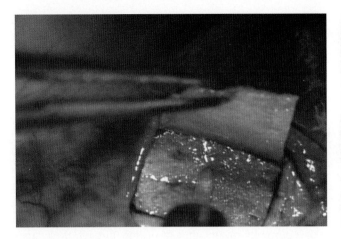

Fig. 14.7 The sapphire blade is used to enter into the anterior chamber under the scleral flap at the level of the scleral spur. An entry parallel to the iris is essential to prevent downward pointing and iris contact of the tip of the shunt

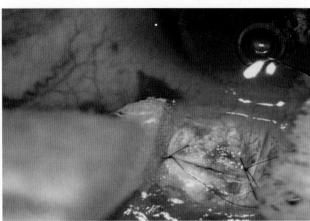

Fig. 14.9 The sutures placed into the scleral flap and surgical sponges evaluating flow out of the site. Note that the Ex-PRESS shunt footplate can be seen through the scleral flap as well as in the anterior chamber

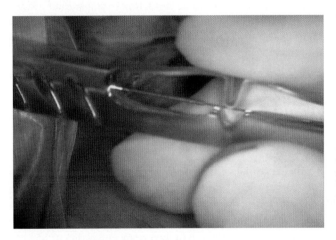

Fig. 14.8 The handle of the Ex-PRESS shunt injector revealing the central metal wire that will be displaced upon compression of the surgeon's index finger on the plastic bridge

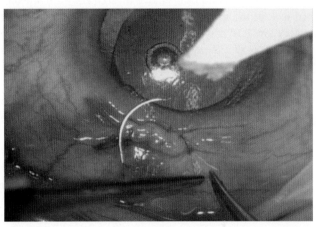

Fig. 14.10 The conjunctiva is closed with 10-0 Vicryl in a running horizontal mattress suture and a slipknot at the end to ensure watertight closure

anterior chamber 90 degrees from its final position in order to be inserted smoothly. This is due to the barb, designed to prevent shunt extrusion, on the underside of the shunt.

After the shunt is inserted, the scleral flap is placed down on top of the Ex-PRESS shunt and the flap sutured as in traditional trabeculectomy. The authors prefer to use a slip-knot technique to adjust suture tension. The flow through the flap is assessed by aspirating viscoelastic from the anterior chamber and capsular bag with a dry technique using a blunt 27-gauge cannula and inflating the anterior chamber subsequently with BSS. With each slipknot, suture tension can be adjusted according to the desired flow observed with infusion into the anterior chamber through the paracentesis incision (Fig. 14.9). When satisfactory flow has been achieved, the conjunctiva is closed as per conventional trabeculectomy methods. The authors prefer to close the posterior conjunctiva to the anterior limbal skirt, fashioned at the outset of the

procedure, with a running 10-0 Vicryl horizontal mattress suture on a vasectomy non-spatulated needle (Fig. 14.10). The conjunctival closure is tied with a slipknot to allow tension of the suture to be adjusted, and the wound ensured to be watertight with light infusion into the anterior chamber.

Postoperative Considerations and Complications

The aim of the Ex-PRESS mini glaucoma shunt is to provide IOP lowering via a subconjunctival reservoir or bleb in a similar fashion to conventional trabeculectomy. As such, the short- and long-term postoperative risk profile and issues of the Ex-PRESS shunt are common to conventional trabeculectomy. The surgeon should maintain vigilance for the development of complications as listed in Table 14.1. These complications and their management are similar to that in conventional trabeculectomy and will not be covered in this chapter. Some of the more common complications and those specific to the Ex-PRESS mini glaucoma shunt will be covered here.

Although the fixed lumen size of the shunt is designed to restrict flow and provide protection against early and late postoperative hypotony with or without a shallow or flat anterior chamber, this complication is still an unfortunate reality of filtering surgery. Despite diligent evaluation of aqueous egress through the scleral flap at the conclusion of surgery, early hypotony remains a potential complication of the Ex-PRESS shunt. This may be in part due to not only flow through the lumen of the shunt but also possibly around the shunt through the slit incision in which it is lying. Postoperative hypotony, especially in the early period, should also prompt careful postoperative assessment for conjunctival leak at the site of wound closure, being cognizant that a very low IOP may mask a conjunctival leak. Early or late hypotony may require pressurization and/or reformation of the anterior chamber with ophthalmic viscosurgical devices (OVDs) and in some cases may even require multiple such postoperative injections at the slit lamp. It is noteworthy that while more viscous and cohesive OVDs, for example, Healon GV or Healon 5, may be more readily cleared through a larger trabeculectomy ostium, the smaller lumen of the Ex-PRESS shunt may result in more difficulty clearing these substances and post-injection IOP spikes should be vigilantly monitored for and possibly expected. For this reason, the authors advise that should anterior chamber pressurization be required, a sequential choice of OVDs be undertaken, starting with agents such as ProVisc or VisCoat (Alcon Laboratories Inc., Fort Worth, TX), and if hypotony, large choroidal effusions, or chamber instability persist, moving to the use of agents such as Healon GV or Healon 5. It is also advisable to begin with small volume injections increasing in an incremental fashion as required. Close follow-up and monitoring, sometimes multiple visits in a day, of these patients is mandatory.

While it is common postoperatively to see the shunt in the anterior chamber directly, regular postoperative gonioscopy to view the shunt is advisable. An elevated IOP postoperatively may indicate an occlusion of the tip of the shunt. Should iris be seen occluding the lumen of the shunt, consideration should be given to mechanical sweeping of the iris away from the tip of the shunt with a 30-gauge needle inserted through the limbus at the slit lamp. An air bubble or a small amount of viscoelastic may be placed in the anterior chamber to prevent recurrence of this event. Sweeping of the iris to break occlusion of the tip of the Ex-PRESS shunt must be done in a timely manner after occurrence. Should the tip be occluded for a prolonged period of time, the lack of flow

into the subconjunctival space is likely to result in episcleral fibrosis, closure of the edges of the scleral flap, and shutdown of the bleb. Thus, in these cases, merely sweeping the iris away from the tip of the Ex-PRESS shunt will be unlikely to restore aqueous outflow. In these cases, a bleb needling with lifting of the scleral flap may be performed concurrently to restore the conduit for aqueous to flow from the anterior chamber to the subconjunctival space. This is performed in a similar fashion to bleb needling performed in trabeculectomy (Fig. 9.7 and Table 9.7). Although the shaft of the shunt has openings also that allow aqueous to enter the shunt, these openings are minute and may not be sufficient to allow an adequate aqueous outflow and IOP lowering effect. No data exists currently on the amount of flow through these small auxiliary openings or its effect on IOP.

While the Ex-PRESS was originally designed for placement directly under the conjunctiva, a common complication with this method of placement was conjunctival erosion with resultant shunt exposure necessitating explantation.[17] Since the adaptation of placing the shunt under a trabeculectomy-style scleral flap, shunt migration and exposure is yet to be reported.

Discussion of Data Related to Combined Surgery

To date, the data available for combined phacoemulsification surgery with the Ex-PRESS shunt are data with shunt implanted directly under the conjunctiva. No data has been published with combined surgery where the Ex-PRESS shunt is placed under a scleral flap. In a study consisting of 35 eyes undergoing combined phacoemulsification and IOL implantation with a subconjunctival Ex-PRESS shunt with an average follow-up of 36.9 ± 18.2 months, the IOP decreased from 19.3 ± 6.3 mmHg preoperatively to 13.3 ± 2.0 mmHg at 48 months postoperatively. The number of medications was reduced by 57%. The shunt, however, was explanted in ten eyes due to shunt migration, conjunctival erosion, or obstruction. In these patients, ten eyes had satisfactory IOP control without medications or complications.[18]

In a retrospective comparative series comparing the Ex-PRESS shunt with conventional trabeculectomy without combined phacoemulsification, there was no statistically significant difference between the IOP lowering of the two procedures, the decrease in number of glaucoma medications, or the change in visual acuity. However, a statistically significant difference was found between the two procedures in early postoperative hypotony and the rate of choroidal effusion with the Ex-PRESS shunt being safer in regards to both complications. While the reduction in IOP was similar for both procedures by 3 months postoperatively, the mean

IOP in the Ex-PRESS shunt group prior to the 3-month time point was significantly higher than that of the trabeculectomy group.[15]

From the best studies and data currently available, the Ex-PRESS shunt appears to provide improved early postoperative safety without compromise in efficacy of IOP lowering when compared to conventional trabeculectomy. However, the Ex-PRESS shunt relies on a subconjunctival filtration bleb to be effective in IOP lowering and thus is prone to the same risks as blebs formed in trabeculectomy. The other advantage to the Ex-PRESS shunt is potential improvement in intraoperative safety. With the small entry incision into the eye, anterior chamber stability and the ability to maintain a relatively stable IOP during surgery are enhanced. This could possibly lower the risk of suprachoroidal hemorrhage, especially in elderly hypertensive patients, or any anterior chamber shallowing event during surgery, which in rare instances may lead to an intraoperative aqueous misdirection type syndrome. Also, the ability to avoid performing a surgical iridectomy may potentially lower the risk of iris bleeding and hyphema intraoperatively and postoperatively, as well as possibly lower the degree of postoperative anterior chamber inflammation.

In summary, the Ex-PRESS mini glaucoma shunt provides glaucoma surgeons with a possibly safer alternative to trabeculectomy, especially for the early postoperative period. While results in combining phacoemulsification and IOL implantation with Ex-PRESS implantation under a partial thickness scleral flap is yet to be published, anecdotal results and outcomes have been similar to conventional phacotrabeculectomy. In patients who are being considered for phacotrabeculectomy, strong consideration should be given for the use of an Ex-PRESS shunt for the potential benefits of an improved early postoperative safety profile, as well as potential for improved control intraoperatively. Issues and precautions surrounding bleb management need to be taken in Ex-PRESS shunt patients as in trabeculectomy due to the common mechanism of subconjunctival reservoir-driven IOP lowering. As well, in the authors' anecdotal experience, the Ex-PRESS shunt in combination with phacoemulsification and IOL placement has been effective in both open angle as well as closed angle glaucoma patients, with no deleterious effects versus conventional phacotrabeculectomy.

Non-penetrating Schlemm's Canaloplasty

Indications for Surgery

The conventional outflow pathway of aqueous humor consists of the uveoscleral, corneoscleral, and juxtacanalicular trabecular meshwork, Schlemm's canal, its collector channels, and then more distally, the episcleral and scleral venous plexi. While conventional trabeculectomy seeks to bypass this physiologic pathway of aqueous outflow, more recent non-penetrating techniques seek to augment flow through the conventional pathway. Because of the non-physiologic nature of subconjunctival filtration surgery and the significant short- and long-term risks, alternate procedures for effective lowering of IOP have been sought to enhance patient safety. Non-penetrating *ab externo* Schlemm's canal surgery first emerged as a procedure called "sinusotomy" in the 1960s.[19–21] This was followed in the 1980s by guarded scleral flaps,[22–24] in the 1990s by viscodilation of Schlemm's canal,[25] and then in the late 1990s and early 2000s by various implants and drainage devices placed under a scleral flap.[26–30] While these procedures sought to improve the safety profile of penetrating trabeculectomy, the means of lowering IOP remained aqueous outflow into a subconjunctival reservoir and thus, the potential complications of blebs followed these procedures.

Early work by Grant in the 1950s and more recent studies have implicated the juxtacanalicular trabecular meshwork and extracellular matrix as the points of major resistance to aqueous outflow in the proximal conventional outflow pathway.[31–33] While collapse of Schlemm's canal is seen in glaucoma patients with elevated IOP,[34] it is unknown whether this is the cause or an effect of the IOP. Once the IOP has elevated, a vicious cycle may be in effect wherein the collapsed Schlemm's canal further reduces aqueous outflow through the canal and collector channels and results in further elevation of IOP. Viscocanalostomy is the procedure by which two cut ends of Schlemm's canal are each intubated with a 44-gauge blunt cannula and inflated with OVD, in an attempt to re-expand the collapsed Schlemm's canal. While this procedure was limited in the degrees of circumference with which the cannula could potentially viscodilate Schlemm's canal, as well as the likely limited duration of time during which the OVD remains distending the canal before absorption, a new technique and device has emerged to maintain mechanical dilation of Schlemm's canal via intracanalicular delivery of a suture.

The iScience device is a flexible microcatheter designed to allow intubation and viscodilation of the entire circumference of Schlemm's canal, as well as allowing delivery of a suture into the canal without ever penetrating the globe. The 45 mm working length 200-micrometer diameter microcatheter is designed to fit into the 300-micrometer Schlemm's canal. It consists of three elements: a central support wire to provide a structural backbone for the device to guide advancement as well as resistance to kinking of the catheter; optical fibers to allow for transmission of a blinking red light from a laser-based micro-illumination system to the tip; and, finally, a true lumen to allow for delivery of

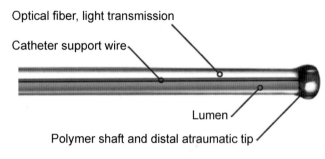

Optical fiber, light transmission

Catheter support wire

Lumen

Polymer shaft and distal atraumatic tip

Fig. 14.11 A schematic diagram of the microcatheter used to cannulate Schlemm's canal. The catheter consists of a bulbous atraumatic tip, a true lumen, a central support wire to add rigidity to the catheter, and an optical fiber to transmit light to the tip

substances such as OVD or trypan blue into Schlemm's canal (Fig. 14.11). The tip of the catheter has a slightly enlarged distal atraumatic smooth bulb at the end of the polymer shaft. The proximal end of the catheter divides into two parts: one for connection into the laser-based micro-illumination light source, and the other for connection into a syringe with OVD, which is attached to a screw-mechanism to provide control of the amount of viscoelastic delivered into the canal. The microcatheter is typically fixated to the surgical drape with tape or Steri-strips (3 M Corp., St. Paul, MN). After the suture is delivered into Schlemm's canal, the tension can be adjusted intraoperatively to provide a mechanical expansion of the canal, allowing increased egress of aqueous humor from the anterior chamber (Fig. 14.12). This procedure, termed *canaloplasty*, attempts to restore conventional outflow of aqueous humor through the trabecular meshwork and Schlemm's canal via a mechanical suture-mediated distension of the canal.

As the intracanalicular suture draws the trabecular meshwork centripetally, albeit by a small amount, canaloplasty is best suited for patients who have open-angle glaucoma or patients whose angles become open after peripheral laser iridotomy or lens extraction (Fig. 14.13). In eyes with narrow angles or iridotrabecular apposition, canaloplasty may exacerbate the situation and should not be considered as a suitable procedure. Open-angle patients with a visually significant cataract, who are considered traditionally for phacotrabeculectomy, should be considered for combined cataract extraction, lens implantation, and canaloplasty. With avoidance of penetration into the globe during surgery, as well as the hypothesized protection against postoperative hypotony because of the primary mechanism of IOP lowering, this procedure allows for improved patient safety both intra- and postoperatively. Studies are currently under way comparing conventional phacotrabeculectomy with combined phacoemulsification with IOL placement and canaloplasty.

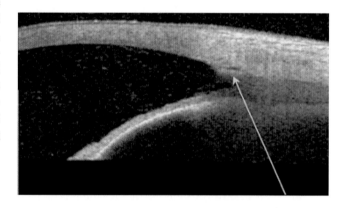

Fig. 14.13 An anterior segment OCT image of the canal, which is distended and expanded by the presence of the intracanalicular suture

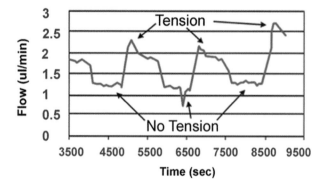

Outflow Facility as a Function of Suture Tension

Perfusion - 20 micron Prolene filament
Alternating - No Tension: Tension

Fig. 14.12 A graph indicating the increase in trans-inner wall flow of aqueous humor when a suture in Schlemm's canal is placed on tension

Instrumentation and Operative Technique

When performing combined phacoemulsification and IOL implantation with canaloplasty, there are considerations that are similar to those discussed in the previous section on the Ex-PRESS shunt. The authors recommend a temporal clear corneal incision for phacoemulsification to avoid any unnecessary manipulation and trauma to superior tissues where the canaloplasty dissection will be performed. In addition, the dissection to unroof Schlemm's canal enters the clear cornea where the trabeculoDescemet window (TDW) is fashioned. A corneal or limbal incision superiorly may interfere with the subsequent glaucoma surgery, thus a temporal incision is advocated. For similar reasons, the sideport incision must be placed carefully with the surgeon cognizant of the intended position of the scleral dissection for the canaloplasty. Again, this incision may be more anterior and closer or farther from the main incision than is customary for the surgeon. The superior conjunctiva and sclera should be examined carefully prior to any incisions to determine the future position of the scleral dissection. Typically, an area between two large ciliary veins is chosen for the performance of canaloplasty to possibly avoid sacrificing these vessels with cautery, keeping in mind that the typical dimensions of the scleral flap are 5 mm circum-limbally by 5 mm posteriorly.

After successful phacoemulsification with IOL implantation, OVD is again left in the anterior chamber and pressurization of the globe achieved with BSS. A suture is placed into the main incision to ensure wound competence in the event of a low postoperative IOP. Acetylcholine should also be instilled into the anterior chamber with a blunt 27-gauge cannula to constrict the pupil. Due to the presence of OVD in the anterior chamber, the superior iris in the area of the anticipated glaucoma procedure may require gentle stroking with the cannula to encourage miosis. The operating microscope and foot pedals are then rotated for the surgeon to sit superiorly to perform the canaloplasty. While topical anesthesia is typically sufficient for the entire procedure, patient cooperation is important to allow for adequate exposure of the superior sclera. In the event that downgaze is difficult for the patient to perform, a traction suture may be placed into the cornea. However, as opposed to the superior cornea, the authors advocate placing the suture into the inferior cornea to avoid distortion and unnecessary tension on the superior cornea where the delicate trabeculodescemet window will be fashioned.

Once adequate exposure has been attained, a conjunctival peritomy is fashioned in the same manner as described previously with the Ex-PRESS shunt. Light cautery is applied to the sclera, attempting to preserve the larger ciliary veins. A scleral flap is then fashioned to the approximate dimensions of 5 mm × 5 mm in a parabolic shape (Fig. 14.14). While any shape of flap may be utilized, the authors prefer a parabolic shape for increased ease of watertight closure at the conclusion of surgery. A crescent blade is then used to dissect the flap forward at an approximately one-third scleral thickness depth. Caution must be exercised especially in cases where the sclera may be thin, as in highly myopic patients. After the dissection is carried forward into clear cornea for approximately 2 mm, the superficial flap is reflected onto the corneal surface and attention is directed toward the creation of a deep scleral flap. This flap should be approximately 1 mm inside from the edge of the superficial dissection and at the base of the deep scleral flap; only a thin approximately 100-micrometer layer of sclera should remain in the bed of the dissection overlying the choroid (Fig. 14.15). It is not uncommon for the bed of the dissection to have some areas of

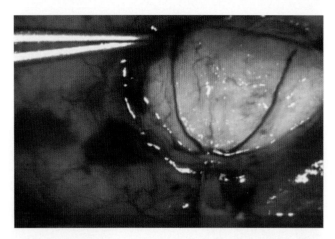

Fig. 14.14 A parabolic scleral flap is fashioned to start canaloplasty

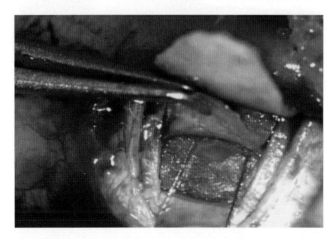

Fig. 14.15 Dissection of the deep scleral flap should occur to almost full thickness scleral depth. Approximately 100 μm should remain. It is common to have some choroidal show in the bed of the dissection

choroidal show. If this occurs, the dissection plane should be re-established on a more superficial level. However, a dissection that occurs at an excessively superficial level presents the risk of the being carried right over Schlemm's canal without actually exposing it. This results in a challenging situation where the surgeon must backtrack and attempt to expose the canal with only a very thin overlying layer of scleral tissue. A much higher risk of perforation into the anterior chamber therefore results, which would require conversion of the procedure to traditional fistulizing trabeculectomy.

As the scleral thickness varies between patients, adjunctive imaging such as an anterior segment optical coherence tomography (Visante™ AS-OCT) scan may be useful in determining the superior scleral thickness, prior to surgery, especially in myopic patients. In these cases, failure to recognize thin sclera prior to surgery may result in an intraoperative surprise in reaching the layer of the choroid prematurely or in penetration into the anterior chamber.

Once the Schlemm's canal is exposed, which should be immediately anterior to the whitened fibers of the scleral spur, fine strands of the outer wall may be seen to peel away and care must be taken to handle the tissues delicately, as excessive traction or manipulation may result in tearing (Fig. 14.16). As the dissection approaches the cornea, the IOP in the eye should be lowered to single digits with dry aspiration of OVD from the previous cataract incisions. This is performed to prevent outward bulging of the Descemet's membrane, risking its perforation, as the dissection is continued into the clear cornea.

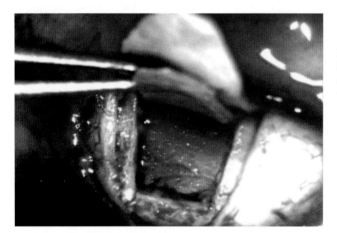

Fig. 14.16 Once the dissection is carried forward adequately, exposure of Schlemm's canal and Descemet's membrane results anterior to the scleral spur

Once the canal has been exposed, a surgical sponge, such as a Merocel (Merocel Corp., North Mystic, CT) or Weck-cel (Medtronic, Jacksonville, FL) slightly wet at the tip, may be used to gently depress the inner wall of Schlemm's canal and Descemet's membrane to bluntly dissect the tissues from the corneal stroma. Great care must be taken as excessive pressure will result in rupture of the fragile trabeculoDescemet's window (TDW). Sharp dissection should be used to release the radial edges of the deep scleral flap. Combined with gentle traction on the deep flap, the TDW gradually becomes exposed (Fig. 14.17). Aqueous humor percolation through the Descemet's membrane may be observed at this point in the procedure. The base of the deep scleral flap should then be scored to provide a plane for excision and a Vannas scissor then used to excise the deep scleral tissue (Figs. 14.18 and 14.19). Once again, excessive traction on the deep scleral flap or sudden movements of the scissor may result in rupture of the TDW. Attention must also be given to not leaving an anterior lip of deep scleral tissue, which may cover the TDW, and so the deep flap must be excised as close as is safely possible to the TDW. If aqueous percolation is inadequate or absent once the TDW has been exposed, the inner wall of Schlemm's canal may be removed and stripped using a Mermoud forceps, leaving bare trabecular meshwork

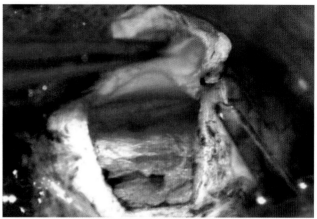

Fig. 14.17 The trabeculodescemet window is fashioned. A slow percolation of aqueous humor through Descemet's membrane is commonly seen. In this figure, pigmentation is visible centrally where the inner wall of Schlemm's canal and trabecular meshwork remain

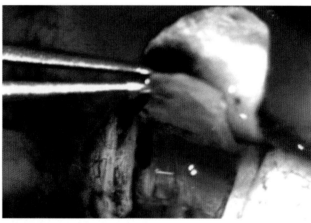

Fig. 14.18 The deep scleral flap is then scored with a blade close to the base of the flap

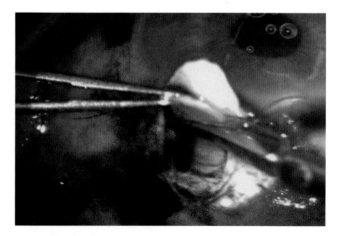

Fig. 14.19 A fine scissor is then used to amputate the deep scleral flap

behind. The cut ends of the canal are then intubated with a viscocanalostomy cannula, which has a 150-micrometer outer bore diameter, and a small amount of high viscosity sodium hyaluronate, such as Healon GV, is gently injected into each side to facilitate the entry and introduction of the iScience device into Schlemm's canal.

With the iScience microcatheter fixated to the surgical drape at the proximal end and connected to the light source and OVD injector at the distal end, the catheter is handled with two non-toothed forceps. If a fixation suture has been placed in the cornea previously, this should be released from the drape at this point in the procedure. Once the tip of the catheter is aligned with one cut end of Schlemm's canal with the angle of entry directly into the lumen, the catheter is introduced and advanced. The microscope light should be dimmed such that the blinking red light at the tip can be easily visualized indicating the progress of the catheter (Fig. 14.20). The catheter should be carefully advanced for the entire circumference of Schlemm's canal, until the tip emerges from the opposite cut end. In a small percentage of cases, complete passage of the catheter is not possible due possibly to strictures or collapse of the canal, or in some cases, a large collector channel tributary. The blinking red light must be closely followed in its progress around Schlemm's canal, as the catheter has been observed to pass into the suprachoroidal space. Early recognition of this phenomenon is critical as the light passes in a posterior direction, and retraction of the catheter should then ensue. Passage may be re-attempted with scleral depression adjacent to the point of posterior passage, the gentle injection of OVD into the canal to attempt to open a stricture, or the catheter may be completely removed and passage attempted in the opposite direction.

After successful passage of the microcatheter, a 10-0 prolene suture with the needles cut off is tied around the catheter a few millimeters away from the bulbous tip. The two loose ends are fixated to the loop securely and the catheter then retracted in the opposite direction in order to deliver the suture into the canal. As the catheter is retracted, the surgical assistant uses the OVD injector to deliver viscoelastic into Schlemm's canal for distension. Care must be taken to not inject an excessive amount of OVD into the canal as a Descemet's detachment may result. During this stage, it is not uncommon to see reflux of heme into the anterior chamber from Schlemm's canal. Once the microcatheter is completely externalized, the suture is then cut to release the device resulting in two intracanicular sutures (Fig. 14.21). The corresponding ends must be identified and then tied together in a slipknot fashion over the TDW. The slipknot is then tightened to achieve the desired tension. While tension on Schlemm's canal is desired (see Fig. 14.12), care must also be taken when performing this step of the procedure, as excessive tension may result in rupture of the TDW. The authors assess the tension on the suture by pulling the knot posteriorly until it can barely reach the scleral spur (Figs. 14.22 and 14.23). The tension created by the intracanalicular suture is thought to produce a surgical pilocarpine-like effect whereby there is enhanced flow of aqueous across the juxtacanalicular trabecular meshwork and inner wall of Schlemm's canal into its collector channels thereby lowering IOP. In this procedure, suture tension has been shown to be important in enhancing aqueous outflow and reducing IOP.[35]

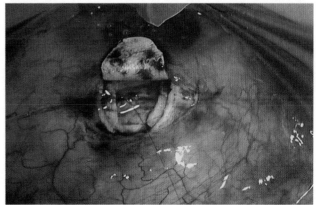

Fig. 14.21 Once the canal has been cannulated completely, a suture is tied to the end of the catheter and the catheter is retracted completely, delivering the suture into the canal

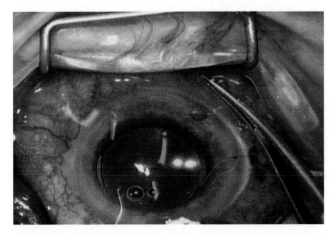

Fig. 14.20 The blinking red light at the tip of the microcatheter indicates to the surgeon the progress of the catheter in Schlemm's canal. Here, the tip of the forceps indicates the location of the tip of the catheter

Once the sutures have been satisfactorily placed in the canal, the superficial scleral flap is reflected back to its anatomical position and sutured in place with five interrupted 10-0 nylon sutures in a watertight fashion. High viscosity OVD, such as Healon GV, is injected under the scleral flap

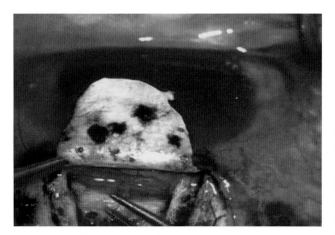

Fig. 14.22 Two sutures will result and each corresponding end should be identified and tied to each other

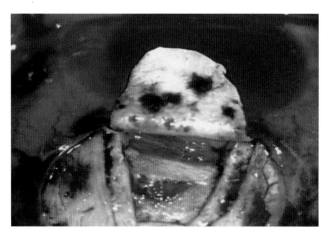

Fig. 14.23 Two suture knots can be seen resting on the trabeculodescemet window causing a slight indentation

Postoperative Considerations and Complications

When performed properly without complication, canaloplasty attempts to lower IOP by augmenting aqueous outflow via the conventional outflow pathway without penetration into the globe during surgery. As a result, many of the complications that patients receiving fistulizing procedures are prone to are avoided in canaloplasty. Postoperatively, while most patients will have a reduction in IOP, occasionally the IOP remains elevated or increases after being at the target in the early postoperative period. In these cases, resistance at the juxtacanalicular meshwork and inner wall of Schlemm's canal may be too great to allow for aqueous outflow, despite the suture distension. In these cases, a YAG laser-induced opening of the TDW may be required to allow for aqueous humor to exit the anterior chamber into the cut ends of Schlemm's canal and the intrascleral lake. While no published data yet exists, the authors feel that should this laser adjunctive procedure be required, it is most likely a time-sensitive procedure, which should be performed prior to closure and fibrosis of the intrascleral lake, typically up to approximately 4–6 weeks postoperatively. Care should be taken to not disrupt the intracanalicular sutures, although inadvertent cutting of these sutures with the laser is not uncommon. The effect of this on IOP and impact on aqueous outflow is unknown at this time. Most often, the YAG laser goniopuncture results in a lowering of the IOP, but occasionally, the IOP will remain elevated even after this adjunctive procedure. In these cases, the treatment options include the resumption of topical medical therapy, needling with lifting of the superficial scleral flap to convert the procedure essentially to a trabeculectomy, or further surgery with a tube shunt or seton device implantation.

The most common intraoperative complication encountered in canaloplasty is perforation of the TDW resulting in a penetrating surgery. The procedure may be converted to a conventional trabeculectomy in this situation. If the perforation is small, the TDW surgical site may be abandoned and an Ex-PRESS shunt placed at the scleral spur (Fig. 14.24). In some instances, depending on the location of the perforation, a collagen wick implant (Aquaflow, Staar Surgical, Monrovia, CA) may be placed in the bed of the dissection with the head of the implant pointing toward, and used as a tamponade of, the perforation (Fig. 14.25).

If iris becomes incarcerated in the perforation, a small surgical iridectomy may be required. Postoperatively, iris adhesion to the TDW may also be seen on gonioscopy, or incarceration may ensue after YAG laser goniopuncture. In these cases, the authors recommend sweeping the iris away from the TDW with a 30-gauge needle inserted through the limbus. To prevent recurrence of iris incarceration, an air bubble

with a viscocanalostomy cannula to distend the potential space vacated by the excision of the deep scleral flap. In addition to the mechanism of IOP lowering being aqueous outflow via the conventional pathway, the potential space in the area of the excised deep scleral flap, commonly termed the scleral lake, may act as a reservoir for aqueous, facilitating its outflow into the episcleral, scleral, and suprachoroidal venous systems as well as the two cut ends of Schlemm's canal. Finally, the conjunctiva is closed in a watertight fashion with running horizontal mattress suture with 10-0 Vicryl on a vasectomy needle, as described earlier in the Ex-PRESS shunt section. Dry aspiration of residual OVD in the anterior chamber should be performed with a blunt 27-gauge cannula to prevent a postoperative spike in IOP. The position of the IOL should be verified to be in the capsular bag during this step as well as with the cannula tip in the anterior chamber. Infusion into the anterior chamber at the end of the case to pressurize the globe should be performed with great care as excessive infusion pressure may also rupture the TDW.

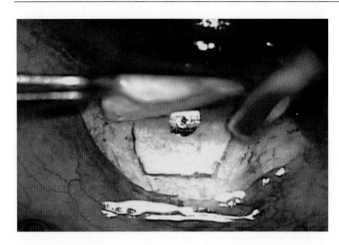

Fig. 14.24 In this case, a perforation of the fine trabeculodescemet window occurred during the dissection of the deep scleral flap. A separate entry is made into the anterior chamber through the deep flap (which is not excised) and an Ex-PRESS shunt inserted. Here the footplate can be seen through the deep scleral flap as well as in the anterior chamber

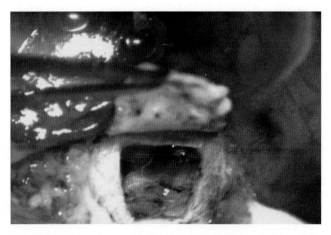

Fig. 14.25 After successful exposure of the trabeculodescemet window in this case, a perforation occurred in the window on the right side, resulting in iris prolapse. A small iridotomy was performed and a collagen wick implant sutured to the bed of the deep scleral dissection with the head of the implant directed at the perforation

or small amount of OVD may be injected into the anterior chamber on top of the iris immediately after sweeping. Argon laser may also be applied onto the superior iris surface in a grid pattern to contract the iris tissue with the aim to prevent recurrence of incarceration. Occasionally, an iris sweep may be required multiple times to ensure that there is no incarceration in the TDW. As previously discussed, patients chosen for canaloplasty should be deemed to have open angles preoperatively, as iris incarceration may occur more frequently in those patients who have iridotrabecular proximity in a narrow angle configuration. This is further accentuated by the centripetal indentation of the inner wall of Schlemm's canal and the trabecular meshwork, which results from the

intracanalicular suture. In addition, peripheral anterior synechiae may form in the narrow angle patient resulting in angle closure. Even patients who have been determined to have indisputable open-angle anatomy prior to surgery have been seen to develop peripheral anterior synechiae (PAS) as well as iris incarceration into microperforations in the TDW.

Careful patient selection is paramount when performing canaloplasty. Careful preoperative gonioscopy—documenting not only angle grade, but iris profile and configuration—is also of importance, and anterior segment imaging such as optical coherence tomography as well as ultrasound biomicroscopy may be useful in aiding the surgeon in making a surgically appropriate decision. Some patients, however, may have a shallow anterior chamber or narrow angle due to a large lens and may have a sufficiently open angle after cataract extraction to perform canaloplasty. In these scenarios, examination of a pseudophakic contralateral eye, or intraoperative gonioscopy, are critical in proper surgical planning.

In cases where conventional pathway outflow combined with aqueous egress through the TDW—punctured postoperatively by YAG laser into the scleral lake—does not result in adequate IOP control, the decision may be made to resume topical therapy in order to achieve the desired IOP target. If this too is insufficient or if there is an intolerance to topical therapy, the procedure may need to be converted to a penetrating filter by first performing laser suture lysis of the nylon sutures in the scleral flap, followed by needle-assisted lifting of the scleral flap, essentially creating a subconjunctival trabeculectomy bleb. Adjunctive antimetabolites such as mitomycin-C may also be used in this scenario (Table 17.1). It has been the authors' experience that a minority of patients require further surgery with implantation of a tube shunt device for definitive adequate IOP control.

Other complications, associated with canaloplasty, include a localized Descemet's detachment or tear (which may result from an injection of excessive OVD into the canal), hyphema, and choroidal effusion. Most of these complications are self-limited and do not require surgical intervention for successful management.[35]

Discussion and Available Data on Outcomes

In surgical procedures designed to augment aqueous outflow through Schlemm's canal, uncertainty exists in the lowest attainable IOP possible because of the possible downstream limitations, namely the episcleral venous pressure. This may lead to a best potential IOP lowering into the mid-teens, but has the benefit of possibly protecting patients against hypotony. It has, however, been the experience of the authors' that IOPs of 10 are attainable in patients who have had canaloplasty. A possible reason for this is that aqueous humor not only egresses from the anterior chamber via the conventional pathway through the trabecular meshwork and Schlemm's canal, but also through a superior TDW. Aqueous egress may be observed through the TDW at the time of surgery. This aqueous humor may flow through both cut ends of Schlemm's canal, as well as into the scleral lake created from the excision of deep sclera during surgery (which will be reviewed in the next section). Then direct flow into the episcleral and scleral veins likely occurs, then flow into the suprachoroidal space, and, finally, subconjunctival flow also may occur resulting in a small bleb despite watertight scleral flap closure. Furthermore, postoperative YAG laser goniopuncture to break the TDW may augment flow through the surgical site into the aforementioned means of drainage, resulting in a lower IOP than would be attainable purely by flow through an enhanced conventional pathway.

Currently, only one peer-reviewed study exists on cataract surgery combined with canaloplasty, although others are ongoing. In this international multicenter prospective study, temporal clear corneal phacoemulsification was combined with canaloplasty in open-angle glaucoma patients with visually significant lens opacities. Inclusion criteria included an IOP of greater than 21 mmHg and open angles. Data from 54 eyes was collected in procedures performed by 11 surgeons at nine sites with a mean preoperative IOP of 24.4 ± 6.1 mmHg and a mean topical glaucoma medication number of 1.5 ± 1.0 per eye. At the 12-month time point, the mean IOP had decreased to 13.7 ± 4.4 mmHg, with the mean medication usage falling to 0.2 ± 0.4 per patient. Surgical complications were low with a total of five eyes suffering from hyphema (3), Descemet's membrane tear (1), and iris prolapse (1). On the first postoperative day, transient elevation of the IOP to more than 30 mmHg was seen in four eyes.[36] In the evaluation of these results, canaloplasty combined with cataract extraction and IOL implantation can be seen to effectively lower IOP while having a low complication profile, avoiding complications associated with filtering bleb surgery such as hypotony, anterior chamber instability, and/or choroidal effusions and hemorrhage.

In summary, combined cataract extraction and IOL implantation with an *ab externo* approach to circumferential dilation and suture placement into Schlemm's canal is an effective procedure in treating those patients who have a visually significant cataract and concurrent open-angle glaucoma. It can result in lowering of IOP and reducing usage of topical glaucoma medications. A low complication profile is also seen with this procedure, especially in relation to visually devastating sequelae such as hypotony and its potential choroidal implications (see Chapter 12). While no direct comparison has been undertaken between combined phacoemulsification and canaloplasty versus conventional phacotrabeculectomy, current studies are ongoing.

Trabecular Micro-bypass Stent

Indications for Surgery

If the point of greatest resistance to aqueous outflow in the conventional pathway is the juxtacanalicular trabecular meshwork,[31,34] a bypass of this resistance allowing aqueous facilitated access to Schlemm's canal and its downstream collector channels would logically lower IOP to the level of the episcleral venous pressure, the further downstream resistance point. In the surgical procedure of goniotomy, a blade inserted through the limbus is used to incise the trabecular meshwork and inner wall of Schlemm's canal to provide access of aqueous humor to Schlemm's canal and the collector channels. While this procedure, as well as trabeculotomy (when visibility through the cornea is poor), has found success in the pediatric patient population,[37] it has not been found to be as effective in the treatment of adult glaucoma patients.[38–40] However, these traditional procedures have given rise to novel *ab interno* devices and procedures to attempt to control elevated IOP. Some of these procedures include goniocurettage,[41] laser trabecular ablation,[42] laser trabeculopuncture,[43] as well as devices that will be discussed in this chapter such as the iStent® and trabecular micro-electrocautery.

The trabecular micro-bypass stent is a device designed to be placed in an *ab interno* fashion through a corneal incision into Schlemm's canal, providing aqueous humor free passage from the anterior chamber into the canal bypassing the major resistance point. The 1-mm-long titanium stent, weighing 0.1 mg, is designed in an L-shape with a short arm "snorkel" designed to sit in the anterior chamber, and a long arm placed into Schlemm's canal. The long arm consists of a half-pipe with a sharp tip to facilitate entry into the canal during surgical placement. The open half-pipe lumen has an outside diameter of 180 μm with three retention barbs on the outside surface to provide stabilization and prevent extrusion from the canal (Fig. 14.26). The open lumen of the stent faces the outer wall while the convex surface rests against the inner wall of Schlemm's canal to allow for aqueous humor to enter the collector channels. It is important to note that the iStent is available in a right-going as well as a left-going orientation. Because the snorkel faces the anterior chamber and points into the vicinity of the iris, it is important when selecting patients for this procedure to determine that the angle is open sufficiently to accommodate the stent without being in close proximity to iris tissue risking its occlusion. Thus, detailed gonioscopic examination preoperatively is essential.

In patients who require an IOP target in the range of high single digits to low double digits with advanced disease and severe visual field loss, the trabecular micro-bypass stent is not the appropriate choice of glaucoma procedure.

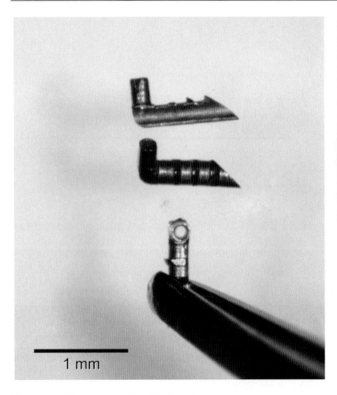

Fig. 14.26 Photograph of the Glaukos iStent

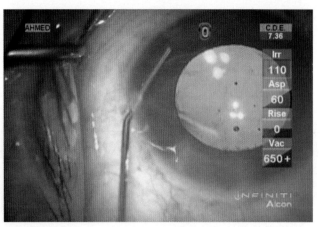

Fig. 14.27 A blunt 27-gauge cannula is used to stroke the iris gently with the injection of a very small amount of acetylcholine to induce miosis in the area of angle surgery

While the major resistance point of the juxtacanalicular meshwork may be overcome by the iStent, the lowest attainable IOP is likely limited by downstream resistance of the episcleral venous pressure, resulting in attainable IOPs likely in the mid-teens. Conversely, in subconjunctival filtration procedures such as trabeculectomy, no downstream resistance exists in the subconjunctival space, and very low, even chronically hypotonous, IOPs are attainable. It is the authors' opinion that patients with mild-to-moderate disease, and preoperative IOPs with borderline or reasonable control on topical medications, are best suited for the Glaukos iStent. In patients with concurrent lens opacity and mild-to-moderate glaucomatous disease who have reasonable control on topical medications, combining the iStent with cataract extraction and IOL implantation is ideal to not only provide the patient with the opportunity for improved IOP control, but also decreased dependence on topical medications.

Instrumentation and Operative Technique

Unlike in canaloplasty or subconjunctival filtration procedures, no manipulation of conjunctiva is required for implantation of the iStent and, thus, the standard cataract incisions with which a surgeon is accustomed are used. At the conclu-sion of clear corneal phacoemulsification and IOL implantation, OVD is allowed to remain in the anterior segment and the authors recommend mechanical stroking of the iris with a blunt 27-gauge cannula and injection of a small amount of Miochol®-E (acetylcholine 1:100, Novartis Ophthalmics, East Hanover, NJ) into the anterior chamber to encourage miosis and bring the iris away from the angle (Fig. 14.27). To achieve hyper-deepening of the anterior chamber and a clear view of the angle, a viscous OVD such as Healon GV should be injected into the angle. Care should be taken not to overinflate the eye and cause an excessively high IOP. This may result in collapse of Schlemm's canal and the inner wall, leading to possibly increased difficulty in implantation of the iStent.

The patient's head should be rotated away from the surgeon with verbal directions to achieve adduction, or alternatively it can be achieved with a toothed forceps held by a surgical assistant. The microscope should then be rotated to a position of between approximately 30° and 45° from the vertical. To visualize angle structures satisfactorily, a gonioprism must be used. The authors' preference is to use a Swan-Jacob lens (Ocular Instuments, Bellevue, WA) to achieve visualization. The iStent is opened from the packaging and arrives preloaded on a lightweight handle with a squeeze mechanism injector at the tip grasping the stent. A button is present on the handle where the index finger of the surgeon is designed to depress, deploying the stent at the tip of the long slender metal shaft, which houses the four grasping prongs holding the snorkel end of the stent (Fig. 14.28). While a 1.5-mm incision is all that is required for insertion of the iStent, when combined with cataract extraction, the cataract incision can be conveniently used with similar principles to using a phacoemulsification handpiece, utilizing the wound as a fulcrum when inserting the stent into the canal. Movements of the surgeon's hands external to

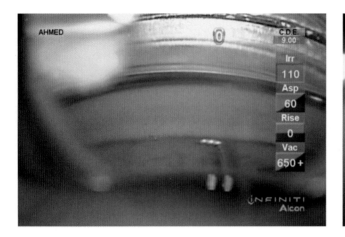

Fig. 14.28 A gonioscopic view of the iStent approaching the angle mounted on the injector shaft

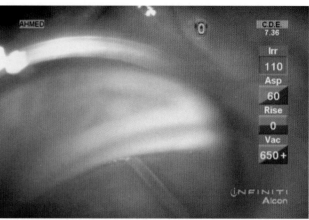

Fig. 14.29 The iStent seen engaging the trabecular meshwork during insertion

the eye should result in movement in the opposite direction intracamerally.

With direct visualization through the gonioprism, the tip of the stent should pierce the trabecular meshwork at an acute angle. The stent is then advanced with a gentle movement in the coronal plane until the long arm of the stent is seen to rest completely in the canal. Because of the common occurrence of reflux of blood from Schlemm's canal, successful initial implantation is the desired result, as repeat attempts at insertion usually take place under hampered visualization and with insufficient trabecular tissue to support the stent. Should visualization be impeded by blood, the stent should be removed and additional OVD should be placed in the angle prior to continuation of implantation. After successful placement, the eye should be slowly and carefully returned to the primary position prior to depressing the button to release the stent. If tension is exerted on the globe while the stent is released, the stent may torque on release, tearing the meshwork, and become dislodged (Figs. 14.29, 14.30, and 14.31). Commonly, the tip of the injector must be used to tap the snorkel into the canal to achieve final satisfactory seating of the shunt. Care must be taken during this step, as this may dislodge a previously well-placed stent. Blood reflux also may be seen emanating from the snorkel, confirming placement in the desired anatomical position. Multiple stents may be placed into the canal, although the effect of multiple stents on IOP is yet unknown, as ongoing studies seek to elucidate this. The IOL position should then be verified at the conclusion of the placement of the stents. Once this has been completed, standard automated irrigation and aspiration can be performed as is typical at the conclusion of cataract extraction and IOL placement. At this stage, it is not uncommon to see a small amount of blood circulating in the anterior chamber. The wounds should be verified

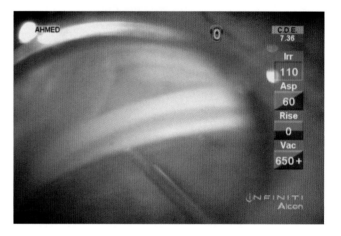

Fig. 14.30 The iStent is released from the injector once it is seated in the canal

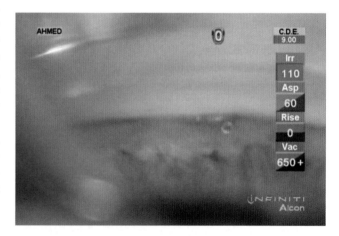

Fig. 14.31 High magnification viewing under the microscope with a gonioprism confirms that the stent is satisfactorily seated in the canal

to be watertight and if not, suture used to ensure adequate closure.

Postoperative Care and Complications

Postoperative complications that are associated with the iStent include transient postoperative hyphema, stent malposition, blockage, and persistently elevated IOP requiring further glaucoma surgery such as trabeculectomy. In management of stent malposition, secondary surgery may be required to remove and/or reposition a stent when it has dislodged significantly. Stent blockage most commonly occurs with fibrin, iris tissue, or, rarely, vitreous. In the case of blockage with fibrin, argon laser may be used or recombinant tissue plasminogen activator may be injected intracamerally in an attempt to dissolve the clot (Table 16.1).[44] When the stent is occluded with iris, a neodymium:YAG laser may be used to separate the iris from the stent. In addition, the authors recommend argon iridoplasty in the area of the stent in an attempt to prevent re-occlusion. If laser intervention fails, mechanical sweeping of the iris with a 30-gauge needle at the slit lamp may be useful in removing iris from the snorkel.

It is important to note that no serious vision-threatening complications have been reported with the iStent. Serious complications that are typically associated with fistulizing procedures, such as hypotony, choroidal effusion, flat anterior chamber, aqueous misdirection syndrome, or suprachoroidal hemorrhage, have not been noted with this device. Furthermore, because of the absence of a subconjunctival bleb, there are no long-term bleb-associated risks such as blebitis, bleb leaks, and dysesthesias. While the attainable IOPs may not be as low as procedures such as trabeculectomy, the safety profile appears to be more favorable for patients with mild-to-moderate disease who would otherwise traditionally have been subject to a higher risk procedure.

Discussion and Available Data

In a study examining the theoretical mathematical effect of aqueous humor dynamics, bypass of the trabecular meshwork with unidirectional flow would increase outflow facility by 13% while bidirectional flow would result in a 26% increase. Furthermore, the higher the initial preoperative IOP, the greater the resultant achieved IOP lowering.[45,46] Other studies placing the stent in cultured human anterior segments in vitro resulted in an IOP reduction from a mean of 21.4 to 12.4 mmHg.[47] The effect of additional stents in this setting, however, was unclear. In theory, when aqueous humor travels through the stent into Schlemm's canal, it travels circumferentially through the canal and exits into the collector channels. However, in a glaucomatous eye with elevated IOP, Schlemm's canal may be collapsed entirely or in segments,

precluding the flow of aqueous into collector channels. Thus, a single stent placed in an area of the canal that is collapsed may have little to no effect on IOP. This further confounds the question of whether multiple stents have an added effect on IOP lowering. It has also been postulated that placement of stents near collector channels, possibly identified by increased pigmentation areas on gonioscopy in the meshwork, may allow for improved IOP lowering. This, however, is yet to be studied.

A recent prospective uncontrolled non-randomized multicenter study was published on combined cataract extraction, IOL implantation, and insertion of a single iStent. Preoperative mean IOP was 21.5 ± 3.7 mmHg with a mean medication number of 1.5 ± 0.7. Postoperatively, at the 6-month time point, the mean IOP was 15.8 ± 3.0 mmHg, with a mean medication number of 0.5 ± 0.8. Statistical significance was found for both the IOP and medication usage reduction. Complications reported in this study included shunt occlusion, malposition, failure to penetrate the canal at the time of surgery, inadequate IOP control requiring trabeculectomy, and a single case of adenoviral conjunctivitis. No serious vision-threatening adverse events were reported.[44]

In summary, cataract extraction combined with implantation of the trabecular micro-bypass iStent resulted in an effective lowering of IOP and decreased dependence on topical glaucoma medications with a low-risk profile. Because the attainable IOP in these cases is likely in the mid-teens, patient selection for this procedure is important. Eyes that require a low target IOP with advanced disease are likely not to reach their target with this procedure, making it better suited for patients with mild-to-moderate disease without excessively high preoperative IOPs. The favorable risk profile of this procedure over traditional penetrating surgery makes this procedure a good choice for these patients. Studies yet need to be undertaken to determine the effect of multiple stents as well as to determine the effect of targeted stent placement on IOP.

Trabecular Micro-electrocautery

Indications for Surgery

A device that is similar to the iStent in terms of mechanism of IOP lowering, surgical approach, and patients best suited for the procedure is the Trabectome micro-electrocautery device. With the same premise of bypassing the juxtacanalicular meshwork point of resistance, the device is designed to cauterize and remove trabecular tissue and the inner wall of Schlemm's canal to allow aqueous humor direct access to the collector channels of the canal. Again, because of the mechanism in which IOP is lowered, attainable postoperative pressure is likely in the mid-teens, making this procedure also most suitable for patients with mild-to-moderate disease with reasonable control on topical medications. In addition, patients should be deemed to have an angle that is open preoperatively. Those who have narrow anatomical angles may be at greater risk for postoperative goniosynechiae after the Trabectome treatment.

The Trabectome is an *ab interno* foot-pedal-activated instrument, which consists of a disposable handpiece composed of a 19-gauge infusion sleeve, 25-gauge aspiration port, and a bipolar electrocautery unit 150 μm away from an insulated footplate. A console allows for control of infusion, aspiration, and electrosurgical energy. The tapered footplate is 800 μm in length from the heel to the tip with a maximum width of 230 μm and thickness of 110 μm at the heel (Fig. 14.32). When viewed in cross-section, the footplate has an elliptical shape with an anterior to posterior width of 5 μm at the tip widening to 50 μm at the heel, while the meridional diameter ranges from 350 to 500 μm, designed with the aim to fit into Schlemm's canal. The tapered footplate design, angled at 90 degrees to the shaft of the instrument, with the pointed tip aids in engaging and penetration into Schlemm's canal. Once the footplate is in the canal, trabecular tissue is directed into the electrocautery unit to be cauterized as the handpiece is advanced in the canal. The smooth edge and insulation of the footplate combined with the cooling effect of the continuous irrigation serve as protection to the outer wall of Schlemm's canal and the collector channel openings from intraoperative injury and trauma.

sions with which the surgeon is accustomed should be used. At the conclusion of cataract extraction and IOL implantation, visualization of the angle should be undertaken in a similar fashion as discussed previously with a goniprism, rotation of the patient's head and microscope, and the eye in mild adduction. OVD need not be aspirated as the Trabectome handpiece possesses both irrigation and aspiration properties and as such may be used to remove remaining viscoelastic at the conclusion of surgery. While the handpiece needs only a 1.6-mm incision to enter the anterior chamber, when performing combined surgery, the main corneal incision may conveniently be used, again, as a fulcrum for the hand piece. Under direct visualization with a gonioprism, the tip of the hand piece engages and enters Schlemm's canal and the foot pedal is depressed to commence tissue ablation. This is carried out in one direction until visibility is no longer available, and then the hand piece may be turned 180° in the eye to ablate in the opposite direction, again, until visualization is not possible (Figs. 14.33, 14.34, and 14.35). Typically, the arc length of ablation is approximately 60°. While the hand piece is activated, the aspiration of tissue debris with continuous irrigation allows the surgeon's view to be clear. However, it is common to observe that when the hand piece is removed and the IOP lowered in the eye, reflux of blood into the anterior chamber is almost always encountered. A clear corneal suture and injection of air into the anterior chamber at the conclusion of surgery appear to correlate with less postoperative hyphema.[48] Conversely, the trabecular ablation may be performed prior to cataract extraction.

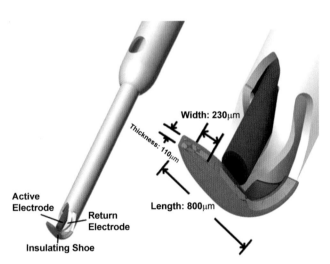

Fig. 14.32 A schematic diagram of the Trabectome handpiece and tip

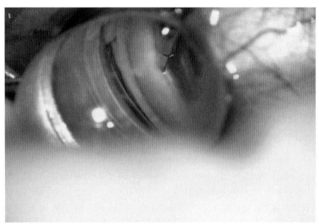

Fig. 14.33 The Trabectome tip incising the trabecular meshwork. Photograph courtesy of Douglas J. Rhee, MD

Instrumentation and Operative Technique

Similar again to the iStent, no conjunctival manipulation is required for the Trabectome and thus standard cataract inci-

Postoperative Considerations and Complications

In the only published data to date with combined cataract extraction with Trabectome treatment, postoperative

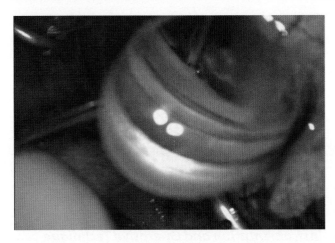

Fig. 14.34 After incision into the canal, reflux of heme is commonly seen. Photograph courtesy of Douglas J. Rhee, MD

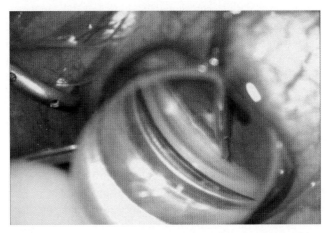

Fig. 14.35 The Trabectome actively ablating trabecular tissue and inner wall of Schlemm's canal. Photograph courtesy of Douglas J. Rhee, MD

complications included transient hyphema, iris and lens capsule injury from the instrument tip, and uncontrolled IOP requiring further glaucoma procedures.[49] Of note, in this study, the Trabectome treatment was performed prior to cataract extraction and IOL implantation. Other potential complications of this procedure that have been reported include peripheral anterior synechiae, transient corneal injury including Descemet's detachment and hemorrhage, corneal epithelial defect, and hypotony.[50] Although one patient has been reported to have hypotony after this procedure, it too has a lower risk profile than traditional filtering surgery, being free of a subconjunctival bleb.

Discussion and Available Data

In patients who received combined cataract extraction with the Trabectome, mean preoperative IOP was 20.0 ±

6.0 mmHg with a mean number of glaucoma medications of 2.65 ± 1.13 decreasing to an IOP of 15.5 ± 2.9 mmHg and a medication usage of 1.44 ± 1.29 at 1 year.[49] These results in conjunction with the favorable risk profile make this procedure a suitable choice for patients with mild-to-moderate glaucomatous disease on medical therapy without excessively high preoperative IOPs. In a similar manner to those patients undergoing the iStent, the angles must be open to minimize postoperative events that could compromise the success of surgery such as goniosynechiae, and proper patient selection is essential to help maximize the potential for successful target IOPs postoperatively. In addition to the lower risk profile involved in these *ab interno* Schlemm's canal procedures, which aim to enhance or restore physiologic aqueous flow, the conjunctiva in these cases is spared from any manipulation should a trabeculectomy be deemed necessary at a later date.

Suprachoroidal Gold Micro-shunt

Indications for Surgery

The uveoscleral outflow pathway for aqueous egress consists of the ciliary body interstitium, the suprachoroidal space, and, ultimately, the scleral vasculature. Reports vary as to the proportion of aqueous outflow that occurs via this pathway versus the conventional pathway. In normal human eyes, anywhere from 20 to 54% of aqueous outflow has been reported to occur via this pathway.[51,52] It is well known that medical augmentation of this pathway is effective in the form of prostaglandin analogues. While various surgical approaches to augmenting suprachoroidal outflow have been attempted, including cyclodialysis cleft creation, suprachoroidal implants, and seton devices, none have produced reliable, effective, and reproducible long-term IOP lowering.

The SOLX gold micro-shunt is a new suprachoroidal device designed for implantation by an *ab externo* technique. Composed of two thin 24-karat gold plates fused together vertically, the 60-micrometer-thick device measures 5.2 mm long, 2.4 mm wide anteriorly, and 3.2 mm wide posteriorly, and houses nine channels connecting the anterior openings to the posterior ones (Figs. 14.36 and 14.37). Two different models of the shunt exist: the GMS (XGS-5) and the GMS Plus (XGS-10). They differ in weight and channel height, with the former weighing 6.2 mg and the latter 9.2 mg. The channels are of 44 micrometer height in the GMS while they are 68 μm thick in the GMS Plus. In both models, the channel width is 25 μm. Aqueous egress is enhanced into the suprachoroidal space either through the shunt or around it. Because of its inert and non-corrosive nature as well as its

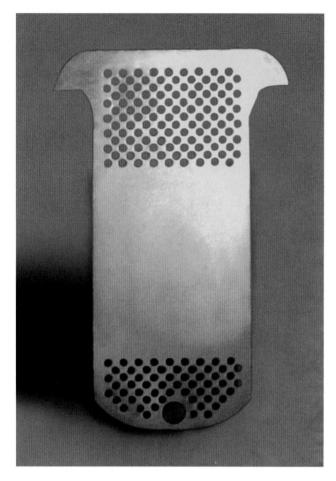

Fig. 14.36 A photograph of the SOLX gold micro-shunt

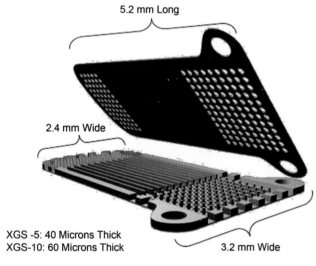

5.2 mm Long

2.4 mm Wide

XGS -5: 40 Microns Thick
XGS-10: 60 Microns Thick

3.2 mm Wide

Fig. 14.37 A schematic diagram of the interior of the shunt with the two plates separated

biocompatibility as a foreign body in the eye, gold was chosen as the material of choice for this implant.[53,54]

While filtration into the suprachoroidal space has a significant potential for hypotony and choroidal effusions or hemorrhage, the shunt design with its thin profile and small microchannels has been designed with patient safety in mind. While the gold shunt may certainly be chosen as the primary glaucoma procedure, especially in those patients who have scarred conjunctiva, or anterior segment trauma or dysgenesis, the current data available has been gathered for patients who have failed at least one prior incisional glaucoma procedure. These results will be discussed in the following sections.

Instrumentation and Operative Technique

When performing combined cataract extraction with gold shunt implantation, phacoemulsification and IOL implantation should proceed as per standard technique. OVD should be left in the anterior segment following IOL implantation followed by a clear corneal suture. If the IOP is low at this point, balanced saline solution may be injected into the anterior chamber to pressurize the eye allowing for a more precise scleral dissection. The conjunctiva should be anesthetized with topical Xylocaine or tetracaine and a corneal traction suture placed if necessary. The gold shunt may be placed in any quadrant of the eye, although from a surgical technique perspective, the temporal 180° offers the most facile area of access for a right-handed surgeon.

A conjunctival peritomy is performed in the same manner as with the Ex-PRESS shunt or canaloplasty, leaving an anterior lip of conjunctiva at the limbus. An approximately 95% scleral thickness cutdown perpendicular to the surface of the sclera is then performed 2 mm posterior to the limbus, observing for a blue hue at the base of the dissection to assess depth (Fig. 14.38). The length of the scleral

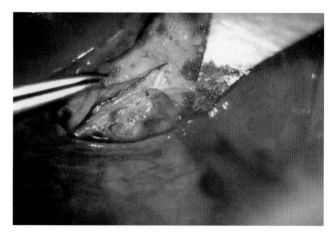

Fig. 14.38 A near full-thickness cutdown into the sclera is performed. Note the hue of choroid at the base of the dissection

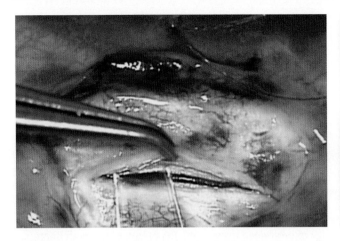

Fig. 14.39 The forceps lifting the superior lip of the incision reveals the layers of the dissection. A scleral tunnel is present at approximately 95% thickness and the full thickness entry perpendicularly into the sclera at the posterior aspect of the dissection

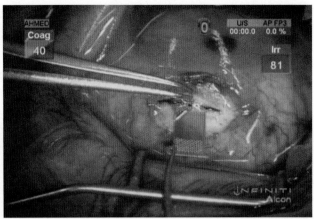

Fig. 14.40 The gold micro-shunt is handled with care at the wings posteriorly with a non-toothed forceps

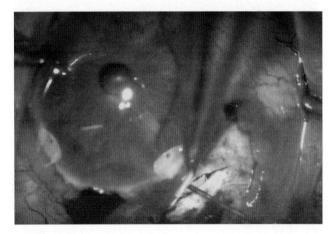

Fig. 14.41 Once the shunt has been inserted, a 27-gauge needle can be used to gently manipulate the body of the shunt into proper position

incision should be approximately 4 mm. Once the depth has been attained satisfactorily over the entire length of the incision, a scleral tunnel is then fashioned toward the limbus. The desired point of entry into the anterior chamber is the scleral spur and thus the dissection need not be carried forward into the clear cornea. Once this has been achieved, a full thickness scleral cutdown is performed, being careful not to injure the choroidal tissue (Fig. 14.39). If the IOP in the eye is too high prior to the full thickness cutdown, choroidal tissue may bulge through the incision resulting in a higher likelihood of injury. As a result, OVD should be removed from the anterior chamber with a dry technique using a blunt cannula through the paracentesis incision. A blunt cannula should also be used to administer non-preserved Xylocaine very gently into the suprachoroidal space. As this space is highly vascular, the cannula should not be placed deep into the incision but merely at the lip of the incision. The anterior chamber should be then evaluated to ensure that the area of intended shunt placement is inflated with OVD. A sharp linear entry is then made into the anterior chamber at the level of the scleral spur. To ensure accurate anatomical placement, a gonioscopic mirror may be utilized intraoperatively to ensure that the entry is not excessively anterior or posterior.

The device is then brought onto the field and removed from the holding apparatus, being very careful not to handle the body of the shunt as the delicate channels may be damaged with grasping of the body. The shunt is then placed into the scleral tunnel and into the anterior chamber (Fig. 14.40). A 27-gauge sharp needle can then be used to guide the posterior aspect of the shunt into the suprachoroidal space, manipulating the body gently (Fig. 14.41). Two positioning holes are also present on the posterior aspect of the shunt, which may be manipulated using an instrument such as a Sinskey hook to properly position the shunt. When properly situated,

the posterior drainage openings should not be visible in the incision but be wholly located in the suprachoroidal space. The shunt may also be pushed posteriorly by using a Sinskey hook through the anterior chamber. A positioning hole is present at the head of the shunt to aid in guiding the implant into place. Intraoperative gonioscopy is a useful adjunct and may be used to verify the proper position of the shunt with the anterior openings fully in the anterior chamber with the shunt entering at the scleral spur. Once satisfactory position has been achieved, the scleral incision is closed with interrupted 10-0 nylon sutures in a watertight fashion as a postoperative bleb is undesirable with this device (Fig. 14.42). The conjunctiva is then closed with 10-0 Vicryl as previously described in the Ex-PRESS shunt section of this chapter (Fig. 14.43). Postoperatively, anterior segment OCT imaging may be used to document a suprachoroidal lake of fluid surrounding the shunt.

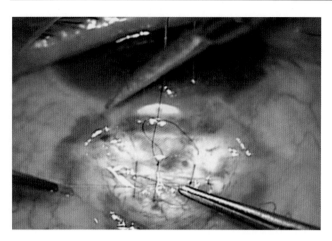

Fig. 14.42 The sclera is closed in a watertight fashion with interrupted 10-0 nylon sutures

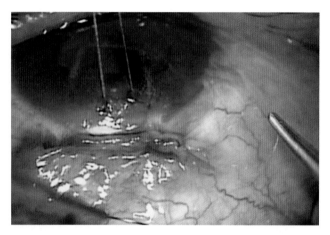

Fig. 14.43 The conjunctiva is closed in a watertight fashion similar to that described previously for the Ex-PRESS shunt and canaloplasty

Postoperative Considerations and Complications

Postoperatively, the reported complications include limited choroidal detachment, shunt-cornea touch, shut-iris touch, shunt exposure, shunt migration, peripheral anterior synechiae formation around the shunt, persistent anterior chamber inflammation, hyphema, hypotony, vitreous hemorrhage, infection, pain, and blurred vision. Uncontrolled IOP requiring the patient to resume topical medications or requiring further surgery has also been observed. On careful gonioscopy, occasionally a fibrous membrane can be seen growing over the shunt in the anterior chamber occluding the anterior orifices. This may prevent aqueous egress through the shunt into the suprachoroidal space. In the event that significant fibrosis occurs around the shunt, if this space also closes, a fairly acute increase in IOP may be observed some time after surgery. While it is an off-label use of the laser,

photo-titration of the flow through the shunt is being studied with the SOLX® 790 nm wavelength Titanium:Sapphire laser.

Discussion and Available Data

Augmentation of suprachoroidal outflow has long been attempted with procedures such as the creation of a cyclodialysis cleft.[55–59] While early control of IOP was good in these procedures, late IOP spikes due to cleft closure and scarring was a significant risk as well as the possibility of prolonged irreversible hypotony. Along with intraoperative issues such as hemorrhage due to the highly vascular nature of uveal tissue, improved control of this procedure was sought with placement of implants into a small cleft. These devices, such as high molecular weight hyaluronic acid, Teflon tube implants, and others such as hydroxyethyl methacrylate capillary strips and even scleral strips have been reported.[60–63] These procedures, however, have yet to demonstrate long-term success in IOP control.

Data has been released by SOLX® on both shunt models in patients who have failed at least one prior incisional glaucoma procedure. In the GMS model, IOP reduced from 27.4 ± 4.7 preoperatively to 18.1 ± 4.7 postoperatively at a 1-year follow-up time point in 39 patients. Topical medication usage decreased in this group from 1.97 ± 0.74 to 1.50 ± 0.94. In the group of 40 patients receiving the GMS Plus, the IOP decreased from 25.5 ± 6.0 to 18.0 ± 2.5 at also a 1-year follow-up, with the medication usage decreasing from 2.25 ± 0.84 to 0.85 ± 0.90. With success defined as IOP control between 5 and 21 mmHg with or without medications, the GMS group had 10 out of 36 patients at final follow-up classified as failures, while the GMS Plus group had 3 out of the final 13 patients as failures.

While FDA trials are currently ongoing for this new suprachoroidal device, the early results show promise in IOP reduction and decrease in dependence on topical medications. However, further studies are required to answer questions such as the optimal size and number of the shunt channels or orifices to control IOP without an increased risk for hypotony, the amount of flow that travels through versus around the shunt, and the role this plays on IOP control.

Summary

Combining cataract surgery with these new glaucoma devices has provided patients with potentially safer alternatives to conventional phacotrabeculectomy discussed in Chapter 6. While studies are ongoing to evaluate these

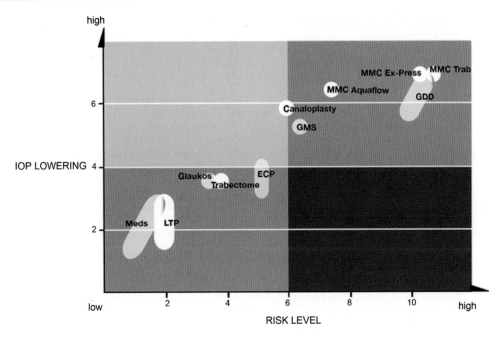

Fig. 14.44 The current treatment landscape in glaucoma with IOP lowering plotted versus risk to the patient

devices in combination with cataract extraction, early results show promise in their efficacy in lowering IOP as well as decreasing dependence on topical medications. Although IOP lowering with these devices may not achieve targets as low as traditional trabeculectomy, the risk profile of these procedures appears to be significantly more favorable and physiologic in their mechanisms of IOP reduction. This has afforded patients the option of undergoing surgery that has a lower risk profile, possibly at an earlier juncture of disease, providing IOP control before the patient develops disease that requires excessively low target IOPs. Patient selection, therefore, is critical in choosing the appropriate procedure if considering a new glaucoma device. Each case should still be considered as a unique situation and in order to maximize success and IOP control, the clinical judgment of the surgeon is critical in determining the amount of IOP reduction required, balanced with the acceptable risk to the patient (Fig. 14.44).

References

1. Stocker F. Combined cataract extraction and scleral cauterization. *Arch Ophthamol.* 1964;72:503.
2. Boyd F. Filtering cautery sclerostomy combined with cataract extraction. *Highlights Ophthalmol.* 1968;11(1):39–77.
3. Maumenee A, Wilkinson CP. A combined operation for glaucoma and cataract. *Am J Ophthamol.* 1971;69:360.
4. Dellaporta A. Combined trepano-trabeculectomy and cataract extraction. *Trans Am Ophthalmol Soc.* 1971;69:113–23.
5. Cairns J. Trabeculectomy. Preliminary report of a new method. *Am J Ophthalmol.* 1968;66(4):673–9.
6. Bindlish R, Condon GP, Schlosser JD, DAntonio J, Lauer KB, Lehrer R. Efficacy and safety of mitomycin-C in primary trabeculectomy: five-year follow-up. *Ophthalmology.* 2002 Jul;109(7):1336–41.
7. Palmer S. Mitomycin as adjunct chemotherapy with trabeculectomy. *Ophthalmology.* 1991 Mar;98(3):317–21.
8. Follow-Up FFSSo-y. The Fluorouracil Filtering Surgery Study Group. *Am J Ophthalmol.* 1989 Dec 15;108(6):625–35.
9. Kupin T, Juzych MS, Shin DH, Khatana AK, Olivier MM. Adjunctive mitomycin C in primary trabeculectomy in phakic eyes. *Am J Ophthalmol.* 1995 Jan;119(1):30–9.
10. Borisuth N, Phillips B, Krupin T. The risk profile of glaucoma filtration surgery. *Curr Opin Ophthalmol.* 1999 Apr;10(2): 112–6.
11. Poley B, Lindstrom RL, Samuelson TW. Long-term effects of phacoemulsification with intraocular lens implantation in normotensive and ocular hypertensive eyes. *J Cataract Refract Surg.* 2008;34:735–42.
12. Shingleton B, Laul A, Nagao K, et al. Effect of phacoemulsification on intraocular pressure in eyes with pseudoexfoliation: single-surgeon series. *J Cataract Refract Surg.* 2008;34:1834–41.
13. Coupin A, Li Q, Riss I. Ex-PRESS Miniature Glaucoma Implant Inserted Under a Scleral Flap in Open-Angle Glaucoma Surgery: A Retrospective Study. *Fr J Glaucoma.* 2007 Jan;30(1):18–23.
14. Dahan E, Carmichael TR. Implantation of a Miniature Glaucoma Device Under a Scleral Flap. *J Glaucoma.* 2005;14(2):98–102.
15. Maris P, Ishida K, Netland PA. Comparison of Trabeculectomy with Ex-PRESS Miniature Glaucoma Device Implanted Under Scleral Flap. *J Glaucoma.* 2007 Jan;16:14–9.
16. Sarkisian SJ. Use of an injector for the Ex-PRESS Mini Glaucoma Shunt. *Ophthalmic Surg Lasers Imaging.* 2007 Sep–Oct;38(5):434–6.
17. Stein J, Herndon LW, Brent Bond J, Challa P. Exposure of Ex-PRESS Miniature glaucoma devices: case series and technique for tube shunt removal. *J Glaucoma.* 2007 Dec;16(8):704–6.
18. Rivier D, Roy S, Mermoud A. Ex-PRESS R-50 miniature glaucoma implant insertion under the conjunctiva combined with cataract extraction. *J Cataract Refract Surg.* 2007 Nov;33(11):1946–52.

19. Krasnov M. Externalization of Schlemm's canal (sinusotomy) in glaucoma. *Br J Ophthalmol*. 1968;43:641–7.

20. Ellingsen B, Grant WM. Trabeculotomy and sinusotomy in enucleated human eyes. *Invest Ophthalmol*. 1972;11:21–8.

21. Johnstone M, Grant WM. Microsurgery of Schlemm's canal and the human aqueous outflow system. *Am J Ophthalmol*. 1973;76:906–17.

22. Koslov V, Bagrov SN, Anisimova SY, et al. [Nonpenetrating deep sclerectomy with collagen][Russian]. *Oftalmokhirurgiia* 1990;3:44–6.

23. Fyodorov S, Ioffe DI, Ronika TI. Deep sclerectomy: technique and mechanism of a new antiglaucomatous procedure. *Glaucoma*. 1984;6:281–3.

24. Zimmerman T, Kooner KS, Ford VJ, et al. Trabeculectomy vs. nonpenetrating trabeculectomy: a retrospective study of two procedures in phakic patients with glaucoma. *Ophthalmic Surg*. 1984;15:734–40.

25. Stegmann R, Pienaar A, Miller D. Viscocanalostomy for open angle glaucoma in black African patients. *J Cataract Refract Surg*. 1999;25:316–22.

26. Sourdille P, Santiago P-Y, Villain F, et al. Reticulated hyaluronic acid implant in nonperforating trabecular surgery. *J Cataract Refract Surg*. 1999;25:332–9.

27. Ambresin A, Shaarawy T, Mermoud A. Deep sclerectomy with collagen implant in one eye compared with trabeculectomy in the other eye of the same patient. *J Glaucoma*. 2002;11:214–20.

28. Sanchez E, Schnyder CC, Sickenberg M, et al. Deep sclerectomy: results with and without collagen implant. *Int Ophthalmol*. 1996/97;20:157–62.

29. Spiegel D, Kobuch K. Trabecular meshwork bypass tube shunt: initial case series. *Br J Ophthalmol*. 2002;86:1228–31.

30. Yablonski M. Trabeculectomy with internal tube shunt: a novel glaucoma surgery. *J Glaucoma*. 2005;14:91–7.

31. Grant W. Further studies on facility of flow through the trabecular meshwork. *AMA Arch Ophthal*. 1958;60(4 part 1):523–33.

32. Ethier C, Kamm RD, Palaszewski BA, et al. Calculations of flow resistance in the juxtacanalicular meshwork. *Invest Ophthalmol Vis Sci*. 1986 Dec;27(12):1741–50.

33. Rosenquist R, Epstein D, Melamed S, et al. Outflow resistance of enucleated human eyes at two different perfusion pressures and different extents of trabeculotomy. *Curr Eye Res*. 1989;8(12):1233–40.

34. Moses R, Grodzki WJ Jr, Etheridge EL, et al. Schlemm's canal: the effect of intraocular pressure. *Invest Ophthalmol Vis Sci*. 1981;20(1):61–8.

35. Lewis R, von Wolff K, Tetz M, et al. Canaloplasty: circumferential viscodilation and tensioning of Schlemm's canal using a flexible microcatheter for the treatment of open-angle glaucoma in adults: interim clinical study analysis. *J Cataract Refract Surg*. 2007 Jul;33(7):1217–26.

36. Shingleton B, Tetz M, Korber N. Circumferential viscodilation and tensioning of Schlemm canal (canaloplasty) with temporal clear corneal phacoemulsification cataract surgery for open-angle glaucoma and visually significant cataract: One-year results. *J Cataract Refract Surg*. 2008;34:443–40.

37. Gramer E, Tausch M, Kraemer C. Time of diagnosis, reoperations and long-term results of goniotomy in the treatment of primary congenital glaucoma: a clincal study. *Int Ophthalmol*. 1996;20:117–23.

38. Luntz M, Livingston DG. Trabeculotomy ab externo and trabeculectomy in congenital and adult-onset glaucoma. *Am J Ophthalmol*. 1977;83:174–9.

39. Herschler J, Davis EB. Modified goniotomy for inflammatory glaucoma. Histologic evidence for the mechanism of pressure reduction. *Arch Ophthalmol*. 1980;98:684–7.

40. Dickens C, Hoskins HD Jr. Epidemiology and pathophysiology of congenital glaucoma. In: Ritch R, Shields MB, Krupin T, eds. The Glaucomas. Vol. 2, 2nd ed. St. Louis: Mosby; 1996: 729–38.

41. Jacobi P, Dietlein TS, Krieglstein GK. Technique of goniocurettage: a potential treatment for advanced chronic open angle glaucoma. *Br J Ophthalmol*. 1997;81:302–7.

42. Hill R, Baerveldt G, Ozler SA, et al. Laser trabecular ablation (LTA). *Laser Surg Med*. 1991;11:341–6.

43. Epstein D, Melamed S, Puliatio CA, Steinert RF. Neodynium: YAG laser trabeculopuncture in open-angle glaucoma. *Ophthalmology*. 1985;92:931–7.

44. Spiegel D, Garcia-Feijoo J, Garcia-Sanchez J, Lamielle H. Coexistent primary open-angle glaucoma and cataract: preliminary analysis of treatment by cataract surgery and the iStent trabecular micro-bypass stent. *Adv Ther*. 2008;25(5):453–64.

45. Zhou J, Smedley GT. A trabecular bypass flow hypothesis. *J Glaucoma*. 2005;14(1):74–83.

46. Zhou J, Smedley GT. Trabecular bypass: effect of Schlemm canal and collector channel dilation. *J Glaucoma*. 2006;15(5):446–55.

47. Bahler C, Smedley GT, Zhou J, Johnson DH. Trabecular bypass stents decrease intraocular pressure in cultured human anterior segments. *Am J Ophthalmol*. 2004;138(6):988–94.

48. Minckler D, Baerveldt G, Alfaro MR, Francis BA. Clinical Results with the Trabectome for tratment of open-angle glaucoma. *Ophthalmology*. 2005;112:962–7.

49. Francis B, Minckler D, Dustin L, et al. Combined cataract extraction and trabeculotomy by the internal approach for coexisting cataract and open-angle glaucoma: Initial results. *J Cataract Refract Surg*. 2008;34:1096–103.

50. Minckler D, Baerveldt G, Ramirez MA, et al. Clinical results with the trabectome, a novel surgical device for treatment of open-angle glaucoma. *Trans Am Ophthalmol Soc*. 2006;104:40–50.

51. Bill A, Phillips CI. Uveoscleral drainage of aqueous humor in human eyes. *Exp Eye Res*. 1971;12:275–81.

52. Toris C, Yablonski ME, Wang YL, et al. Aqueous humor dynamics in the aging human eye. *Am J Ophthalmol*. 1999;127:407–12.

53. Sen S, Ghosh A. Gold as an intraocular foreign body. *Br J Ophthalmol*. 1983;67:398–9.

54. Eisler R. Mammalian sensitivity to elemental gold (Au). *Biol Tr Elem Res*. 2004;100:1–17.

55. Suguro K, Toris CB, Pederson JE. Uveoscleral outflow following cyclodialysis in the monkey eye using a fluorescent tracer. *Invest Ophthalmol Vis Sci*. 1985;26:810–3.

56. Jordan J, Dietlein TS, Dinslage S, et al. Cyclodialysis ab interno as a surgical approach to intractable glaucoma. *Graefe's Arch Clin Exp Ophthalmol*. 2007;245:1071–6.

57. Shields M, Simmons RJ. Combined cyclodialysis and cataract extraction. *Ophthalmic Surg*. 1976;7(2):62–73.

58. Gallin M, Baras I. Combined cyclodialysis cataract extraction: a review. *Ann Ophthalmol*. 1975;7(2):271–5.

59. Gills J Jr, Paterson CA, Paterson ME. Action of cyclodialysis utilizing an implant studied by manometry in the human eye. *Exp Eye Res*. 1967;6:75–8.

60. Klemm M, Balazs A, Draeger J, Wiezorrek R. Experimental use of space-retaining substances with extended duration: functional and morphological results. *Graefes Arch Clin Exp Ophthalmol*. 1995;233(9):592–7.

61. Nesterov A, Batmanov YE, Cherkasova IN, Egorov EA. Surgical stimulation of the uveoscleral outflow: experimental studies on enucleated human eyes. *Acta Ophthalmologica*. 1979;57(3):3.

62. Pinnas G, Boniuk M. Cyclodialysis with teflon tube implants. *Am J Ophthalmol*. 1969;68(5):879–83.

63. Krejci L. Cyclodialysis with hydroxyethyl methacrylate capillary strip. *Ophthalmologica*. 1972;164:113–21.

Chapter 15

Cataract Surgery in Patients with Exfoliation Syndrome

Anastasios G.P. Konstas, Nikolaos G. Ziakas, Miguel A. Teus, Dimitrios G. Mikropoulos, and Vassilios P. Kozobolis

Introduction: Update on Exfoliation Syndrome

Exfoliation syndrome (XFS) was first described in 1917 by the Finnish ophthalmologist John Lindberg[1] and currently affects 60–70 million people worldwide.[2–4] Of these, 15–17 million have increased intraocular pressure (IOP) and 5–6 million are estimated to suffer from exfoliative glaucoma (XFG), a form of secondary open-angle glaucoma that develops as a consequence of XFS and is considered the most common identifiable cause of open-angle glaucoma worldwide.[2] Its aggressive course and worldwide prevalence makes it critical for ophthalmologists to be familiar with the full clinical spectrum of the disease.[5–10] However, significant barriers to the successful diagnosis and management of XFS and XFG still exist. As XFS is a slowly progressive disease with subtle signs, early diagnosis is difficult.[3,7,9,11] Indeed, the condition may remain undetected until the clinical signs become more apparent or when cataract or XFG develop. With increasing life expectancy, it is important that efforts are focused on improving the management of patients with exfoliation and alleviating the burden of visual loss and complications during cataract surgery in patients with XFS and XFG.[7,8]

Pathophysiology

Both XFS and XFG are age-related conditions characterized by the systemic synthesis and progressive accumulation of a fibrillar extracellular material (exfoliation material) in many ocular and systemic tissues. Exfoliation material synthesis may relate to disturbed elastin metabolism.[12] The

discovery in 2007 of the role played by lysyl oxidase-like protein 1 (LOXL1) gene polymorphism in the development of the condition has shed more light on its genetic background.[13] LOXL1 is a member of a gene family that plays an important role in elastin metabolism. Specific mutations of the LOXL1 gene are strongly associated with the development of XFS and XFG. It is hypothesized that dysfunction of the LOXL1 gene may lead to the progressive accumulation exfoliation material. This may explain the histological findings and several XFS-related complications.[12]

Ultrastructurally, exfoliation deposits consist of electron dense, fibrillar, elastotic material.[5] Histochemically, XFM consists of a core protein surrounded by glycoconjugates, giving it a glycoprotein/proteoglycan structure.[5,6,12] Exfoliation aggregates can be seen both intracellularly during synthesis, and as extracellular deposits. Though intraocular and extraocular deposits are not morphologically or biochemically identical, both represent the same type of abnormal fibrillopathy.[12] Recent data suggest that the exfoliation-related biochemical changes are influenced by increased oxidative stress,[14] which as a part of a vicious circle, is enhanced by the exfoliation-induced tissue damage. Development of nuclear cataract is more common in patients with XFS/XFG and may be related to the increased oxidative stress in the anterior segment of the affected eye.[3,14]

Clinical Implications

Exfoliation material is not only synthesized and accumulated in different tissues, but by disturbing extracellular matrix metabolism it can induce alterations in function. These XFS-related degenerative changes are clinically important, may result in surgical complications during phacoemulsification surgery,[11,15,16] and, consequently, must be known by all ophthalmologists. Prevention of surgical complications in cataract surgery is a key aim of successful XFS management. Existing evidence shows that XFS is an important risk factor for vitreous loss.[3,7,9,11] Although the ultimate impact of

A.G.P. Konstas (✉)
AHEPA Hospital, 1st University Department of Ophthalmology,
Thessaloniki 54636, Greece
e-mail: konstas@med.auth.gr

XFS/XFG in cataract surgery is currently not known (since there are limited controlled data on the subject) there is some evidence to show that detection of exfoliation signs in the cataract patient, together with the appropriate management during surgery, can improve surgical outcome.

On routine biomicroscopic examination of the eye, without dilatation of the pupil, the diagnosis of XFS can be missed[5,11] and the prevalence can be underestimated.[4,9] The diagnostic sensitivity increases when the condition is sought by an experienced observer who is fully aware of the full diagnostic spectrum of the disease.[7] See Table 15.1. Although the clinical description of fully developed XFS is well established, little is known about the early changes, which are less well defined.[17] For example, exfoliation aggregates can be identified by transmission electron microscopy within eyes in which it is not clinically apparent.[10,17] These factors result in an artificially low prevalence of the condition. More efficient diagnostic techniques and a new classification scheme may be key components in improving detection in the future.

Table 15.1 Clinical manifestations of pseudoexfoliation

- Cataract
- Exfoliation aggregates on anterior segment tissues
- Poor dilation
- Weak zonules/zonular laxity
- Glaucoma
- Corneal endotheliopathy
- Possibly vascular disease

Although not well described, there appears to be a significant association between XFS and cataract formation. There is a high prevalence of XFS in eyes coming to cataract surgery and a high prevalence of cataract in eyes with XFS[7,15,16] compared with age-matched eyes without XFS. The etiologic relationship between the two disorders remains unclear. Koliakos et al.[14] observed a significantly reduced level of ascorbic acid in the aqueous humor of patients with XFS. Since ascorbic acid plays an important role in protecting the lens from ultraviolet irradiation, this finding may provide a logical explanation for the greater incidence of cataract formation and posterior capsular opacification after cataract extraction in eyes with XFS.

The clinical diagnosis of XFS or XFG is based on the incidental finding of "dandruff-like" exfoliation material upon the pupillary margin, or "sugar frosting" of the anterior lens capsule.[2,3] Generally these are the most consistent signs of the condition. In the fully developed condition,[3] complete or sometimes incomplete distinct exfoliation zones may be visualized after pupillary dilatation: a relatively homogeneous, subtle central disc corresponding to the diameter of the pupil; a granular, often layered, peripheral zone; and a clear intermediate area separating the two (Fig. 15.1). Several variations may arise, however, due to the differences in the

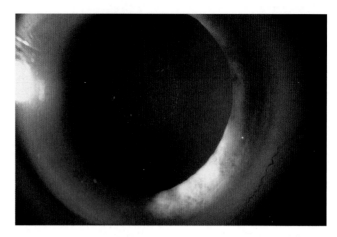

Fig. 15.1 A slit lamp photo of a dilated pupil revealing the lens with the zones associated with pseudoexfoliation syndrome. Courtesy of Tom Monego, Dartmouth Hitchcock Medical Center (DHMC), Lebanon, NH

quantity and rate of deposition of exfoliation material, different stages in the disease process, and the varied anatomic relationship and proximity of the posterior iris surface to the anterior lens.[5,7] The peripheral granular zone is thought to be a pathognomonic clinical sign and thus the most reliable sign assisting the diagnosis. Early in the course of the disease, subtle striations of exfoliation material and/or pigment "sunflower" deposits may be discerned on the surface of the lens.[3] The diagnosis of the condition is more difficult in the presence of cataract. In a histological study, XFS was diagnosed in 33% of cataractous lenses, whereas only 16% of the cases had been diagnosed clinically prior to cataract surgery.[18] After cataract extraction, exfoliation material may be found deposited upon the anterior vitreous face or on vitreous strands when the face is ruptured, on the posterior capsule, and on intraocular lenses, indicating that the presence of the lens is unnecessary for its continued formation.[2,9,10]

Exfoliation deposits may be detected early on the ciliary processes and zonules. Zonular aggregates may in fact predate the development of the peripheral granular zone upon the lens surface.[5,6] It is well documented that XFS can cause zonular fragility, which may lead to lens subluxation and surgical complications during phacoemulsification. The zonules are sometimes heavily coated with exfoliation material and, in extreme cases, severely damaged and broken.[9] An additional mechanism may also be the degeneration induced to the zonular attachments to the lens, or ciliary body. Currently, the zonular fragility, thinning of the equatorial lens capsule, and reduced dilation of the pupil in XFS are thought to be responsible for the increased complication rate during cataract surgery, as well as the postoperative decentration of intraocular lenses even years after uncomplicated cataract surgery.[9] In a small number of cases, exfoliation-induced corneal degenerative changes may impact the number and shape of corneal endothelial cells, which may ultimately lead to corneal decompensation[5] even after uncomplicated phacoemulsification, or following marked elevation of IOP.[11]

Degenerative ischemic changes in the iris are also induced by XFS and result in reduced pupillary dilatation. These changes induced by massive exfoliation deposits around iris vessel walls lead to micro-occlusions, formation of ghost vessels, and secondary micro-neovascularization.[3,5,12] These ultrastructural and functional alterations result in increased vascular permeability and impairment of the blood-aqueous barrier function, which can lead to increased incidence of posterior synechiae formation and a higher incidence and duration of inflammation after intraocular surgery. Retrobulbar perfusion may also be impaired in XFS and XFG.[8,9]

There is evidence to suggest that XFS is a systemic disorder.[19–21] Patients with XFS may exhibit systemic vascular involvement[20,21] and it has been postulated that XFS may contribute to increased morbidity. There are reports of impaired regulation of heart function and reduced precapillary perfusion.[20] There are conflicting reports suggesting an increased prevalence of ischemic heart disease in XFS, but the prevalence of diabetes mellitus is only half of that seen in age-matched controls or in patients with primary open-angle glaucoma and there is no evidence that XFS/XFG lead to increased mortality.[19] Further controlled evidence is required to elucidate the precise systemic risk induced by XFS.

Elevated IOP with or without glaucomatous damage occurs in approximately 25% of people with XFS or about 6–10 times the rate in eyes without XFS.[6–10] When XFG develops, it is associated with worse untreated 24-h IOP characteristics and a worse prognosis than primary open-angle glaucoma.[22,23] Due to the unfavorable pressure characteristics, more aggressive medical therapy is needed and it is generally more difficult to reach the predetermined target IOP in XFG.[11,23] Thus, adjunctive medical therapy, laser treatment, and surgery are more often necessary in XFG. However, the best first-line and stepwise therapy in XFG remains controversial.[11] Therefore, it is important to determine in the future the optimum choices for successful therapy in XFG.

Intraocular Pressure Changes After Phacoemulsification in Eyes with XFS

The common coexistence of cataract and raised IOP in XFS often poses management dilemmas concerning the optimal surgical approach. Accurate estimation of the magnitude of potential IOP reduction in response to cataract surgery in XFS or XFG would be useful in determining whether to do phacoemulsification alone or combine

the surgery with trabeculectomy. Several studies have noted a decrease in IOP following phacoemulsification in eyes with and without XFS.[24–27] A number of studies were retrospective and have examined the effect of phacoemulsification on IOP levels in patients with and without XFS. Suzuki et al.[28] reported a decrease in IOP after surgery in patients without preexisting disease. Patients with increased preoperative IOP with or without glaucoma but no XFS may also exhibit meaningful postoperative IOP drops.[25,29] Three studies have reported that XFS patients with a normal preoperative IOP manifested a decrease in IOP postoperatively that was significantly greater than similarly matched controls without XFS, with the effect sustained up to a 2-year follow-up.[26,30,31] In the study by Merkur et al., postoperative IOP changes from baseline in the XFS group were –1.8, –4.5, and –2.3 mmHg at 3, 6, and 12 months, respectively. In the study by Shingleton, IOP declined from a mean of 16.8 to 13.9 mmHg in the XFS group and from 16.3 to 14.4 mmHg in the control group at 2 years.[34]

These observations have been confirmed in a large prospective multicenter cohort study by Damji et al.[32] This study demonstrated that patients with XFS have a greater IOP lowering effect following phacoemulsification than those without XFS. The IOP reduction was significantly greater in the exfoliation group at all time points out to 2 years. In the subgroup analyses, IOP lowering was –1.85 mmHg at 2 years in the XFS patients versus –0.62 mmHg in the controls. Importantly, patients with XFG also exhibited a more pronounced IOP lowering than those with POAG (–3.15 mm versus –1.54 mmHg, respectively) after 2 years. It is interesting that the IOP lowering effect in the XFS group was closely related to the irrigation volume utilized at the time of surgery. The authors speculated that this may be because of one or more of the following factors: washing out of exfoliation material and pigment from the anterior segment, deepening of the anterior chamber angle, and low-grade inflammation leading to enhanced aqueous outflow.

It has been argued that patients with XFS undergoing phacoemulsification experience a greater decrease in IOP postoperatively in comparison with patients without XFS because phacoemulsification eliminates iridolenticular friction and thus significantly reduces the release of pigment from the iris and exfoliation material from the lens and iris. The procedure also removes loose exfoliation material and pigment from the clogged outflow system, and thus may lead to further IOP lowering in patients with XFS or XFG.[33,34] It has been hypothesized that the removal of exfoliation material and pigment is the mechanism for this recorded IOP lowering with subsequent improved outflow. The term "trabecular aspiration" (TA) was introduced by Jacobi and Krieglstein in 1994, who employed a special aspiration system.[33–35] Trabecular debris and pigment was cleared with a suction force of 100–200 mmHg.

They concluded that trabecular aspiration combined with phacoemulsification was significantly more effective than cataract surgery alone in reducing postoperative IOP and the necessity for anti-glaucoma medications, but not as effective as phacotrabeculectomy. Cimetta et al.[36] performed phacoemulsification with exfoliation material aspiration with IOP reduction lasting up to 1 year postoperatively. Other possibilities that contribute to IOP lowering include upregulation of matrix metalloproteinases, biochemical or blood-aqueous barrier alterations with release of prostaglandins,[37] or other physiological processes that alter and improve trabecular or uveoscleral outflow.

Whether to perform cataract surgery alone or combine it with a trabeculectomy is an important clinical decision when treating patients who have XFG and a visually significant cataract. The advantages of a combined procedure are the prevention of IOP spikes and better long-term IOP control postoperatively. However, combined cataract surgery and trabeculectomy in XFG may lead to a higher rate of complications including hypotony, suprachoroidal hemorrhage, and endophthalmitis.

The data being accumulated to date are consistent with the notion that in many patients with early to moderate XFG, phacoemulsification alone is a reasonable option for better IOP management. This approach has the advantage of faster visual rehabilitation and fewer surgical complications. How long the beneficial effect of cataract surgery on IOP lowering lasts is currently unknown and merits further investigation.

Operative Techniques and Considerations for Phacoemulcification in Eyes with XFS

Cataract surgery in the presence of XFS is generally considered to be a challenge as it has been associated with an increased incidence of intraoperative complications. The risks were first described for extracapsular cataract extraction[38–43] and later for phacoemulsification.[30,44–47] In XFS, lysosomal proteinases destroy the normal basement membrane structure of the non-pigmented epithelium of the ciliary body and anterior lens capsule. This loosens the zonule–lens capsule complex and causes adhesions between the zonules and non-pigmented epithelium.[9,48] The rotational and antero-posterior forces created during surgery may lead to total separation of these weakened zonules, resulting in vitreous loss. As discussed previously, other factors thought to contribute to the increased incidence of intraoperative complications during cataract surgery in eyes with XFS are a poorly dilating pupil, corneal endothelial changes, and blood–aqueous barrier breakdown.[49–52]

Preoperative Examination

In most cases, exfoliation material can be observed with careful slit-lamp examination after pupil dilatation, even in the early stages of XFS. The presence of XFS or XFG poses an increased risk during and after cataract surgery, particularly if undetected. Zonular weakness and poor trabecular outflow with elevated IOP may pose specific intraoperative problems. Hence, preoperative documentation of XFS, which often may otherwise go undetected, is key to successful cataract surgery. Signs indicative of weak zonules are listed in Table 15.2. However, only slight phacodonesis andor an iridolenticular gap may be seen. Kuchle et al.[47] found a correlation between a shallow anterior chamber and zonular instability, which indicates that reduced anterior chamber depth with normal axial length should alert the surgeon to possible zonular laxity. Reduced chamber depth in a highly myopic eye is virtually pathognomonic of zonular laxity. It is important to study anterior chamber depth when seated and lying prone, since this would give a measure of zonular laxity, particularly after paralysis of accommodation. In patients with XFG elevated IOP, especially in elderly patients, may increase the risk of perioperative complications and, specifically, increase the risk of choroidal hemorrhage.[53]

Table 15.2 Signs of weak zonules

- Distinct phacodonesis
- Iridodonesis
- Vitreous prolapse
- Lens subluxation
- Shallow anterior chamber

Management of Small Pupil in XFS

A small pupil is a problem frequently encountered during phacoemulsification in eyes with XFS. Maximal pupil dilatation is significantly less in XFS eyes compared to normal eyes.[30] Mechanical dilatation of the smallest pupils (e.g., <4 mm in diameter) is an efficient and commonly used technique, although it may lead to micro-ruptures of the sphincter, increased postoperative inflammation, and, sometimes, result in a permanently dilated pupil.[41,54,55] In these cases, bimanual stretching with Y-hooks, iris retractor hooks (Fig. 3.4), Beehler pupil dilator (Fig. 3.3), or polymethylmethacrylate (PMMA) pupil dilator rings (Figs. 3.5, 3.6, 3.7 and 3.8) are useful. Akman et al.[56] compared these four methods of pupil dilatation in XFS eyes undergoing phacoemulsification and concluded that all of them were effective. The two most time consuming devices, iris retractor hooks and PMMA pupil dilator rings, were also best at keeping the pupil dilated during surgery. The dilator ring caused the least iris trauma. See also Chapter 3.

Surgical Considerations in the Presence of Zonular Weakness

Capsulorrhexis and Hydrodissection

It is important to avoid overinflating the anterior chamber with viscoelastics when loose zonular support is suspected. Movement of the entire lens-capsule complex during anterior capsulotomy is always a sign of severe zonular laxity; the lens may be so loose that completion of the capsulorrhexis (CCC) by the usual means may be impossible because of lack of resistance and stability of the lens. However, the insertion of a retractor (iris or modified retractor) after the creation of an initial capsulotomy can provide a counterforce against which the CCC can usually be performed. Multiple grasps of the capsular flap may be helpful in overcoming the problem and completing the capsulorrhexis. CCC should be performed with the least possible downward pressure on the lens and avoiding any centripetal traction on the flap. The most obvious signs of zonular weakness include subluxation of the entire nucleus with visualization of the lens equator. However, mild zonular laxity resulting in the development of anterior capsule striae adjacent to the capsular flap during capsulorrhexis is more commonly seen. The location of these striae also indicates the weak region of the zonules. The CCC should be neither too small nor too large. Too small a diameter will add further stress to loose zonules during manipulation of the nucleus in the bag, whereas too large a diameter may engage the zonular attachments. The final capsulorrhexis size should be larger than that in non-XFS eyes, in order to reduce future shrinkage of the anterior capsule, due to the fibrosis produced by the remaining epithelial cells. Centripetal forces induced by anterior capsule contraction may aggravate zonular weakness and lead to late dislocation of the intraocular lens (IOL) within the capsular bag.[57,58]

Hydrodissection and/or hydrodelineation must be performed carefully to avoid downward pressure on the lens whenever zonular fragility is suspected. Access to rotating the nucleus and epinucleus is important for performing the maneuver as gently as possible during surgery.[59] However, the degree of dissection must be balanced against the fact that too aggressive an injection of fluid can lead to further zonular weakness. Alternatively, the entire nucleus should be hydrodissected and luxated anteriorly for supracapsular phacoemulsification to minimize zonular stress in XFS. However, in choosing this approach, care should be taken not to damage the endothelial cells.

Phacoemulsification and Cortex Aspiration

Phacoemulsification must follow the same principle of not stretching the zonulae. During surgery, extreme deepening of the anterior chamber at the onset of infusion may be indicative of zonular laxity. However, this phenomenon is more commonly seen in highly myopic eyes. It is generally advisable to perform phacoemulsification with a lower infusion pressure and, therefore, lower aspiration flow rate and vacuum levels in these eyes, although this will slow down the emulsification process. During sculpting of the nucleus, a tendency of the lens to move with the sculpted tip—that is, away from the surgical incision—is a clear sign of inadequate zonular strength. Ultrasonic power should be increased and stabilization of nuclear position by placement of a lens chopper, or a similar instrument, over the equator opposite the phaco incision to stabilize the position of the nucleus should be considered. During nucleus rotation, a tendency of the nucleus to return toward its previous location when released by the rotating instrument can be an ominous sign of zonular dehiscence. This indicates that the entire capsule has rotated somewhat with the nucleus, and subsequently returned to its normal anatomic location when the rotary force was discontinued. Therefore, rotation of the nucleus should be performed gently or even avoided, if possible. The surgeon should maintain centration of the nucleus during rotation with bimanual rotation, using both the phaco tip and a second instrument such as a phaco chopper or spatula whenever possible. Segmentation of the nucleus should be accomplished as gently as possible. Deep sculpting enables the nucleus to be cracked with less effort. Chopping techniques are preferred instead of the classic "divide and conquer" method, as all forces are directed to the center of the nucleus with minimal induced stress on the capsule and zonules.[60] Finally, another sign of zonular deficiency, visible as nucleus volume decreases, is inward collapse of the lens capsule with possible inadvertent aspiration by the phaco tip.

Aspiration of the cortex is one of the steps that stress the zonules the most. After nucleus removal, tangential stripping of lens cortex from the capsular fornices may prevent further zonular dehiscence. In extreme circumstances, it may be necessary to position the distal end of a second instrument, such as a blunt spatula, against the capsular fornix to create counteraction as cortex is removed. At any time during cortex removal, peripheral posterior capsule striae may straddle an area of zonular dehiscence. The longest striae demarcate the area of dehiscence. Also, a forward shift of the posterior capsule caused by infusion fluid accumulation behind the posterior capsule (infusion misdirection) may occur. This phenomenon is more common in eyes with exfoliation and other causes of zonular laxity than in normal eyes.

Intraocular Lens Implantation

Implantation of the IOL before finishing aspiration, when little residual cortex is left, will help to stabilize the capsular bag and reduce zonular stress. It is important to place both haptics either in the bag or in the sulcus, to equally distribute the pressure on the zonules. In the case of a capsular break, the IOL should be placed in the ciliary sulcus, provided there is sufficient capsular support. Additional prolapse of the lenticulus behind the capsulorrhexis optimizes centration. If not, an angle-supported IOL, an iris-claw IOL, or an IOL fixed to the scleral wall may be utilized.[61] An angle-supported anterior chamber IOL should probably not be chosen in the case of eyes with XFG or in the presence of corneal endothelial cell abnormalities.[62]

When deciding the type of IOL for in the bag implantation, the surgeon should take into account the higher incidence of capsular fibrosis in XFS. Typically the choice of intraocular lens (IOL) does not differ between eyes with and without XFS. Heparin surface modified posterior chamber intraocular lenses were postulated to result in a lower incidence of postoperative fibrinoid reaction, less frequent pigment, and cellular deposits on the intraocular lenses,[63] but this observation requires further confirmation. Therefore, hydrophobic acrylic IOLs, which are associated with less anterior capsular fibrosis compared to PMMA, silicone, and hydrogel lenses, are preferably used.[44] Also, theoretically, the PMMA haptics of the three-piece acrylic IOLs provide higher rigidity against contraction of the capsule.[64] Achieving IOL centration and long-term stability can be challenging in eyes with significant zonular dehiscence. Foldable acrylic IOLs with long haptics and an optic diameter not smaller than 6 mm should preferably be used, in case some lens decentration occurs postoperatively. Injectors that allow the haptics to unfold directly into the capsular bag without the need to dial in the haptics minimize the zonular stress that occurs during haptic placement. Plate-haptic style IOLs are a poor choice as they have a greater tendency for postoperative decentration and capsular contraction. Some surgeons advocate placing the haptics perpendicularly to the dialysis to expand the partially collapsed capsular bag. However, the IOL then relies on zonular support from only one haptic. Haptic orientation parallel to the dialysis provides better zonular support, yet will induce an oval formation of the bag and perhaps increases the chance for decentration away from the dialysis. Cionni et al.[65] recommend placing the IOL into the bag and gently rotating the IOL into the axis that provides the best possible centration. Complicated cataract surgery with loss of integrity of the capsular bag can lead to immediate dislocation of the IOL. However, spontaneous dislocation of the IOL within the capsular bag following uncomplicated surgery usually occurs many months postoperatively.

Special Techniques, Instrumentation, and Devices for the Management of Severe Zonular Weakness in XFS

Severe zonular deficiency with phacodonesis or frank lens dislocation poses a particular surgical challenge. In such cases, multiple iris hooks, with which most surgeons are familiar, engaged to the CCC edge may be used to stabilize the capsular bag during phacoemulsification[66,67] (Fig. 15.2a). However, the relatively short length of the hook and the single plane design may cause them to slip off the capsule during manipulation of the nucleus. In addition, the short iris retractors do not extend into the capsular fornix and, therefore, do not offer support to this region. A hook designed for stabilization of the capsule is also described[68] (Fig. 15.2b). When the lens is completely loose, this technique should be exchanged for intracapsular cataract surgery.

Stabilization of the lens-zonule complex during surgery in XFS with zonular weakness is helpful and can be accomplished using a capsular tension ring (CTR) to provide support to the lens capsule[69,70] (Fig. 15.3). These rings are manufactured in different sizes, to better fit in the capsular bag. When inserted into the capsular sac, a CTR provides a circumferentially expanding force to the capsular equator and distributes the forces equally all over the zonular apparatus.[65,71] The capsule is, therefore, less likely to be attracted to the phaco tip, and increased stability of the lens may be obtained. The stage of the operation at which a CTR is implanted should be considered individually in every case. In general, CTRs may be inserted at any time during PCE.[72] Bayraktar et al.[59] reported less zonular dialysis in XFS eyes when a CTR was used. In his study, the CTRs were inserted before phacoemulsification. Others prefer to insert the ring after the epinucleus and cortical remnants have been removed, thereby avoiding entrapment of cortical material by the CTR against the capsular bag. Removal of the trapped cortex can be difficult and, in fact, attempts to do so can cause further zonular dehiscence. However, the cortical clean-up may be performed successfully when inserting the CTR before surgery if the ring is inserted just beneath the lens capsule and not between the cortical fibers. Meticulous cortical cleaving hydrodissection, as described by Fine,[73] and a viscoelastic injection along the path of the CTR may help separate the lens capsule from the cortex.[59] A study on cadaver eyes compared CTR implantation before and after nucleus extraction and found that early implantation gave significantly increased capsular torque and displacement compared with implantation after the nucleus had been extracted.[74] In our opinion, the rings should be used only when they are really needed, and placing them as late as possible during surgery is advisable. Capsular tension rings

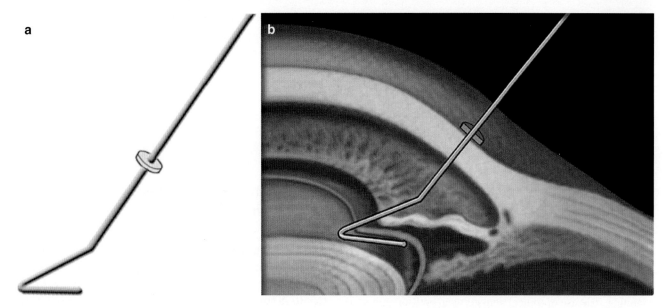

Fig. 15.2 Hooks designed to stabilize the capsule. (**a**, **b**) Mackool Cataract Support System MH-105. Courtesy of FCI Ophthalmics, Marshfield Hills, MA

can also be used to help prevent intraoperative posterior capsule rupture by keeping the posterior capsule taut, preventing its anterior bulging and protecting it from being aspirated by phaco or irrigation/aspiration tips during phacoemulsification and cortical aspiration.[75] Finally, in theory, the CTR would counter the postoperative contraction of the anterior capsule, thus reducing shrinkage of the CCC and the risk of IOL dislocation. However, there is no real evidence to support this and several late dislocations with the IOL in the bag have been reported specifically in eyes with XFS.[58] Moreno-Montanes et al.[76] described a useful surgical technique for removing the CTR after phacoemulsification in cases of posterior capsular rupture to prevent CTR dislocation into the vitreous cavity.

Modified endocapsular rings that can also be sutured to the sclera are available (e.g., the Cionni design)[77] and should be used in eyes with more significantly loose zonules as they offer greater capsular stability and centration. Such rings contain a small strut with a distal eyelet (Fig. 15.4). Prior to inserting the ring, a double-armed 10-0 prolene suture can be passed through the eyelet. After ring insertion, both needles are passed through the appropriate region of the ciliary sulcus and tied to each other under a scleral flap to establish permanent positioning of the endocapsular ring and surrounding capsule.

Although the use of a CTR has been of great help to avoid complications due to loose zonulae, it does not always achieve lens stability and also may be hazardous, as its insertion can create further zonular damage. Nonetheless, expansion of the capsule sac is often desirable either during or after lens removal, and these devices enhance implant centration and reduce postoperative pseudophacodonesis.

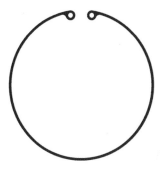

Fig. 15.3 Photo of a Morscher MR 1400 capsular tension ring. Courtesy of FCI Ophthalmics, Marshfield Hills, MA

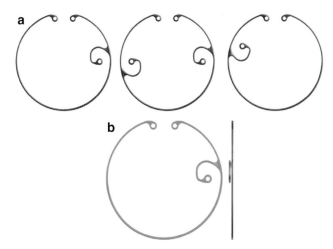

Fig. 15.4 Modified capsular tension rings: Cionni rings (**a**) MRiL and (**b**) M2L. Courtesy of FCI Ophthalmics, Marshfield Hills, MA

Perioperative and Postoperative Complications in Cataract Surgery in Eyes with XFS

Preoperative Evaluation

As mentioned previously, it is mandatory to look for exfoliation material, which can be observed with high magnification by careful slit-lamp examination after pupil dilatation. Several sophisticated procedures, such as Scheimpflug photography,[78] or ultrasound biomicroscopy of the zonules can enhance diagnostic accuracy.[79] In eyes with XFS or XFG, it is important to carefully assess the corneal endothelium and to check for signs of zonular fragility. An estimate of pupillary dilatation should also be carried out the day surgery is decided, to allow for better risk assessment and for surgical planning. The use of topical non-steroidal anti-inflammatory drugs (NSAIDs) (e.g., diclofenac or ketorolac) may be advisable but more information is needed for their efficacy in enhancing preoperative dilatation of the pupil.

Extracapsular Cataract Extraction

Phacoemulsification has become the gold standard in cataract surgery. Nevertheless, extracapsular cataract extraction (ECCE) can still be selected in some settings and especially in some cases with XFS and phacodonesis. Published evidence has demonstrated a higher incidence of complications with ECCE in eyes with XFS. In a prospective study, Katsimpris et al.[80] evaluated XFS eyes with small pupils and phacodonesis, and reported a much higher incidence of posterior capsule rupture and vitreous loss with ECCE surgery compared with phacoemulsification. In another prospective clinical trial of 1000 ECCE surgeries,[39] the only significant risk factors for vitreous loss were the presence of XFS and small pupil size, which underscores the importance of adequate surgical mydriasis in cataract surgery. The increased force needed to extrude the lens nucleus through a small pupil as well as the risk of posterior capsule breaks with the capsulotomy techniques in XFS eyes may explain the high frequency of complications during surgery in ECCE. Ruotsalainen and Tarkkanen[81] reported that posterior capsular rupture during ECCE cataract surgery was 5–13 times greater in eyes with XFS compared to eyes without XFS. They considered that the posterior capsule is of normal thickness in XFS and attributed the higher complication rate in these eyes to zonular fragility.

Exfoliation syndrome (XFS) is not a contraindication for posterior chamber lens implantation and, providing sufficient support exists, posterior chamber lenses may be placed in the ciliary sulcus even in the presence of small capsular tears. Overall, there is convincing evidence to suggest that in ECCE intraoperative and postoperative complications, including zonular disruption, crystalline lens and IOL dislocation, vitreous loss, increased intraocular pressure, and trauma to other ocular structures, occur more frequently in eyes with XFS than in eyes without.[82]

Intraoperative Complications with Phacoemulsification in XFS

There is controversy in the published literature concerning the rate of intraoperative complications with phacoemulsification in eyes with XFS. The reason for the conflicting reports in complication rates may be explained by differences in how common and how advanced XFS was in the surgical cohorts of these studies. For example, in studies that did not observe an increased rate of complications with XFS, none of the cases had phacodonesis.[55,83,84] As previously stated, in eyes with XFS, the lens tends to be harder and requires an increased emulsification time, which can result in more challenging surgery. In several eyes with advanced XFS, weakened zonular stability may lead to phacodonesis and these patients are at a higher risk for vitreous loss. The increased rigidity of the iris in XFS could also conceal iridodonesis in the presence of phacodonesis.[85] Further, a small anterior chamber depth (less than 2.5 mm) may indicate zonular instability in eyes with XFS or XFG and should alert the cataract surgeon to the possibility of surgical complications.[47,82]

The data being accumulated are consistent with the notion that the most serious complications in XFS are attributable to zonular weakness. With careful planning the incidence of complications in XFS may be reduced in experienced hands.[86] Importantly, a number of factors in XFS predispose to capsular rupture, of which the most important appear to be inadequate mydriasis and the concomitant or consequent zonular dehiscence. Other factors such as areas of capsular degeneration, iridolenticular synechiae, or difficulty with cortical aspiration may also play a smaller role. It is not disputed that zonular stress is increased when dilatation of the pupil is inadequate in cataract surgery. The preoperative use of anti-inflammatory drugs may improve dilatation and thus reduce complications, but this requires further elucidation with an adequately powered controlled trial.

The ciliary sulcus becomes smaller with age and this should be born in mind with respect to the size of sulcus implanted IOLs.[87] Little is currently known concerning the scale of severity for XFS, yet the risk of complications should be related to the severity of the condition. Parmar et al. described a central bulge in the anterior lens capsule of some patients with XFS. They believed that an association of this central bulge with an increased zonular fragility may exist and consequently pose a higher risk for intraoperative zonular dialysis.[88] No proper classification system has been developed as yet to facilitate clinical characterization of the condition and optimum evaluation of the likely magnitude of surgical risk. Such a scale would provide a better understanding of the various stages of the exfoliation process and the impact of the condition to the ocular structures.

The influence of cataract stage on the surgical risk has not been adequately determined in XFS, but there is some evidence that the posterior capsule complication rate increases as the level of cataract maturity increases and the preoperative visual acuity decreases.[89] Vision blue may provide better visualization in eyes with XFS and advanced cataract.

In a clinical trial by Scorolli and coauthors,[46] XFS was associated with a statistically significant increase in intraoperative complications (vitreous loss, capsular break, zonular break) during cataract surgery. The aim of this study was to determine the rate of intraoperative complications induced by XFS in 1052 consecutive patients who underwent phacoemulsification. The odds ratio for intraoperative complications (vitreous loss, capsular break, zonular break) was estimated to be 5:1 when XFS was present. These authors concluded that XFS was associated with a statistically significant increase in intraoperative complications during cataract surgery.

In XFS cases with inadequate pupil dilatation, hard lens nucleus, endothelial cell abnormalities, or reduced zonular support, gentle manipulation of the nucleus in phacoemulsification is mandatory. As to which method to choose, the best advice is probably that everyone sticks to their own favored procedure.[15] It is also important to point out that clinically, most patients with XFS reveal only unilateral ocular involvement. The nature of the disorder suggests that XFS is clinically asymmetric rather than unilateral. Hammer et al. performed an ultrastructural study of the contralateral eyes in patients with unilateral XFS and reported that ultrastructural alterations consistent with the condition were observed in the anterior segment tissues of all apparently not-involved fellow eyes. The involvement of both eyes in clinically unilateral XFS should warn clinicians when they operate on these fellow eyes for potential complications.[90]

Nevertheless, the majority of published studies indicate a significantly reduced complication rate in XFS eyes when phacoemulsification is performed compared with ECCE. This suggests that phacoemulsification is a safer procedure in eyes with XFS.[31] Additionally, there is a lower incidence and less severity of an inflammatory response with phacoemulsification compared to ECCE, and in most eyes XFS itself does not significantly increase the risk of inflammation.[45,86]

Reports in the literature concerning the incidence of intraoperative complications during phacoemulsification in eyes with XFS are controversial. In a large series of phacoemulsification procedures, Hyams et al.[55] evaluated 137 eyes with XFS—but excluded XFS eyes with marked phacodonesis or lens subluxation—and 1364 control eyes and reported no significant difference in the rate of intraoperative complications between the two groups with exfoliation (5.8%) and without (4.0%). Specifically, the authors did not detect a difference in the incidence of capsular breaks, vitreous loss, and zonular ruptures without vitreous loss in the two groups. Capsular break was recorded in 2.9% in both groups, zonular tear 2.9% in the XFS group versus 1.1% in the control group, and vitreous loss in 1.5% in the XFS group versus 2% in the non-XFS group. It is important to point out, however, that this study had a power of 90% to detect a difference in complications of 10% between the XFS and the control group. This study was in agreement with previous reports by Dosso and coauthors[30] and Shastri and Vasavada,[83] in which they observed similar rates of intraoperative complications with and without XFS. The evidence from these two studies, however, is inconclusive due to the small samples investigated: 20 cases in the former and 45 cases in the latter report. In another controlled study of 1210 phacoemulsification surgeries, intraoperative complications were similar between the XFS and the control group.[91] This led the authors to conclude that the preoperative presence of XFS had no direct influence on the complication rate of phacoemulsification cataract surgery.

Subsequent reports have shown that the prevalence of XFS may not influence the surgical outcome. A retrospective study[31] reported that the overall rate of vitreous loss was 4% (7/297) in the XFS cohort compared to 0% (0/427) in the non-XFS group, but again, due to the low prevalence of the condition, the study had insufficient power to demonstrate a significant difference between the two groups.

The same group[92] in a more recent retrospective report on 1000 consecutive patients who underwent cataract surgery by the same surgeon, compared intraoperative and postoperative complications, best corrected visual acuity, IOP, and glaucoma medication use between 137 eyes with clinically apparent XFS and fellow eyes without evidence of XFS in those patients undergoing bilateral cataract surgery. They did not observe significant differences between the two groups. The eyes with XFS had a significantly greater IOP reduction after surgery than the fellow eyes without XFS. The XFS group required more glaucoma medications overall and needed more glaucoma medications at 3–5 years than preoperatively.

Akinci et al.[93] were in general agreement with the previous studies and concluded that patients with XFS who undergo phacoemulsification cataract surgery can achieve results almost similar to patients without XFS. However, they suggested that IOP control in the early postoperative period is more important in patients with XFS. Another controlled study[84] suggested that XFS does not impact the incidence of intraoperative complications nor the rate of late intraocular lens dislocation. The authors compared 67 cases with XFS versus 1670 control cases. There were no cases of intraocular lens dislocation over a mean follow-up period of 54.1 months. Although the authors considered that caution is still advised in patients with XFS who undergo phacoemulsification, surgical results can be achieved similar to patients without XFS. Although the view that XFS is not a significant risk factor in cataract surgery is supported by several investigations, most of the literature on the subject is difficult to assess critically due to a number of methodology errors and biases. As reviewed by Drolsum and coworkers,[45] XFS is a risk factor for phacoemulsification cataract surgery in ethnic cohorts with high prevalence of XFS and when all cases of XFS are diagnosed and included in the cohorts under investigation. At the present time there is no agreement on this subject, and large prospective adequately powered studies with conclusive evidence are required to elucidate this topic.

Corneal Changes in XFS

A feature stressed by some writers is that patients with XFS may have reduced corneal endothelial reserve. Awareness of this factor may help minimize the degree of intraoperative endothelial cell loss and avoid postoperative corneal failure. Preoperative assessment in selected eyes with XFS or XFG should therefore include careful clinical evaluation of endothelial status and corneal health assessment along with preoperative counseling of patients considered at risk of corneal decompensation. Performance of endothelial cell count is an important evaluation in these patients. During surgery the use of a viscoelastic material that coats and protects the corneal endothelial surface or higher viscosity hyaluronate may help in these patients,[53] but further controlled data are required.

In contrast, Kaljurand et al.[94] claimed that XFS per se does not have a negative influence on endothelial cell loss. They compared in a small prospective series 27 consecutive patients with and 26 patients without XFS scheduled for cataract surgery, and they evaluated the influence of cataract surgery to cornea endothelium and thickness. They monitored corneal endothelial cells preoperatively and postoperatively at 1 day and 1 month after surgery using non-contact specular microscopy. According to these authors there were no significant preoperative differences in endothelium morphology between the two study groups. The mean endothelial cell loss 1 month after surgery was 18.1% in the XFS group and 11.6% in the control group ($P = 0.06$). Phaco time and volume of balanced salt solution (BSS) values were significantly greater in patients with XFS, but according to the authors had no significant influence on endothelial cell loss. By regression analysis, only phaco power and

age had a significant influence on endothelial cell loss count. Only by increasing overall phacoemulsification time, XFS exerted a negative influence on corneal endothelium. Still, the authors concluded that XFS in certain cases may significantly increase the risk of endothelial cell loss.

Postoperative Complications

After surgery, careful monitoring is important in patients with XFS for the early detection and treatment of complications occurring in the early postoperative period. Inflammation and postoperative IOP spikes and, in the long term, secondary cataract development/capsular opacification and IOL decentration are reported to be more common in XFS. The higher rate of postoperative inflammation together with the impaired trabecular meshwork and blood–ocular barrier defect present in XFS result in an increased risk of postoperative IOP elevation in XFS eyes. Postoperative IOP spikes should therefore be expected and ideally be prevented by monitoring IOP and using prophylactic ocular and systemic hypotensive agents,[53] especially in XFG patients with compromised optic nerve function. Patients with XFS without evidence of ocular hypertension or glaucoma are at higher risk to develop IOP elevation postoperatively than patients with normal eyes.[93] The postoperative IOP spikes seem to be more pronounced after the ECCE technique, which is likely to increase the subsequent tissue reaction—given the area and degree of surgical trauma—with exaggerated breakdown of the blood–aqueous barrier and subsequent obstruction of the trabecular meshwork.[15]

Shastri and Vasavada,[83] after performing phacoemulsification cataract extraction, recorded IOP higher than 22 mmHg in 22.6% of XFS eyes and 13.3% of control eyes as measured on the first postoperative day, but this difference was not statistically significant. An increased risk of early IOP rise was also observed by Pohjalainen et al.[27] However, these observations have not been confirmed by another study.[26] This discrepancy may be explained by differences in inclusion criteria and surgical techniques. Several surgeons believe that some of the early postoperative IOP spikes can be attributed to the type of viscoelastic material that had been used. A meticulous removal of the viscoelastic material at the end of the procedure should be performed and may decrease the incidence and severity of postoperative spikes. On the other hand, as mentioned previously, IOP reduction has been recorded after phacoemulsification in both normal and glaucomatous eyes,[95] while some reports indicate that the IOP reduction over time is greater in XFS patients.[26,30,31]

Finally, careful follow-up after cataract surgery is necessary in patients with XFS, particularly those with in-the-sulcus IOL implantation, to monitor the development of XFG.[96]

Inflammation after cataract extraction—especially after ECCE—is more common in eyes with XFS than in those without, and a transient fibrinoid reaction, attributed to the concomitant breakdown of the blood-aqueous barrier, may occur.[97] Evidence of blood-aqueous barrier impairment in XFS and especially XFG has been suggested by studies using fluorescein angiography, fluorophotometry,[98] and the laser flare-cell meter.[99] The abnormal blood–aqueous barrier is an integral part of the condition.

Importantly, eyes with XFS may show evidence of a further breakdown in the blood–aqueous barrier in the immediate postoperative period, manifested as increased aqueous flare, cells, fibrinous inflammatory reaction, posterior synechiae formation, and a more prolonged recovery time after surgery. Several authors suggest a more intense postoperative treatment with topical dexamethasone, which may be beneficial along with more prolonged therapy and, in rare selected cases, systemic corticosteroid therapy.[51,52] The mechanical stretching of small pupils intraoperatively may also further increase postoperative inflammation. A high correlation between aqueous flare measurements and aqueous protein concentration in eyes with XFS has been described by Kuchle et al.[99]

Intraocular Lens Dislocation

Several studies have reported that anterior capsule contraction in XFS and the potentially weakened zonules can lead to late intraocular lens decentration.[57,100] Furthermore, the development of "in the bag" IOL dislocation is a recognized late complication of cataract surgery in XFS. In XFS, zonular weakness predisposes to zonular dehiscence secondary to capsular fibrosis, which can lead to IOL dislocation within the bag. It is important to recognize areas of zonular weakness and to consider prophylactic support with a capsular tension ring (CTR) at the time of surgery.[101] Indeed, dislocation or simple decentration of the IOL within the bag can occur several years after uneventful surgery. This complication is due to progressive zonular disintegration and capsular shrinkage.[58,100,102–104]

Scherer et al.[105] described two patients with XFS in whom late spontaneous in-the-bag intraocular lens (IOL) and capsular tension ring (CTR) dislocation occurred 3 and 6 years following cataract surgery. The patients had CTRs inserted because of phacodonesis due to zonular fragility. In both cases, removal of the IOL and CTR within the capsular bag was performed uneventfully and an anterior chamber IOL was implanted. Capsular tension ring implantation in XFS-associated zonular weakening does not guarantee long-term zonular stability and capsular bag/IOL position in these patients after cataract surgery.

Several mechanisms may be involved in postoperative capsule dislocation such as preoperative zonular weakness, surgical trauma to the zonules, capsule contraction syndrome, and postoperative trauma. The exact contribution of each mechanism probably varies on a case-by-case basis. Dislocation of intraocular lenses within the capsular bag is a late complication of cataract surgery and is reported with increasing frequency in recent years. The presence of XFS, uveitis, myopia, and other diseases associated with progressive zonular weakening and capsular contraction are the commonest predisposing conditions.[104,106] Subluxation of the IOL can occur if the zonules break or the capsular bag dislocates. From this point of view, choice of IOL is therefore important in eyes with XFS.

According to some authors, the diameter of the capsulorrhexis should be at least 5 mm in order to minimize zonular stress, supporting the hypothesis that a large diameter helps to prevent the contraction of the anterior capsule in XFS.[57,107] On the other hand, several authors have recorded no relationship between CCC size and shrinkage.[108] It should be noted, however, that XFS has been reported as the cause in more than 50% of all late in-the-bag IOL dislocations. The incidence of this late postoperative complication should be expected to increase in the years to come.[104] Remember, the use of a capsular tension ring (CTR) does not guarantee protection from late capsule fibrosis, shrinkage, and dislocation.[104,105,109,110]

Capsule Contraction Syndrome

The degree of anterior capsule contraction is believed to be related to many factors, including the state of lens capsule and zonules of the patient, concurrent ocular pathology, IOL material and composition, and surgical complications. CCS is common in patients with XFS and in eyes with a history of uveitis. Indeed, the degree of anterior capsule contraction varies substantially between each individual, although it has been shown that the contraction is more pronounced in eyes with ocular pathologies such as retinitis pigmentosa, exfoliation syndrome, and diabetic retinopathy.[57,111] The hypothesis that capsule contraction syndrome is much more common after capsulorrhexis because of an exaggerated reduction in capsular opening and capsular bag diameter after cataract extraction was supported by several authors.[57,111] According to Hayashi,[57] this anterior capsule opening contraction was more extensive in the XFS eyes than in the control eyes, thus resulting in a high Nd:YAG laser anterior capsulotomy rate. IOL tilt was also more frequent in the XFS eyes than in the control eyes. In cases of pronounced fibrosis and shrinkage of the anterior capsule without decentration of an in-the-bag IOL, Nd:YAG laser radial anterior capsulotomy is recommended.[110]

Anterior Capsular Phimosis

Anterior capsular phimosis (ACP) is now a well-recognized complication following phacoemulsification and intraocular lens implantation. Risk factors for ACP among others (diabetes mellitus, retinitis pigmentosa, and uveitis) include XFS, while intraoperative complications and intraocular lens design and material may also play a role. A case of severe capsular phimosis following implantation of a hydrophobic acrylic intraocular lens with polymethyl methacrylate haptics in a patient with XFS has recently been described by Venkatesh and coworkers.[112]

Posterior Capsular Opacification

Posterior capsular opacification (PCO) and secondary cataract (SC) could be considered to be another potential complication of cataract surgery in eyes with XFS. In a retrospective study, carried out by Kuchle et al.[113] over a period of 2 years, PCO and secondary cataract was recorded in 45% of XFS eyes versus 24% in the controls. This increased risk for PCO and SC in XFS eyes may be due, among other factors, to the impaired blood–aqueous barrier, to increased inflammatory activity, and to hypoxia of the anterior chamber, which may subsequently facilitate migration of lens epithelial cells. However, during the last decade, the postoperative inflammatory response in eyes that have undergone phacoemulsification surgery is much lower than that recorded after ECCE, as is the frequency of secondary cataract in general. This is due to improvements in IOL design and material, as well as due to the new phaco technology and improved surgical techniques.[114,115] Therefore, even in XFS eyes the risk of developing secondary cataract is probably lower today than it was some years ago.

Combined Cataract and Glaucoma Surgery in XFG Patients

It is well known that cataracts (mainly nuclear and subcapsular) are commonly associated with XFS[116,117] and that eyes with XFS or XFG are more prone to have complications during cataract surgery.[42,118] Clinicians face quite frequently the coexistence of XFG and cataract in the same eye. For those eyes, surgery may be indicated either because of inadequate control of XFG (uncontrolled IOP or visual field defect progression) and/or because of visually significant cataract. There are several possible surgical approaches for an eye with XFG with visually significant cataract: either phacoemulsification and IOL implantation alone or combined cataract–glaucoma surgery. Generally speaking, when

there is little or moderate optic nerve head damage, and the IOP is reasonably well controlled with medical therapy, cataract surgery with temporal corneal incision alone is indicated. There are several advantages of this approach. First, the conjunctiva is not affected by this approach, saving the conjunctiva from scarring, which is clinically important if filtering surgery is needed in the future. Second, visual recovery occurs more promptly. As described previously, the IOP control is expected to be better after cataract extraction, especially in eyes with XFG. Importantly, the additional surgical complications due to the filtering procedure are avoided. In addition, it is well established that the hypotensive efficacy of combined cataract and glaucoma surgery is less than that of filtering surgery alone.[119,120] This fact is probably due to the inflammatory reaction caused by cataract extraction and its detrimental effect on bleb development. This has also been demonstrated when cataract surgery is performed in eyes with a pre-existing filtering bleb.[121] See Chapter 16.

Nevertheless, one of the commonest complications of cataract surgery is an acute IOP increase in the early post-op period,[122] and although this IOP increase is usually self-limited, it may lead to irreversible visual field loss, especially in eyes with pre-existing severe optic nerve damage. This is why combined cataract and glaucoma surgery should be considered in XFG eyes with poor IOP control and/or severe glaucoma damage. In that scenario, a careful evaluation of the optic nerve and visual field status is mandatory in the preoperative exam of every XFG patient with coexisting glaucoma and cataract. Visual field tests using stimulus size V, instead of the usual size III, may be helpful[123] in order to document changes in functional visual field, which are otherwise rarely sought in patients with glaucoma.

General Surgical Techniques for a Combined Approach

It is widely accepted that conventional phacoemulsification and intraocular lens (IOL) implantation is the best approach for cataract surgery nowadays. On the other hand, there are several glaucoma surgical procedures that may be employed together with cataract surgery in XFG eyes. Direct trabecular aspiration at the time of cataract surgery has been shown to be beneficial in terms of IOP control in XFG eyes,[124] with a better safety profile than phacotrabeculectomy, and better IOP control than cataract surgery alone for at least 2 years after surgery. These procedures have been shown to be effective when associated with cataract surgery. Combined tube implant and filtration surgery is usually reserved for refractory glaucoma cases.[125]

Although several combined procedures are available, a short comment is provided here for the commonest surgical choices of phacotrabeculectomy and combined phaco-deep sclerectomy.

There is no consensus on which filtering procedure (trabeculectomy, deep sclerectomy, or viscocanalostomy) offers the best risk/benefit ratio in combined procedures specifically in XFG. A recent report suggests better IOP control after combined surgery with deep sclerectomy than after standard phacotrabeculectomy.[126] Another, non-controlled study[127] suggests a low complication rate after combined cataract and non-penetrating filtering surgery in XFG eyes, but there is limited information on the long-term success of these procedures.

For combined surgery, it appears that there is no difference between a one site and two site approach[131], unless the surgeon chooses to perform a non-penetrating procedure. In this case, a two-site approach is mandatory. The filtering procedure is performed as usual, generally after the cataract surgery and IOL implantation have been performed. There is no consensus regarding the efficacy of antimetabolites in combined cataract-filtering procedures. The use of antimetabolites (mitomycin C or 5-fluorouracil [5-FU]) seem to significantly increase the success rate in a large follow-up study of phacotrabeculectomy,[128] although other authors question its benefit.[129] It may offer some advantages in terms of IOP control[128]; the effect seems to be less than that seen in primary filtering procedures.[130] So there is no clear evidence to recommend its widespread use. Generally, little controlled information exists on the success of antimetabolites in combined surgery in eyes with XFG.

Regarding the preference for either penetrating surgery (conventional trabeculectomy) or a non-penetrating procedure (deep sclerectomy or viscocanalostomy) in combined procedures there are very little data in the literature for XFG. Both procedures show significant IOP lowering, but there is limited evidence for any difference between them. Nevertheless, given the fact that combined phacotrabeculectomy is the standard procedure that has passed the "test of time," the non-penetrating approach has to prove its efficacy and/or safety in the combined approach before it is recommended in XFG.

Postoperative Care and Complications

There is some evidence to suggest that a combined procedure in XFG is associated with more complications than seen in eyes with POAG.[128] The postoperative care of combined procedures is virtually the same as that employed after a filtering procedure in XFG, and the surgeon may use any of the well-known maneuvers either to increase the filtration (laser suture lysis, massage, 5-FU injections) or to decrease it (bandage contact lens, ocular patching, etc.). Inflammation

may be more prominent in eyes with XFG and thus steroids should be used for a longer period. Avoidance of a postoperative flat anterior chamber is important because the endothelium may already be damaged by cataract surgery, and the optic of the IOL may be more harmful to the corneal endothelium than the anterior lens capsule of a phakic eye.

Summary

Cataract surgery alone is the recommended approach for eyes with well-controlled XFG and mild or moderate glaucoma damage. A significantly lower IOP is expected after cataract surgery alone, although potentially harmful IOP peaks may appear in the early post-op. Careful preoperative evaluation of the glaucoma status is mandatory in these cases. Combined cataract and filtering procedures offer improved IOP control in the short term than cataract surgery alone, although the hypotensive effect is significantly lower than expected for a filtering procedure when performed alone, in the mid to long term.

References

1. Tarkkanen A, Kivela T. John G. Lindberg and the discovery of exfoliation syndrome. *Acta Ophthalmol Scand.* 2002;80(2): 151–154.
2. Ritch R. Exfoliation syndrome and occludable angles. *Trans Am Ophthalmol Soc.* 1994;92:845–944.
3. Ritch R, Konstas AG, Schlotzer-Schrehardt U. Exfoliation syndrome and exfoliative glaucoma. In: Shaarawy T, Sherwood M, Hitchings R, Crowston J, eds. *Glaucoma.* Amsterdam: Elsevier; 2009.
4. Ringvold A. Epidemiology of the pseudo-exfoliation syndrome. *Acta Ophthalmol Scand.* 1999;77(4):371–375.
5. Ritch R, Schlotzer-Schrehardt U. Exfoliation syndrome. *Surv Ophthalmol.* 2001;45(4):265–315.
6. Vesti E, Kivela T. Exfoliation syndrome and exfoliation glaucoma. *Prog Retin Eye Res.* 2000;19(3):345–368.
7. Ritch R, Schlotzer-Schrehardt U, Konstas AG. Why is glaucoma associated with exfoliation syndrome? *Prog Retin Eye Res.* 2003;22(3):253–275.
8. Ritch R. The management of exfoliative glaucoma. *Prog Brain Res.* 2008;173:211–224.
9. Naumann GO, Schlotzer-Schrehardt U, Kuchle M. Pseudoexfoliation syndrome for the comprehensive ophthalmologist. Intraocular and systemic manifestations. *Ophthalmology.* 1998;105(6):951–968.
10. Konstas AG, Tsironi S, Ritch R. Current concepts in the pathogenesis and management of exfoliation syndrome and exfoliative glaucoma. *Compr Ophthalmol Update.* 2006;7(3): 131–141.
11. Holló G, Konstas AG, eds. *Exfoliation Syndrome and Exfoliative Glaucoma.* Savona: Dogma S.r.l.; 2008:1–161.
12. Schlotzer-Schrehardt U. Molecular pathology of pseudoexfoliation syndrome/glaucoma—new insights from LOXL1 gene associations. *Exp Eye Res.* 2009;88:776–785.

13. Thorleifsson G, Magnusson KP, Sulem P, et al. Common sequence variants in the LOXL1 gene confer susceptibility to exfoliation glaucoma. *Science.* 2007;317(5843):1397–400.

14. Koliakos GG, Konstas AG, Schlotzer-Schrehardt U, et al. Ascorbic acid concentration is reduced in the aqueous humor of patients with exfoliation syndrome. *Am J Ophthalmol.* 2002;134(6): 879–883.

15. Drolsum L, Ringvold A, Nicolaissen B. Cataract and glaucoma surgery in pseudoexfoliation syndrome: a review. *Acta Ophthalmol Scand.* 2007;85(8):810–821.

16. Sekeroglu MA, Bozkurt B, Irkec M, et al. Systemic associations and prevalence of exfoliation syndrome in patients scheduled for cataract surgery. *Eur J Ophthalmol.* 2008;18(4):551–555.

17. Prince AM, Streeten BW, Ritch R, Dark AJ, Sperling M. Preclinical diagnosis of pseudoexfoliation syndrome. *Arch Ophthalmol.* 1987;105(8):1076–1082.

18. Krause U, Tarkkanen A. Cataract and pseudoexfoliation. A clinicopathological study. *Acta Ophthalmol (Copenh).* 1978;56(3):329–334.

19. Tarkkanen A. Is exfoliation syndrome a sign of systemic vascular disease? *Acta Ophthalmol.* 2008;86(8):832–836.

20. Visontai Z, Horváth T, Kollai M, Holló G. Decreased cardiovagal regulation in exfoliation syndrome. *J Glaucoma.* 2008;17(2):133–138.

21. Mitchell P, Wang JJ, Smith W. Association of pseudoexfoliation syndrome with increased vascular risk. *Am J Ophthalmol.* 1997;124(5):685–687.

22. Konstas AG, Mantziris DA, Stewart WC. Diurnal intraocular pressure in untreated exfoliation and primary open-angle glaucoma. *Arch Ophthalmol.* 1997;115(2):182–185.

23. Konstas AG, Hollo G, Astakhov YS, et al. Factors associated with long-term progression or stability in exfoliation glaucoma. *Arch Ophthalmol.* 2004;122(1):29–33.

24. Wirbelauer C, Anders N, Pham DT, Wollensak J, Laqua H. Intraocular pressure in nonglaucomatous eyes with pseudoexfoliation syndrome after cataract surgery. *Ophthalmic Surg Lasers.* 1998;29(6):466–471.

25. Suzuki R, Kuroki S, Fujiwara N. Ten-year follow-up of intraocular pressure after phacoemulsification and aspiration with intraocular lens implantation performed by the same surgeon. *Ophthalmologica.* 1997;211(2):79–83.

26. Merkur A, Damji KF, Mintsioulis G, Hodge WG. Intraocular pressure decrease after phacoemulsification in patients with pseudoexfoliation syndrome. *J Cataract Refract Surg.* 2001;27(4):528–532.

27. Pohjalainen T, Vesti E, Uusitalo RJ, Laatikainen L. Intraocular pressure after phacoemulsification and intraocular lens implantation in nonglaucomatous eyes with and without exfoliation. *J Cataract Refract Surg.* 2001;27(3):426–431.

28. Suzuki R, Tanaka K, Sagara T, Fujiwara N. Reduction of intraocular pressure after phacoemulsification and aspiration with intraocular lens implantation. *Ophthalmologica.* 1994;208(5):254–258.

29. Yalvac I, Airaksinen PJ, Tuulonen A. Phacoemulsification with and without trabeculectomy in patients with glaucoma. *Ophthalmic Surg Lasers.* 1997;28(6):469–475.

30. Dosso AA, Bonvin ER, Leuenberger PM. Exfoliation syndrome and phacoemulsification. *J Cataract Refract Surg.* 1997;23(1):122–125.

31. Shingleton BJ, Heltzer J, O'Donoghue MW. Outcomes of phacoemulsification in patients with and without pseudoexfoliation syndrome. *J Cataract Refract Surg.* 2003;29(6):1080–1086.

32. Damji KF, Konstas AG, Liebmann JM, et al. Intraocular pressure following phacoemulsification in patients with and without exfoliation syndrome: a 2 year prospective study. *Br J Ophthalmol.* 2006;90(8):1014–1018.

33. Jacobi PC, Krieglstein GK. Trabecular aspiration: clinical results of a new surgical approach to improve trabecular facility in glaucoma capsulare. *Ophthalmic Surg.* 1994;25(9):641–645.

34. Jacobi PC, Krieglstein GK. Trabecular aspiration. A new mode to treat pseudoexfoliation glaucoma. *Invest Ophthalmol Vis Sci.* 1995;36(11):2270–2276.

35. Jacobi PC, Dietlein TS, Krieglstein GK. Bimanual trabecular aspiration in pseudoexfoliation glaucoma: an alternative in nonfiltering glaucoma surgery. *Ophthalmology.* 1998;105(5):886–894.

36. Cimetta DJ, Cimetta AC. Intraocular pressure changes after clear corneal phacoemulsification in nonglaucomatous pseudoexfoliation syndrome. *Eur J Ophthalmol.* 2008;18(1):77–81.

37. Althaus C, Demmer E, Sundmacher R. Anterior capsular shrinkage and intraocular pressure reduction after capsulorhexis. *Ger J Ophthalmol.* 1994;3(3):154–158.

38. Skuta GL, Parrish RK 2nd, Hodapp E, Forster RK, Rockwood EJ. Zonular dialysis during extracapsular cataract extraction in pseudoexfoliation syndrome. *Arch Ophthalmol.* 1987;105(5): 632–634.

39. Guzek JP, Holm M, Cotter JB, et al. Risk factors for intraoperative complications in 1000 extracapsular cataract cases. *Ophthalmology.* 1987;94(5):461–466.

40. Moreno J, Duch D, Lajara J. Pseudoexfoliation syndrome: clinical factors related to capsular rupture in cataract surgery. *Acta Ophthalmol (Copenh).* 1993;71(2):181–184.

41. Drolsum L, Haaskjold E, Davanger M. Results and complications after extracapsular cataract extraction in eyes with pseudoexfoliation syndrome. *Acta Ophthalmol (Copenh).* 1993;71(6):771–776.

42. Alfaiate M, Leite E, Mira J, Cunha-Vaz JG. Prevalence and surgical complications of pseudoexfoliation syndrome in Portuguese patients with senile cataract. *J Cataract Refract Surg.* 1996;22(7):972–976.

43. Chitkara DK, Smerdon DL. Risk factors, complications, and results in extracapsular cataract extraction. *J Cataract Refract Surg.* 1997;23(4):570–574.

44. Fine IH, Hoffman RS. Phacoemulsification in the presence of pseudoexfoliation: challenges and options. *J Cataract Refract Surg.* 1997;23(2):160–165.

45. Drolsum L, Haaskjold E, Sandvig K. Phacoemulsification in eyes with pseudoexfoliation. *J Cataract Refract Surg.* 1998;24(6):787–792.

46. Scorolli L, Scorolli L, Campos EC, Bassein L, Meduri RA. Pseudoexfoliation syndrome: a cohort study on intraoperative complications in cataract surgery. *Ophthalmologica.* 1998;212(4): 278–280.

47. Küchle M, Viestenz A, Martus P, Händel A, Jünemann A, Naumann GO. Anterior chamber depth and complications during cataract surgery in eyes with pseudoexfoliation syndrome. *Am J Ophthalmol.* 2000;129(3):281–285.

48. Schlotzer-Schrehardt U, Naumann GO. A histopathologic study of zonular instability in pseudoexfoliation syndrome. *Am J Ophthalmol.* 1994;118(6):730–743.

49. Repo LP, Naukkarinen A, Paljärvi L, Teräsvirta ME. Pseudoexfoliation syndrome with poorly dilating pupil: a light and electron microscopic study of the sphincter area. *Graefes Arch Clin Exp Ophthalmol.* 1996;234(3):171–176.

50. Wirbelauer C, Anders N, Pham DT, Wollensak J. Corneal endothelial cell changes in pseudoexfoliation syndrome after cataract surgery. *Arch Ophthalmol.* 1998;116(2):145–149.

51. Küchle M, Nguyen NX, Hannappel E, Naumann GO. The blood-aqueous barrier in eyes with pseudoexfoliation syndrome. *Ophthalmic Res.* 1995;27(Suppl 1):136–142.

52. Schumacher S, Nguyen NX, Küchle M, Naumann GO. Quantification of aqueous flare after phacoemulsification with intraocular lens implantation in eyes with pseudoexfoliation syndrome. *Arch Ophthalmol.* 1999;117(6):733–735.

53. Conway RM, Schlötzer-Schrehardt U, Küchle M, Naumann GO. Pseudoexfoliation syndrome: pathological manifestations of relevance to intraocular surgery. *Clin Exp Ophthalmol.* 2004;32(2):199–210.

54. Drolsum L, Davanger M, Haaskjold E. Risk factors for an inflammatory response after extracapsular cataract extraction and posterior chamber IOL. *Acta Ophthalmol (Copenh).* 1994;72(1):21–26.

55. Hyams M, Mathalone N, Herskovitz M, Hod Y, Israeli D, Geyer O. Intraoperative complications of phacoemulsification in eyes with and without pseudoexfoliation. *J Cataract Refract Surg.* 2005;31(5):1002–1005.

56. Akman A, Yilmaz G, Oto S, Akova YA. Comparison of various pupil dilatation methods for phacoemulsification in eyes with a small pupil secondary to pseudoexfoliation. *Ophthalmology.* 2004;111(9):1693–1698.

57. Hayashi H, Hayashi K, Nakao F, Hayashi F. Anterior capsule contraction and intraocular lens dislocation in eyes with pseudoexfoliation syndrome. *Br J Ophthalmol.* 1998;82(12):1429–1432.

58. Jehan FS, Mamalis N, Crandall AS. Spontaneous late dislocation of intraocular lens within the capsular bag in pseudoexfoliation patients. *Ophthalmology.* 2001;108(10):1727–1731.

59. Bayraktar S, Altan T, Küçüksümer Y, Yilmaz OF. Capsular tension ring implantation after capsulorhexis in phacoemulsification of cataracts associated with pseudoexfoliation syndrome. Intraoperative complications and early postoperative findings. *J Cataract Refract Surg.* 2001;27(10):1620–1628.

60. Nordlund ML, Marques DM, Marques FF, Cionni RJ, Osher RH. Techniques for managing common complications of cataract surgery. *Curr Opin Ophthalmol.* 2003;14(1):7–19.

61. Dick HB, Augustin AJ. Lens implant selection with absence of capsular support. *Curr Opin Ophthalmol.* 2001;12(1):47–57.

62. Drolsum L. Long-term follow-up of secondary flexible, open-loop, anterior chamber intraocular lenses. *J Cataract Refract Surg.* 2003;29(3):498–503.

63. Ravalico G, Tognetto D, Baccara F. Heparin-surface-modified intraocular lens implantation in eyes with pseudoexfoliation syndrome. *J Cataract Refract Surg.* 1994;20(5):543–549.

64. Chang DF. Prevention of bag-fixated IOL dislocation in pseudoexfoliation. *Ophthalmology.* 2002;109(11):1951–1952.

65. Cionni RJ, Osher RH. Endocapsular ring approach to the subluxed cataractous lens. *J Cataract Refract Surg.* 1995;21(3):245–249.

66. Lee V, Bloom P. Microhook capsule stabilization for phacoemulsification in eyes with pseudoexfoliation-syndrome-induced lens instability. *J Cataract Refract Surg.* 1999;25(12):1567–1570.

67. Santoro S, Sannace C, Cascella MC, Lavermicocca N. Subluxated lens: phacoemulsification with iris hooks. *J Cataract Refract Surg.* 2003;29(12):2269–2273.

68. Nishimura E, Yaguchi S, Nishihara H, Ayaki M, Kozawa T. Capsular stabilization device to preserve lens capsule integrity during phacoemulsification with a weak zonule. *J Cataract Refract Surg.* 2006;32(3):392–395.

69. Hara T, Yamada Y. "Equator ring" for maintenance of the completely circular contour of the capsular bag equator after cataract removal. *Ophthalmic Surg.* 1991;22(6):358–359.

70. Hasanee K, Butler M, Ahmed II. Capsular tension rings and related devices: current concepts. *Curr Opin Ophthalmol.* 2006;17(1):31–41.

71. Sun R, Gimbel HV. In vitro evaluation of the efficacy of the capsular tension ring for managing zonular dialysis in cataract surgery. *Ophthalmic Surg Lasers.* 1998;29(6):502–505.

72. Menapace R, Findl O, Georgopoulos M, Rainer G, Vass C, Schmetterer K. The capsular tension ring: designs, applications, and techniques. *J Cataract Refract Surg.* 2000;26(6):898–912.

73. Fine IH. Cortical cleaving hydrodissection. *J Cataract Refract Surg.* 1992;18(5):508–512.

74. Ahmed II, Cionni RJ, Kranemann C, Crandall AS. Optimal timing of capsular tension ring implantation: Miyake-Apple video analysis. *J Cataract Refract Surg.* 2005;31(9):1809–1813.

75. Gimbel HV, Sun R, Heston JP. Management of zonular dialysis in phacoemulsification and IOL implantation using the capsular tension ring. *Ophthalmic Surg Lasers.* 1997;28(4):273–281.

76. Moreno-Montanes J, Heras H, Fernandez-Hortelano A. Extraction of endocapsular tension ring after phacoemulsification in eyes with pseudoexfoliation. *Am J Ophthalmol.* 2004;138(1):173–175.

77. Cionni RJ, Osher RH. Management of profound zonular dialysis or weakness with a new endocapsular ring designed for scleral fixation. *J Cataract Refract Surg.* 1998;24(10):1299–1306.

78. Goder GJ, Rechlin RG. The exfoliation in the Scheimpflug photography. *Acta Ophthalmol Suppl.* 1988;184:44–47.

79. Inazumi K, Takahashi D, Taniguchi T, Yamamoto T. Ultrasound biomicroscopic classification of zonules in exfoliation syndrome. *Jpn J Ophthalmol.* 2002;46(5):502–509.

80. Katsimpris JM, Petropoulos IK, Apostolakis K, Feretis D. Comparing phacoemulsification and extracapsular cataract extraction in eyes with pseudoexfoliation syndrome, small pupil, and phacodonesis. *Klin Monatsbl Augenheilkd.* 2004;221(5):328–333.

81. Ruotsalainen J, Tarkkanen A. Capsule thickness of cataractous lenses with and without exfoliation syndrome. *Acta Ophthalmol (Copenh).* 1987;65(4):444–449.

82. Ritch R, Schlotzer-Schrehardt U. Exfoliation (pseudoexfoliation) syndrome: toward a new understanding. Proceedings of the First International Think Tank. *Acta Ophthalmol Scand.* 2001;79(2):213–217.

83. Shastri L, Vasavada A. Phacoemulsification in Indian eyes with pseudoexfoliation syndrome. *J Cataract Refract Surg.* 2001;27(10):1629–1637.

84. Nagashima RJ. Decreased incidence of capsule complications and vitreous loss during phacoemulsification in eyes with pseudoexfoliation syndrome. *J Cataract Refract Surg.* 2004;30(1):127–131.

85. Bartholomew RS. Lens displacement associated with pseudocapsular exfoliation. A report on 19 cases in the Southern Bantu. *Br J Ophthalmol.* 1970;54(11):744–750.

86. Busic M, Kastelan S. Pseudoexfoliation syndrome and cataract surgery by phacoemulsification. *Coll Antropol.* 2005;29(Suppl 1):163–166.

87. Auffarth GU, Blum M, Faller U, Tetz MR, Völcker HE. Relative anterior microphthalmos: morphometric analysis and its implications for cataract surgery. *Ophthalmology.* 2000;107(8):1555–1560.

88. Parmar P, Salman A. Anterior "lenticonus" in exfoliation syndrome. *Indian J Ophthalmol.* 2005;53(3):193–194.

89. Bayramlar H, Hepsen IF, Yilmaz H. Mature cataracts increase risk of capsular complications in manual small-incision cataract surgery of pseudoexfoliative eyes. *Can J Ophthalmol.* 2007;42(1):46–50.

90. Hammer T, Schlotzer-Schrehardt U, Naumann GO. Unilateral or asymmetric pseudoexfoliation syndrome? An ultrastructural study. *Arch Ophthalmol.* 2001;119(7):1023–1031.

91. Menkhaus S, Motschmann M, Kuchenbecker J, Behrens-Baumann W. Pseudoexfoliation (PEX) syndrome and intraoperative complications in cataract surgery. *Klin Monatsbl Augenheilkd.* 2000;216(6):388–392.

92. Shingleton BJ, Nguyen BK, Eagan EF, Nagao K, O'Donoghue MW. Outcomes of phacoemulsification in fellow eyes of patients with unilateral pseudoexfoliation: single-surgeon series. *J Cataract Refract Surg.* 2008;34(2):274–279.

93. Akinci A, Batman C, Zilelioglu O. Phacoemulsification in pseudoexfoliation syndrome. *Ophthalmologica*. 2008;222(2): 112–116.

94. Kaljurand K, Teesalu P. Exfoliation syndrome as a risk factor for corneal endothelial cell loss in cataract surgery. *Ann Ophthalmol (Skokie)*. 2007;39(4):327–333.

95. Mathalone N, Hyams M, Neiman S, Buckman G, Hod Y, Geyer O. Long-term intraocular pressure control after clear corneal phacoemulsification in glaucoma patients. *J Cataract Refract Surg*. 2005;31(3):479–483.

96. Park KA, Kee C. Pseudoexfoliative material on the IOL surface and development of glaucoma after cataract surgery in patients with pseudoexfoliation syndrome. *J Cataract Refract Surg*. 2007;33(10):1815–1818.

97. Wålinder PE, Olivius EO, Nordell SI, Thorburn WE. Fibrinoid reaction after extracapsular cataract extraction and relationship to exfoliation syndrome. *J Cataract Refract Surg*. 1989;15(5): 526–530.

98. Brooks AM, Gillies WE. Fluorescein angiography and fluorophotometry of the iris in pseudoexfoliation of the lens capsule. *Br J Ophthalmol*. 1983;67(4):249–254.

99. Küchle M, Nguyen NX, Hannappel E, Beck W, Ho ST, Naumann GO. Tyndallometry with the laser flare cell meter and biochemical protein determination in the aqueous humor of eyes with pseudoexfoliation syndrome. *Ophthalmologe*. 1994;91(5): 578–584.

100. Davison JA. Capsule contraction syndrome. *J Cataract Refract Surg*. 1993;19(5):582–589.

101. Kumar A, Freeman M, Kumar V, Ramanathan US. In the bag IOL dislocation following uncomplicated phacoemulsification. *Cont Lens Anterior Eye*. 2008;31(2):103–106.

102. Auffarth GU, Tsao K, Wesendahl TA, Sugita A, Apple DJ. Centration and fixation of posterior chamber intraocular lenses in eyes with pseudoexfoliation syndrome. An analysis of explanted autopsy eyes. *Acta Ophthalmol Scand*. 1996;74(5):463–467.

103. Gross JG, Kokame GT, Weinberg DV. In-the-bag intraocular lens dislocation. *Am J Ophthalmol*. 2004;137(4):630–635.

104. Gimbel HV, Condon GP, Kohnen T, Olson RJ, Halkiadakis I. Late in-the-bag intraocular lens dislocation: incidence, prevention, and management. *J Cataract Refract Surg*. 2005;31(11):2193–204.

105. Scherer M, Bertelmann E, Rieck P. Late spontaneous in-the-bag intraocular lens and capsular tension ring dislocation in pseudoexfoliation syndrome. *J Cataract Refract Surg*. 2006;32(4):672–675.

106. Breyer DR, Hermeking H, Gerke E. Late dislocation of the capsular bag after phacoemulsification with endocapsular IOL in pseudoexfoliation syndrome. *Ophthalmologe*. 1999;96(4): 248–251.

107. Kimura W, Yamanishi S, Kimura T, Sawada T, Ohte A. Measuring the anterior capsule opening after cataract surgery to assess capsule shrinkage. *J Cataract Refract Surg*. 1998;24(9): 1235–1238.

108. Gonvers M, Sickenberg M, van Melle G. Change in capsulorhexis size after implantation of three types of intraocular lenses. *J Cataract Refract Surg*. 1997;23(2):231–238.

109. Waheed K, Eleftheriadis H, Liu C. Anterior capsular phimosis in eyes with a capsular tension ring. *J Cataract Refract Surg*. 2001;27(10):1688–1690.

110. Moreno-Montanes J, Sanchez-Tocino H, Rodriguez-Conde R. Complete anterior capsule contraction after phacoemulsification with acrylic intraocular lens and endocapsular ring implantation. *J Cataract Refract Surg*. 2002;28(4):717–719.

111. Kato S, Suzuki T, Hayashi Y, et al. Risk factors for contraction of the anterior capsule opening after cataract surgery. *J Cataract Refract Surg*. 2002;28(1):109–112.

112. Venkatesh R, Tan CS, Veena K, Ravindran RD. Severe anterior capsular phimosis following acrylic intraocular lens implantation in a patient with pseudoexfoliation. *Ophthalmic Surg Lasers Imaging*. 2008;39(3):228–229.

113. Küchle M, Amberg A, Martus P, Nguyen NX, Naumann GO. Pseudoexfoliation syndrome and secondary cataract. *Br J Ophthalmol*. 1997;81(10):862–866.

114. Nishi O, Nishi K, Osakabe Y. Effect of intraocular lenses on preventing posterior capsule opacification: design versus material. *J Cataract Refract Surg*. 2004;30(10):2170–2176.

115. Dewey S. Posterior capsule opacification. *Curr Opin Ophthalmol*. 2006;17(1):45–53.

116. Hietanen J, Kivelä T, Vesti E, Tarkkanen A. Exfoliation syndrome in patients scheduled for cataract surgery. *Acta Ophthalmol (Copenh)*. 1992;70(4):440–446.

117. Puska P, Raitta C. Exfoliation syndrome as a risk factor for optic disc changes in nonglaucomatous eyes. *Graefes Arch Clin Exp Ophthalmol*. 1992;230(6):501–504.

118. Avramides S, Traianidis P, Sakkias G. Cataract surgery and lens implantation in eyes with exfoliation syndrome. *J Cataract Refract Surg*. 1997;23(4):583–587.

119. Shields MB. Combined cataract extraction and glaucoma surgery. *Ophthalmology*. 1982;89(3):231–237.

120. Noben KJ, Linsen MC, Zeyen TG. Is combined phacoemulsification and trabeculectomy as effective as trabeculectomy alone? *Bull Soc Belge Ophtalmol*. 1998;270:85–90.

121. Rebolleda G, Munoz-Negrete FJ. Phacoemulsification in eyes with functioning filtering blebs: a prospective study. *Ophthalmology*. 2002;109(12):2248–2255.

122. McCartney DL, Memmen JE, Stark WJ, et al. The efficacy and safety of combined trabeculectomy, cataract extraction, and intraocular lens implantation. *Ophthalmology*. 1988;95(6): 754–763.

123. Teus MA, C.M.A., Sánchez J. Effect of stimulus size on the computerized visual field in glaucomatous patients. *Arch Soc Esp Ophthalmol*. 1996;70:497–501.

124. Jacobi PC, Dietlein TS, Krieglstein GK. Comparative study of trabecular aspiration vs. trabeculectomy in glaucoma triple procedure to treat pseudoexfoliation glaucoma. *Arch Ophthalmol*. 1999;117(10):1311–1318.

125. Nassiri N, Nassiri N, Yarandi SS, Mohammadi B, Rahmani L. Combined phacoemulsification and Ahmed valve glaucoma drainage implant: a retrospective case series. *Eur J Ophthalmol*. 2008;18(2):191–198.

126. Lüke C, Dietlein TS, Lüke M, Konen W, Krieglstein GK. A prospective trial of phaco-trabeculotomy combined with deep sclerectomy versus phaco-trabeculectomy. *Graefes Arch Clin Exp Ophthalmol*. 2008;246(8):1163–1168.

127. Hassan KM, Awadalla MA. Results of combined phacoemulsification and viscocanalostomy in patients with cataract and pseudoexfoliative glaucoma. *Eur J Ophthalmol*. 2008;18(2): 212–219.

128. Rockwood EJ, Larive B, Hahn J. Outcomes of combined cataract extraction, lens implantation, and trabeculectomy surgeries. *Am J Ophthalmol*. 2000;130(6):704–711.

129. Ruderman JM, Fundingsland B, Meyer MA. Combined phacoemulsification and trabeculectomy with mitomycin-C. *J Cataract Refract Surg*. 1996;22(8):1085–1090.

130. Shin DH, Hughes BA, Song MS, et al. Primary glaucoma triple procedure with or without adjunctive mitomycin. Prognostic factors for filtration failure. *Ophthalmology*. 1996;103(11): 1925–1933.

131. Buys YM, et al. Prospective randomized comparison of one- version two-site Phacotrabeculectomy two-year results. *Ophthalmol*. 2008;115(7):1130–1133.

Chapter 16

Cataract Surgery in the Presence of a Functioning Trabeculectomy Bleb

Hylton R. Mayer and James C. Tsai

Introduction

Performing cataract surgery in an eye with a preexisting trabeculectomy bleb raises unique challenges for the ophthalmic surgeon. Addressing the spectrum of bleb morphologies and the anatomic setting in which the cataract exists requires careful attention to detail and an array of surgical skills. Successful preoperative planning, intraoperative execution, and postoperative care can optimize the functional outcome of the bleb and the short- and long-term visual outcome for the patient.

The development of visually significant cataracts in glaucoma patients who have had previous trabeculectomy surgery is common and expected[1-8] (Fig. 16.1). Cataracts and glaucoma share many similar pathogenic origins, including well-documented risk factors such as age, diabetes, steroid use, and trauma.[9-25] In addition, glaucoma and/or elevated intraocular pressure (IOP) and the treatments for glaucoma—including medications, laser, and surgery—have been shown to increase the development of cataracts.[26-29] Conversely, the presence of a cataract can initiate and/or exacerbate ocular hypertension and glaucoma.

Indications for Surgery

The most common indication for cataract extraction is a visually significant cataract, though defining what a visually significant cataract is can be nebulous. In general, cataract surgery is considered when a patient is unable to perform his/her usual activities of daily living due to a decrease in visual function, and when this decrease can be attributed

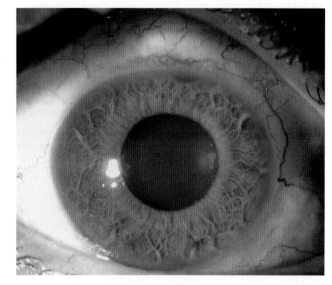

Fig. 16.1 A low, moderately vascular bleb in the presence of a nuclear sclerotic cataract and pseudoexfoliation syndrome. Courtesy of Dr. James C. Tsai

to the cataract. In patients with advanced glaucoma, it may be difficult to determine how much diminished visual function is a result of glaucomatous optic neuropathy and how much visual loss is related to the cataract. Glaucoma patients may also have other ocular morbidities, such as irregular astigmatism related to previous surgery or ocular surface disease, and visual reduction related to peripheral iridectomies or retinal pathology. All glaucoma patients with complaints of decreased vision should initially be refracted to determine their best-corrected visual acuity. It is often useful to have patients clarify the nature of their visual disability. Anecdotally, patients with cataractous visual loss often describe blurry or hazy vision, while patients with glaucomatous visual loss may describe dimmer or darker vision. Visual field testing is a critical step to determine whether vision loss is related to glaucoma progression. Potential acuity meters (PAM) or illuminated near pinhole assessment of visual acuity may also assist in determining visual potential.[30] Assessing visual field loss and identifying

H.R. Mayer (✉)
Department of Ophthalmology, Yale University School of Medicine, New Haven, CT 06510, USA
e-mail: hylton.mayer@yale.edu

alternative causes for visual dysfunction should aid in avoiding unnecessary surgeries as well as improving expectations for patients who have a visually significant cataract in the presence of field defects encroaching on or affecting fixation. In spite of compromised visual function due to glaucoma, cataract removal may reduce refractive errors, glare, and subjective dimming, while enhancing contrast sensitivity. The improvement of general visual function has been shown to improve quality of life as well as reduce morbidity and mortality.[31–37]

Instrumentation and Operative Techniques

The location, functionality, and morphology of the preexisting trabeculectomy bleb are especially relevant when planning cataract extraction after trabeculectomy. In addition, preoperative gonioscopy to visualize and assess the sclerostomy and angle structures may also be helpful for surgical planning. In the presence of an intact bleb, clear corneal cataract surgery likely represents a safer technique compared with a scleral tunnel, as there is less conjunctival manipulation, lowering the risk of bleeding and/or bleb disruption. Decreasing vascular tissue manipulation may also reduce the inflammation that may predispose a bleb to scarring and failure.[38,39] Temporal clear corneal (TCC) cataract incisions have increased in popularity in recent years and may be considered the most reasonable technique for cataract removal in the presence of a bleb. Compared to a superior clear corneal incision, TCC reduces the risk of injuring blebs—especially large, cystic avascular blebs—from incidental damage by the keratome or other surgical instruments. If a suture is required to close the cataract wound, there is less chance for disruption or irritation of an existing bleb. While there is controversy regarding the risk of endophthalmitis in TCC incisions compared with superior incisions, there has been no definitive evidence to support one incision over the other, and most surgeons believe that a properly constructed TCC incision has a low risk of endophthalmitis. The authors prefer a biplanar near-clear temporal corneal incision with a 2.75-mm keratome that results in a square or nearly square corneal tunnel. The wound should be watertight with the IOP at a supraphysiologic level and should not leak with gentle pressure along the posterior border of the wound. If there is any suggestion of wound instability, low IOP due to filtration into the bleb, or if ocular massage is anticipated in the postoperative period, a 10-0 nylon suture is used to reinforce the wound. Wound leaks divert flow from the bleb and cause a bleb to flatten, which can lead to adhesions between the conjunctiva and episclera and failure.

Identifying specific risk factors for individual eyes can help to improve visual outcomes and promote bleb function.

Patients who are using systemic alpha-1 blockers, such as tamsulosin (Flomax), are at an increased risk for intraoperative floppy iris syndrome (IFIS), characterized by iris billowing, prolapse, and miosis (Table 3.1).[40] Reasonable preoperative and intraoperative management strategies, used in combination or alone, include preoperative atropine 1% bid, intraoperative pharmacologic dilation with epinephrine and/or lidocaine (epi-Shugarcaine), the use of dense viscoelastics, such as sodium hyaluronate 23 mg/ml (Healon 5, Advanced Medical Optics, Santa Ana, CA), and mechanical pupil expanders such as iris hooks.[41] See Chapter 3.

Patients with pseudoexfoliation syndrome, a history of topical miotic use, or eyes with posterior synechiae often require iris manipulation to achieve an adequate pupil opening. In many instances, adequate dilation can be achieved with pupil stretching and viscodilation, such as by using opposing Kuglen hooks and a dense viscoelastic (Fig. 3.2). Iris hooks may also be effective in this setting and have the added benefit of reducing the progressive miosis that may occur through the course of the case (Figs. 3.4 and 18.5). Care should be taken when placing hooks to avoid damage to the existing bleb. The use of iris hooks or other iris manipulation may increase inflammation, and has been shown to decrease bleb function[42,43] Other studies, however, have not found the use of iris hooks to have an increased association with bleb dysfunction.[44–46] The authors do not hesitate to use iris hooks when they are felt to be necessary to enable safe and efficient cataract removal.

Manipulation of the pupil may result in fibrin formation. If fibrin blocks filtration postoperatively, and IOP cannot be controlled or if bleb failure is likely due to impaired flow into the bleb, then intracameral tissue plasminogen activator (TPA) can be utilized.[47,48] See Table 16.1.

Table 16.1 Intracameral tissue plasminogen activator (TPA) for anterior chamber fibrinolysis (off-label use)

Alteplase (Actilyse, Genentech, South San Francisco, CA)
- Alteplase is available as 2, 50, and 100 mg dry powder vials.
- Use balanced salt solution to dilute alteplase to 125 μg/ml.
- Following sterile preparation and technique remove 0.2 ml of aqueous and inject 0.2 ml of dilute alteplase (125 micrograms/ml) for a total intracameral dose of 25 micrograms.
- It can be given in 0.1 ml increments—up to twice if needed.
- Residual, reconstituted alteplase can be frozen at −20°C for 12 months for use at a later date by the pharmacy or physician

The authors do not hesitate to use iris hooks when they are felt to be necessary to enable safe and efficient cataract removal.

As with any preoperative cataract surgery evaluation, meticulous care should be taken to assess for zonular instability or absence, as well as for the presence of vitreous in the anterior chamber. Occasionally, zonular disruption and even vitreous loss can occur during the creation of a peripheral iridectomy during trabeculectomy surgery. Aside from the altered phacodynamics associated with vitreous in the anterior chamber and instability of the capsular bag associated with zonular disruption, disruption of the anterior hyaloid face may predispose the eye to infusion misdirection syndrome during cataract surgery or aqueous misdirection postoperatively.[49,50]

Typically, cataract surgery in the presence of a bleb can be performed without any alteration to the surgeon's standard technique. Care should be taken with the prep, placement of the lid speculum, and use of the second instrument to avoid damage to the bleb, especially if it is thin and cystic. An adequately sized capsulorhexis should be created to avoid capsular phimosis and the inflammation associated with a Nd:YAG laser capsulotomy. Rarely, excess filtration during phacoemulsification may decrease chamber stability, requiring either an increase in bottle height or more frequent use of viscoelastics to improve phacodynamics. Occasionally, filtration into the bleb and subconjunctival space can cause significant chemosis, pooling of balanced salt solution (BSS) on the cornea, and a disruption of the surgeon's view. In the setting of significant chemosis, it may be necessary to create one or two small incisions through the conjunctiva and Tenon's capsule 90–180° away from the bleb in order to express fluid from the subconjunctival space.[51] If these cut-down incisions are made through vascular tissue and far from the bleb, there should be little risk of postoperative leakage affecting bleb function. Upon removal of viscoelastics, after the insertion of the lens, and prior to completion of the surgery, it is reasonable to make a special effort to aspirate in the area of the sclerostomy to make certain there are no retained lenticular fragments that may increase inflammation and/or compromise bleb function.[52] A Seidel test with a sterile fluorescein strip, at the end of the procedure, can ensure that the bleb is still intact and that no surgical repair is required (Fig. 9.4).

The advent of multifocal and accommodative intraocular lenses (IOL) has added a degree of complexity to the issue of lens selection. Polymethyl methacrylate (PMMA), silicone, and acrylic IOLs each have specific advantages and disadvantages. In a uveitic population, silicone IOLs were associated with greater postoperative inflammation, but no clinically significance differences in visual outcomes. Acrylic and silicone lenses have been favored recently, since they can be folded or injected, allowing the surgeon to use a smaller phaco incision. While multifocal lenses are occasionally used in patients with mild glaucoma, multifocal lenses are relatively contraindicated in patients with advanced glaucoma because of the reduction in contrast sensitivity and uncertain influence on visual field performance.[54,55] An accommodative IOL, such as the Crystalens (Bausch & Lomb, Rochester, NY), may be a reasonable option for a patient motivated to reduce spectacle dependence, as no reduction in contrast sensitivity was observed in the Crystalens' Food and Drug Administration trials. The

best IOL option for glaucoma patients may be an aspheric monofocal IOL, which has been shown to improve perifoveal threshold levels by 4 dB when compared to standard IOLs.[56,57] While there has been some concern that blue-light filtering IOLs unnecessarily limit available light to patients with already compromised visual systems, studies have not shown a difference in visual function, including performance on short wavelength automated perimetry (SWAP—blue on yellow perimetry) between non-filtering and blue-filtering IOLs.[58–60] The authors' preference is to use a one-piece, blue-light filtering, injectable aspheric acrylic lens (Alcon SN60WF-IQ; Alcon, Fort Worth, TX).

If vitreous prolapse and/or loss occurs during cataract surgery, complete anterior vitrectomy is necessary to prevent vitreous from compromising the functioning trabeculectomy. The site of the vitrectomy ports should be placed away from the bleb. Dilute intracameral triamcinolone can be used, off-label, to identify vitreous strands, improving the efficiency of anterior vitrectomy, while helping to decrease postoperative inflammation.[61] See Table 16.2.

Table 16.2 Visualizing anterior chamber vitreous

Dilute intracameral triamcinolone to visualize anterior chamber vitreous

- Withdraw 0.2 ml of preserved triamcinolone 40 mg/ml
- Inject triamcinolone into a 5-μm syringe filter to capture particles
- Rinse particles with 2 ml of balanced salt solution (BSS)
- Re-suspend particles with 5 ml of BSS
- Re-capture particles on syringe filter by injecting and discarding the 5 ml of BSS through filter
- Withdraw 2 ml of BSS for final suspension of rinsed triamcinolone particles, for a final concentration of 4 mg/ml
- Inject rinsed triamcinolone 4 mg/ml into anterior chamber.
- BSS can be used to irrigate excess triamcinolone from the anterior chamber
- Preservative-free triamcinolone 40 mg/ml (Triesence, Alcon, Fort Worth, TX) does not require rinsing and can be diluted with BSS to 4 mg/ml.

If a sulcus IOL is required, care should be taken to avoid haptic placement in the area of the peripheral iridectomy where the haptic could migrate into the anterior chamber or sclerectomy, or compromise angle structures (Fig. 16.2). Anterior chamber IOLs (ACIOLs) are generally avoided in patients with functioning trabeculectomies as the IOL footplates may mechanically disrupt the sclerectomy, induce peripheral anterior synechiae that can obstruct the sclerectomy, and/or increase inflammation that may lead to bleb fibrosis and failure. If there is inadequate support for a posterior chamber lens, the authors believe the patient should be left aphakic and an attempt made at a trial of a gas permeable contact lens. If the bleb is cystic and avascular or likely to be damaged by the presence of a contact lens, or the contact lens is not well tolerated, a secondary ACIOL or suture-fixated IOL may be a reasonable option.

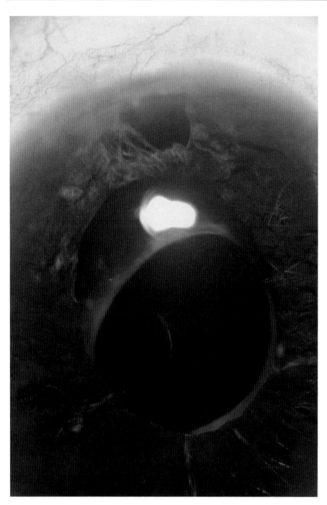

Fig. 16.2 The blue haptic of a three-piece IOL prolapsing through a surgical peripheral iridectomy. Courtesy of Dr. Hylton R. Mayer

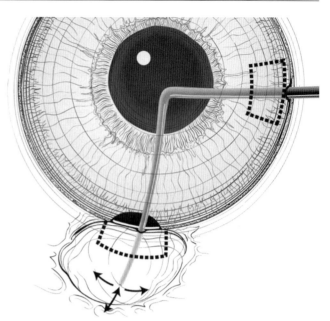

Fig. 16.3 Surgeon's view: *Ab interno* bleb revision. (**a**) A goniolens can be used intraoperatively to view the sclerostomy. (**b**) A cyclodialysis spatula or iris sweep can be used to probe the sclerectomy and raise the scleral flap from an internal approach

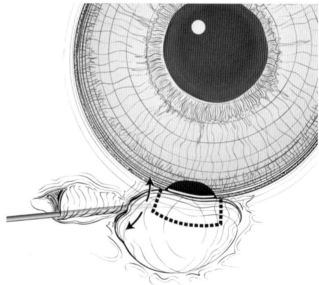

Fig. 16.4 Surgeon's view: *Ab externo* bleb revision. A 25- or 27-gauge needle enters under the conjunctiva about 5 mm from the avascular bleb and lyses subconjunctival adhesions with small sweeping motions. Courtesy of Dr. Hylton R. Mayer

When performing cataract surgery on a dysfunctional or marginally functional bleb concomitant bleb revision can improve filtration. *Ab interno* bleb revision can be performed using a blunt cannula or cyclodialysis spatula to identify the sclerostomy and raise the flap from within the anterior chamber (Fig. 16.3).[62] Intraoperative gonioscopy can be used to verify the sclerostomy site and the placement of the spatula. After the scleral flap is elevated, BSS can be injected into the anterior chamber to assess filtration. The bleb should easily and broadly elevate. It is best to make small changes to the scleral flap with each attempt to avoid hyperfiltration and hypotony, though it may require multiple efforts to achieve adequate filtration.

Ab externo bleb revision may be performed alone or in combination with *ab interno* bleb revision. To perform *ab externo* bleb revision, a 25- or 27-ga needle is tunneled from a point in the vascular conjunctiva, 5 mm or more from the area of the bleb (Fig. 16.4, Fig. 9.7 and Table 9.7.). Balanced salt solution, preservative-free 1% lidocaine, or viscoelastic

can be injected as the needle is advanced to elevate the conjunctiva and to aid in the delineation of the conjunctival adhesions. Small sweeping motions tangential to the globe are made to cut through scar tissue in the area of the dysfunctional bleb. If adequate visibility through the conjunctiva exists, the needle can be used to elevate the flap, or even enter into the anterior chamber under the flap. BSS can be used to assess filtration, and lysis of fibrosis can be repeated as necessary to obtain an appropriate bleb.

Intracameral trypan blue (Vision Blue, Dutch Ophthalmic, Exeter, NH) may also help delineate areas of fibrosis or decreased filtration within the trabeculectomy bleb[63,64] Concomitant intraoperative pharmacotherapy with antifibrotic agents, such as 5-fluorouracil (5-FU) or mitomycin C (MMC) may promote bleb function and survival in patients undergoing cataract surgery who have a functioning bleb and/or in patients undergoing bleb needling revision (Table 17.1).[65–69] Corticosteroids have been demonstrated to improve outcomes in glaucoma filtering surgery and assist in controlling inflammation after cataract surgery, especially in eyes with functioning filtering blebs.[70,71] Subconjunctival, sub-Tenon's, or intravitreal corticosteroid injections after cataract surgery may help to control perioperative inflammation and promote bleb survival.[72] Recently anti-vascular endothelial growth factor (anti-VEGF) agents, such as bevacizumab or ranibizumab, have been reported to decrease bleb vascularity and reduce bleb fibrosis.[73–75]

Surgical goniosynechialysis may be an appropriate intervention at the time of cataract removal.[76–78] Most reports indicate that synechiae of 6 months duration or less are more amendable to synechialysis than more chronic synechiae.[71,77–79] Goniosynechialysis can be performed with a direct goniolens, such as a Barkan's lens, using a needle or cystotome to break the irido-angle adhesions.[79] Alternatively, micro-grasping forceps can also be used to pull the iris from the angle, while using an indirect mirror.[80] Reports indicate that peripheral anterior synechialysis can improve IOP and decrease the number of necessary medications.[76–80] Synechialysis may, however, increase the risk for hemorrhage, pigment release, and inflammation, which may decrease bleb function or survival. The authors rarely perform goniosynechialysis in combination with cataract surgery in the setting of a functional bleb.

Postoperative Care

The postoperative medication regimen minimally deviates from standard phacoemulsification surgery. The authors routinely use topical prophylactic antibiotics and non-steroidal drops, as well as topical steroid drops, such as prednisolone 1%, given every 2 h while awake for the first week. If topical corticosteroid therapy fails to control postoperative inflammation, the authors may use 20–40 mg of sub-Tenon's triamcinolone or a short course of oral prednisone (Table 16.3). While many surgeons forgo non-steroidal drops for routine cataracts, non-steroidal medication may help decrease inflammation induced by iris manipulation.[81]

Table 16.3 Steroids for post-surgical inflammation control

Type of steroid	Typical dose	Typical duration of effect[a]	Relative potency (compared with prednisone)
Oral prednisone	1 mg/kg	1 day (commonly used for ~2 weeks)	1
Subconjunctival dexamethasone (1)	2.5 mg	1–2 days	6.5
Intravitreal triamcinolone	2–4 mg	12 weeks	1.25
Sub-Tenon's triamcinolone	20–40 mg	16 weeks	1.25

[a]Duration of effect is a function of drug solubility and local tissue factors such as vascularity and fluid turnover (vitreous present or absent).

Topical prostaglandin analogues and miotics are typically withheld, until inflammation is controlled, but other IOP lowering drops are continued as prior to surgery, unless a bleb revision was performed. Patients are seen on post-op day one and at post-op week one, though patients with high or low IOPs are typically seen at shorter intervals.

As discussed in the "Instrumentation and Operative Techniques" section, subconjunctival 5-FU, MMC, or anti-VEGF agents may be useful to promote bleb functionality postoperatively if the IOP rises or the bleb develops increased vascularity and/or decreased dimensions. Inadvertent entry of MMC into the eye should be avoided to prevent damage to the corneal endothelium and/or ciliary body. In the setting of threatened or realized bleb failure, the authors prefer a series of five subconjunctival injections of 5 mg of 5-FU injected adjacent to the bleb, administered over the course of a few weeks. Care should be taken to irrigate the eye thoroughly after the 5-FU injection to avoid corneal epithelial toxicity.

Results/Outcomes

The outcomes of cataract extraction with intraocular lens placement in the presence of a functional trabeculectomy have been repeatedly evaluated, both in the extracapsular cataract extraction (ECCE) era and in the phacoemulsification (phaco) era (Table 16.4). Most studies indicate that ECCE decreases the functionality of the trabeculectomy bleb, evident by an increase in postoperative IOP.[42,43,45,82–86] Reports on the affect of phaco on functioning blebs are more varied, with some studies indicating decreased bleb function, [46,81,86–90] some indicating minimal to no affect on filtration, [91–94] and other studies demonstrating improved IOP control after phaco.[44,85] Based on the varied reports, one may conclude that the effect of cataract

Table 16.4 Summary of reports on the effect of cataract removal on IOP

Author	Date	Study type	Number of eyes	Mean follow-up (mo)	Procedure	IOP effect
Dickens[82]	1996	Retrospective	23	48	ECCE	+3.5
Manoj[84]	2000	Retrospective	34	44	ECCE	+0.32
Halikiopoulos[85]	2001	Retrospective	31	36	ECCE	+4.1
Casson[91]	2002	Retrospective	28	35	ECCE	+2.8
Seah[42]	1996	Retrospective	22	9	ECCE/Phaco	+8
Yamagami[81]	1994	Retrospective	45	18	ECC/Phaco	+2.2
Chen[83]	1998	Retrospective	58	21	ECCE	+1.6
Manoj[84]	2000	Retrospective	21	15	Phaco	−0.61
Park[44]	1997	Retrospective	40	57	Phaco	−0.2
Casson[91]	2002	Retrospective	28	25	Phaco	+0.5
Crichton[90]	2001	Retrospective	69	22.2	Phaco	+0.55
Ehrnrooth[93]	2005	Retrospective	46	25	Phaco	+0.9
Rebolleda[46]	2002	**Prospective**	49	19.6	Phaco	+1.57
Shingleton[86]	2003	Retrospective	58	12	Phaco	1.9
Derbolav[92]	2002	Retrospective	48	23	Phaco	+1.6
Halikiopoulos[85]	2001	Retrospective	24	36	Phaco	+2.9
Inal[89]	2005	**Prospective**	30	27	Phaco	+3.2
Swamynathan[87]	2004	**Prospective**	29	20	Phaco	+3.7

surgery on filtering blebs in unpredictable. However, Spaeth and Fellman have observed that preoperative bleb morphology and function likely plays a significant role in postoperative IOP control, identifying that partially functional blebs often have a 50% increase in IOP postoperatively, whereas large, cystic, avascular blebs with preoperative IOPs under 10 mmHg without medication rarely have an increase in IOP after cataract extraction.[95]

Complications

Mild to moderate inflammation following uncomplicated cataract surgery is expected. Bleb dysfunction and failure following post-cataract extraction is most likely related to inflammatory mediated fibrosis.[96] The fibrosis may occur at the sclerectomy, within the scleral flap, or within the bleb. Uncontrolled or excessive postoperative inflammation can also exacerbate glaucoma via progressive peripheral anterior synechia or posterior synechia with iris bombe. Uncommon potential causes for bleb failure following cataract surgery include bleb leak, retained lenticular fragments within the sclerectomy, iris incarcerated in the sclerectomy, and aqueous misdirection. Further complications can be due to manipulations of filtering blebs, intentionally or inadvertently, resulting in induced refractive errors, bleb dysesthesias, overhanging blebs, bleb leak, hypotony and its sequelae, hyphema, and a lifetime risk of endophthalmitis.

Postoperative IOP spikes may exacerbate poorly controlled glaucoma. Significant loss of vision after trabeculectomy, or "snuffing out" vision, is a feared complication following any invasive procedure in patients with advanced glaucoma, and has been a concern of surgeons operating on patients with advanced glaucoma. Although "snuffing out" is a controversial topic and exceedingly rare, significant loss of vision following a seemingly uncomplicated trabeculectomy has been reported. Postoperative vision loss, in the absence of identifiable ocular pathology, has been proposed to be due to ganglion cell loss related to IOP elevation or shifts in the cribriform plate, non-arteric anterior ischemic optic neuropathy, or occult maculopathy.[97–100] When considering surgery in a patient with advanced glaucoma, the informed consent process should include an informed discussion about the potential for progression of glaucoma and/or loss of vision.

Summary

Anterior segment surgeons will inevitably encounter patients with functioning filtering blebs who have visually significant cataracts. The surgeon should be prepared to manage ocular conditions including intraocular scarring, miosis, and/or pseudoexfoliation. Cataract surgery may present an opportunity to perform a bleb needling revision, a somewhat effective intervention to revitalize and/or optimize fibrotic blebs. Crystalline lens removal in patients with filtering blebs can be safely performed, but patients and surgeons should be aware that the surgery may hasten bleb failure, especially in marginally functioning blebs. Careful preoperative evaluation and planning can establish realistic patient expectations and prepare the surgeon for minor perioperative adjustments and interventions that can promote long-term visual function.

References

1. D'Ermo F, Bonomi L, Doro D. A critical analysis of the long-term results of trabeculectomy. *Am J Ophthalmol* 1979; 88:829–835.

2. Mills KB. Trabeculectomy: a retrospective long-term follow-up of 444 cases. *Br J Ophthalmol* 1981; 65:790–795.

3. Watson PG, Jakeman C, Oztur M, et al. The complications of trabeculectomy (a 20-year follow-up). *Eye* 1990;4:425–438.

4. Tornqvist G, Drolsum LK. Trabeculectomies: a longterm study. *Acta Ophthalmol* 1991; 69:450–454.

5. Popovic V, Sjostrand J. Long-term outcome following trabeculectomy: Retrospective analysis of intraocular pressure regulation and cataract formation. *Acta Ophthalmol* 1991;69:299–304.

6. Advanced Glaucoma Intervention Study (AGIS) Investigators. Advanced Glaucoma Intervention Study: 8. Risk of cataract formation after trabeculectomy. *Arch Ophthalmol* 2001;119: 1771–1779.

7. Molteno ACB, Bosma NJ, Kittelson JM. Otago glaucoma surgery outcome study: long-term results of trabeculectomy—1976 to 1995. *Ophthalmology* 1999;106:1742–1750.

8. Musch DC, Gillespie BW, Niziol LM, et al. Cataract extraction in the collaborative initial glaucoma treatment study: Incidence, risk factors, and the effect of cataract progression and extraction on clinical and quality-of-life outcomes for the collaborative initial glaucoma treatment study (CIGTS) group. *Arch Ophthalmol* 2006;124(12):1694–1700.

9. Shaffer RN, Rosenthal G. Comparison of cataract incidence in normal and glaucomatous population. *Am J Ophthalmol* 1970;69:368–371

10. Bernth-Petersen P, Bach E. Epidemiologic aspects of cataract surgery. III: frequencies of diabetes and glaucoma in a cataract population. *Acta Ophthalmol* 1983;61:406–416.

11. Lee AJ, Rochtchina E, Wang JJ, et al. Does smoking affect intraocular pressure? Findings from the Blue Mountains Eye Study. *J Glaucoma* 2003; 12:209–212.

12. van Heyningen R, Harding JJ. A case-control study of cataract in Oxfordshire some risk factors. *Br J Ophthalmol* 1988;72:804–808.

13. Harding JJ, Harding RS, Egerton M. Risk factors for cataract in Oxfordshire diabetes, peripheral neuropathy, myopia, glaucoma and diarrhoea. *Acta Ophthalmol* 1989;67:510–517.

14. Harding JJ, Egerton M, van Heyningen R, et al. Diabetes, glaucoma, sex, and cataract analysis of combined data from two case control studies. *Br J Ophthalmol* 1993;77:2–6.

15. Klein BE, Klein R, Moss SE. Incident cataract surgery the Beaver Dam Eye Study. *Ophthalmology* 1997;104:573–580.

16. Mitchell PG, Smith W, Chey T, et al. Open-angle glaucoma and diabetes: the Blue Mountains Eye Study, Australia. *Ophthalmology* 1997;104:712–718.

17. Cumming RG, Mitchell PG. Alcohol, smoking, and cataracts the Blue Mountains Eye Study. *Arch Ophthalmol* 1997;115:1296–1303.

18. Cumming RG, Mitchell PG, Leeder SR. Use of inhaled corticosteroids and the risk of cataracts. *N Engl J Med* 1997;337:8–14.

19. Mitchell PG, Hourihan F, Sandbach J, et al. The relationship between glaucoma and myopia the Blue Mountains Eye Study. *Ophthalmology* 1999; 106:2010–2015.

20. Mitchell PG, Cumming RG, Mackey DA. Inhaled corticosteroids, family history, and risk of glaucoma. *Ophthalmology* 1999;106:2301–2306.

21. Lim R, Mitchell PG, Cumming RG. Refractive associations with cataract the Blue Mountains Eye Study. *Invest Ophthalmol Vis Sci* 1999;40:3021–3026.

22. Rowe NG, Mitchell PG, Cumming RG, et al. Diabetes, fasting blood glucose and age-related cataract the Blue Mountains Eye Study. *Ophthalmic Epidemiol* 2000;7:103–114.

23. Cumming RG, Mitchell PG, Lim R. Iris color and cataract the Blue Mountains Eye Study. *Am J Ophthalmol* 2000;130: 237–238.

24. Weih LM, Mukesh BN, McCarty CA, et al. Association of demographic, familial, medical, and ocular factors with intraocular pressure. *Arch Ophthalmol* 2001;119:875–880.

25. Leske MC, Wu SY, Nemesure B, et al. Barbados Eye Studies Group, Risk factors for incident nuclear opacities. *Ophthalmology* 2002;109:1303–1308.

26. Klein BE, Klein R, Linton KL. Intraocular pressure in an American community. The Beaver Dam Eye Study. *Invest Ophthalmol Vis Sci* 1992;33:2224–2228.

27. Lichter PR, Musch DC, Gillespie BW, et al. Interim clinical outcomes in the Collaborative Initial Glaucoma Treatment Study comparing initial treatment randomized to medications or surgery. *Ophthalmology* 2001;108:1943–1953.

28. Klein BE, Klein R, Lee KE, et al. Drug use and five-year incidence of age-related cataracts the Beaver Dam Eye Study. *Ophthalmology* 2001;108:1670–1674.

29. Chandrasekaran S, Cumming RG, Rochtchina E, et al. Associations between elevated intraocular pressure and glaucoma, use of glaucoma medications, and 5-year incident cataract: the Blue Mountains Eye Study. *Ophthalmology* 2006;113: 417–424.

30. Hofeldt AJ, Weiss MJ. Illuminated near card assessment of potential acuity in eyes with cataract. *Ophthalmology* 1998;105: 1531–1536.

31. Fletcher A, Vijaykumar V, Selvaraj S, et al. The Madurai Intraocular Lens Study III: Visual functioning and quality of life outcomes. *Am J Ophthalmol* 1998;125:26–35.

32. Wang JJ, Mitchell P, Simpson JM, et al. Visual impairment, age-related cataract, and mortality. *Arch Ophthalmol* 2001;119: 1186–1190.

33. McGwin G, Owsley C, Gauthreaux S. The association between cataract and mortality among older adults. *Ophthalmic Epidemiol* 2003;10:107–119.

34. Knudtson MD, Klein BE, Klein R. Age-related eye disease, visual impairment, and survival: the Beaver Dam Eye Study. *Arch Ophthalmol* 2006;124:243–9.

35. Owsley C, McGwin G, Scilley K, et al. Impact of cataract surgery on health-related quality of life in nursing home residents. *Br J Ophthalmol* 2007;91:1359–1363.

36. Sach TH, Foss AJ, Gregson RM, et al. Falls and health status in elderly women following first eye cataract surgery: an economic evaluation conducted alongside a randomised controlled trial. *Br J Ophthalmol* 2007;91:1675–1679.

37. Hodge W, Horsley T, Albiani D, et al. The consequences of waiting for cataract surgery: a systematic review. *CMAJ* 2007;176: 1285–1290.

38. Eakins KE. Prostaglandin and non-prostaglandin mediated breakdown of the blood-aqueous barrier. *Exp Eye Res* 1977;25:483–498.

39. Ernest PH, Tipperman R, Eagle R, et al. Is there a difference in incision healing based on location? *J Cataract Refract Surg* 1998;24:482– 486.

40. Chang DF, Campbell JR. Intraoperative floppy iris syndrome associated with tamsulosin (Flomax). *J Cataract Refract Surg* 2005;31:664–673.

41. Shugar JK. Intracameral epinephrine for prophylaxis of IFIS [letter]. *J Cataract Refract Surg* 2006;32:1074–1075.

42. Seah SK, Jap A, Prata JA, et al. Cataract surgery after trabeculectomy. *Ophthalmic Surg Lasers* 1996;27:587–594.

43. Chen PP, Weaver YK, Budenz DL, et al. Trabeculectomy function after cataract extraction. *Ophthal* 1998;105:1928–1935.

44. Park HJ, Kwon YH, Weitzman M, et al. Temporal corneal phacoemulsification in patients with filtered glaucoma. *Arch Ophthalmol* 1997;115:1375–1380.

45. Casson RJ, Riddell CE, Rahman R, et al. Long-term effect of cataract surgery on intraocular pressure after trabeculectomy: extracapsular extraction versus phacoemulsification. *J Cataract Refract Surg* 2002;28:2159–2164.

46. Rebolleda G, Muñoz-Negrete FJ. Phacoemulsification in eyes with functioning filtering blebs: a prospective study. *Ophthalmology* 2002;109:2248–2255.

47. Ozeveren F, Eltutar K. Therapeutic application of tissue plasminogen activator for fibrin reaction after cataract surgery. *J Cataract Refract Surg* 2004;30:1727–1731.

48. Wedrich A, Menapace R, Ries E, et al. Intracameral tissue plasminogen activator to treat severe fibrinous effusion after cataract surgery. *J Cataract Refract Surg* 1997; 23:873–877

49. Mackool RJ, Sirota M. Infusion misdirection syndrome. *J Cataract Refract Surg* 1993;19:671–672

50. Ruben ST, Tsai JC, Hitchings RA. Malignant glaucoma and its management. *Br J Ophthalmol* 1997;81:163–167.

51. Liyanage SE, Angunawela RI, Little BC. Conjunctival sweeping with a squint hook to reduce chemosis. *J Cataract Refract Surg* 2007;33:1691–1693.

52. Swan K. Reopening of nonfunctioning filters-simplified surgical techniques. *Trans Am Acad Ophthalmol Otolaryngol* 1975;79:342–348.

53. Elgohary MA, McCluskey P, Towler HM, et al. Outcome of phacoemulsification in patients with uveitis. *Br J Ophthalmol* 2007;91:916–21.

54. Vingolo EM, Grenga P, Iacobelli L, et al. Visual acuity and contrast sensitivity: AcrySof ReSTOR apodized diffractive versus AcrySof SA60AT monofocal intraocular lenses. *J Cataract Refract Surg* 2007;33:1244–1247.

55. Martínez PA, Gómez FP, España AA, et al. Visual function with bilateral implantation of monofocal and multifocal intraocular lenses: a prospective, randomized, controlled clinical trial. *J Refract Surg* 2008;24:257–264.

56. Cuthbertson FM, Dhingra S, Benjamin L. Objective and subjective outcomes in comparing three different aspheric intraocular lens implants with their spherical counterparts. *Eye* May 9, 2008 [Epub ahead of print].

57. Tzelikis PF, Akaishi L, Trindade FC, et al. Spherical aberration and contrast sensitivity in eyes implanted with aspheric and spherical intraocular lenses: a comparative study. *Am J Ophthalmol.* 2008;145:827–833.

58. Marshall J, Cionni RJ, Davison J, et al. Clinical results of the blue-light filtering AcrySof Natural foldable acrylic intraocular lens. *J Cataract Refract Surg* 2005;31:2319–2323.

59. Kara-Júnior N, Jardim JL, de Oliveira Leme E, et al. Effect of the AcrySof Natural intraocular lens on blue-yellow perimetry. *J Cataract Refract Surg* 2006;32:1328–1330.

60. Landers J, Tan TH, Yuen J, et al. Comparison of visual function following implantation of Acrysof Natural intraocular lenses with conventional intraocular lenses. *Clin Experiment Ophthalmol* 2007;35:152–15.

61. Burk SE, Da Mata AP, Snyder ME, et al. Visualizing vitreous using Kenalog suspension. *J Cataract Refract Surg* 2003;29:645–651.

62. Kasahara W, Sibayan SH, Montenegro MH et al. CE with internal bleb revision. *Ophthal Surg Lasers* 1996;27:361–366

63. Agrawal S, Agrawal J, Agrawal TP. Use of trypan blue to confirm the patency of filtering surgery. *J Cataract Refract Surg* 2005;31:235–237.

64. Dada T, Muralidhar R, Sethi HS. Staining of filtering bleb with trypan blue during phacoemulsification. *Eye* 2006;20: 858–859.

65. Johnstone MA, Ziel CJ. Cataract surgery in the presence of a filtering bleb with postoperative 5-fluorouracil (5-FU). *Invest Ophthalmol Vis Sci* 1992;33:948.

66. Pasternack JJ, Wand M, Shields MB, Abraham D. Needle revision of failed filtering blebs using 5-Fluorouracil and a combined ab-externo and ab-interno approach. *J Glaucoma* 2005;14:47–51.

67. Shetty RK, Wartluft L, Moster MR. Slit-lamp needle revision of failed filtering blebs using high-dose mitomycin C. *J Glaucoma* 2005;4:52–56.

68. Gutiérrez-Ortiz C, Cabarga C, Teus MA. Prospective evaluation of preoperative factors associated with successful mitomycin C needling of failed filtration blebs. *J Glaucoma* 2006;15: 98–102.

69. Sharmal TK, Arora S, Corridan PG. Phacoemulsification in patients with previous trabeculectomy: role of 5-fluorouracil. *Eye* 2007;21:780–783.

70. Starita RJ, Fellman RL, Spaeth GL, et al. Short- and long-term effects of postoperative corticosteroids on trabeculectomy. *Ophthalmol* 1985;92:938–946.

71. Araujo SV, Spaeth GL, Roth SM, et al. A ten-year follow-up on a prospective, randomized trial of postoperative corticosteroids after trabeculectomy. *Ophthalmol* 1995;102:1753–1759.

72. Hosseini H, Mehryar M, Farvardin M. Focus on triamcinolone acetonide as an adjunct to glaucoma filtration surgery. *Medical Hypotheses* 2007;68:401–403.

73. Kahook MY, Schuman JS, Noecker RJ. Needle Bleb Revision of Encapsulated Filtering Bleb With Bevacizumab. *Ophthalmic Surg Lasers Imaging* 2006;37:148–150.

74. Kitnarong N, Chindasub P, Metheetrairut A. Surgical outcome of intravitreal bevacizumab and filtration surgery in neovascular glaucoma. *Adv Ther* 2007;25:438–443.

75. Jonas JB, Spandau UH, Schlichtenbrede F. Intravitreal bevacizumab for filtering surgery. *Ophthalmic Res* 2007;39:121–122.

76. Shingleton BJ, Chang MA, Bellows AR, et al. Surgical goniosynechialysis for angle-closure glaucoma. *Ophthalmology* 1990;97:551–556.

77. Tanihara H, Nishiwaki K, Nagata M. Surgical results and complications of goniosynechialysis. *Graefes Arch Clin Exp Ophthalmol* 1992;230:309–313.

78. Teekhasaenee C, Ritch R. Combined phacoemulsification and goniosynechialysis for uncontrolled chronic angle-closure glaucoma after acute angle-closure glaucoma. *Ophthalmology* 1999;106:669–674

79. Campbell DG, Vela A. Modern goniosynechialysis for the treatment of synechial angle-closure glaucoma. *Ophthalmology* 1984;91:1052–1060

80. Chen T, Pongpun PR, Walton DS. Goniosynechiolysis. In: Chen T (ed) Surgical Techniques in Ophthalmology: Glaucoma Surgery. Saunders Elsevier, China. 2008.

81. van Haeringen NJ, van Sorge AA, Carballosa Coré-Bodelier VM. Constitutive cyclooxygenase-1 and induced cyclooxygenase-2 in isolated human iris inhibited by S(+) flurbiprofen. *J Ocul Pharmacol Ther* 2000;16:353–361.

82. Yamagami S, Araie M, Mori M, et al. Posterior chamber intraocular lens implantation in filtered or nonfiltered glaucoma eyes. *Jpn J Ophthalmol* 1994;38:71–79.

83. Dickens MA, Cashwell LF. Long-term effect of cataract extraction on the function of an established filtering bleb. *Ophthalmic Surg Lasers* 1996;27:9–14.

84. Chen PP, Weaver YK, Budenz DL, et al. Trabeculectomy function after cataract extraction. *Ophthalmology* 1998;105: 1928–1935.

85. Manoj B, Chako D, Khan MY. Effect of extracapsular cataract extraction and phacoemulsification performed after trabeculectomy on intraocular pressure. *J Cataract Refract Surg* 2000;26:75–78.

86. Halikiopoulos D, Moster MR, Azuara-Blanco A, et al. The outcome of the functioning filter after subsequent cataract extraction. *Ophthalmic Surg Lasers.* 2001;32:108–117.

87. Shingleton BJ, O'Donoghue MW, Hall PE. Results of phacoemulsification in eyes with preexisting glaucoma filters. *J Cataract Refract Surg* 2003;29:1093–1096.

88. Swamynathan K, Capistrano AP, Cantor LB, et al. Effect of temporal corneal phacoemulsification on intraocular pressure in eyes with prior trabeculectomy with an antimetabolite. *Ophthalmology* 2004;111:674–678.

89. Ehrnrooth P, Lehto I, Puska P, et al. Phacoemulsification in trabeculectomized eyes. *Acta Ophthalmol Scand* 2005;83:561–566.

90. Inal A, Bayraktar S, Inal B, et al. Intraocular pressure control after clear corneal phacoemulsification in eyes with previous trabeculectomy: a controlled study. *Acta Ophthalmol Scand* 2005;83:554–560.

91. Crichton ACS, Kirker AW. Intraocular pressure and medication control after clear corneal phacoemulsification and Acry-Sof posterior chamber intraocular lens implantation in patientswith filtering blebs. *J Glaucoma* 2001;10:38–46.

92. Casson R, Rahman R, Salmon JF. Phacoemulsification with intraocular lens implantation after trabeculectomy. *J Glaucoma* 2002;11:429–433.

93. Derbolav A, Vass C, Menapace R, Schmetterer K, Wedrich A. Long-term effect of phacoemulsification on intraocular pressure after trabeculectomy. *J Cataract Refract Surg* 2002;28:425–430.

94. Ehrnrooth P, Lehto I, Puska P, Laatikainen L. Phacoemulsification in trabeculectomized eyes. *Acta Ophthalmol Scand* 2005;83: 561–566.

95. Spaeth GL, Fellman RL. Cataract extraction in patients with glaucoma. In: Duane's Ophthalmology, CD-ROM Edition. Clinical volume 6, chapter 16, 2001, Lippincott Williams & Wilkins.

96. Lama PJ, Fechtner RD. Antifibrotics and wound healing in glaucoma surgery. *Surv Ophthalmol* 2003;48:314–346.

97. Kolker AE. Visual prognosis in advanced glaucoma: a comparison of medical and surgical therapy for retention of vision in 101 eyes with advanced glaucoma. *Trans Am Ophthalmol Soc* 1977;75:539–555.

98. Aggarwal SP, Hendeles S. Risk of sudden visual loss following trabeculectomy in advanced primary open-angle glaucoma. *Br J Ophthalmol* 1986;70:97–99.

99. Levene RZ. Central visual field, visual acuity, and sudden visual loss after glaucoma surgery. *Ophthalmic Surg* 1992;23: 388–394.

100. Law SK, Nguyen AM, Coleman AL, et al. Severe Loss of Central Vision in Patients Advanced Glaucoma Undergoing Trabeculectomy. *Arch Ophthalmol* 2007;125: 1044–1050.

Chapter 17

Cataract Extraction in Eyes with Prior GDD Implantation

Ramesh Ayyala and Brian Mikulla

Introduction

Glaucoma patients with prior glaucoma drainage device (GDD) implantation can develop visually significant cataracts and may need cataract surgery. Cataract surgery when properly performed will result in significant visual improvement with minimal effect on the IOP control. The literature review on this topic is rather sparse.[1–3]

Sa et al. evaluated the effect of temporal clear corneal phacoemulsification on intraocular pressure (IOP) in eyes after Ahmed glaucoma valve insertion.[1] They retrospectively evaluated the medical records of 13 patients with prior Ahmed valve implantation who underwent cataract surgery. They reported no significant increase in the IOP in eyes with prior Ahmed glaucoma valve insertion. However, some eyes experienced an IOP elevation 1 month after phacoemulsification and required additional glaucoma medication.[1] A retrospective review of 23 cataract surgeries in eyes with prior AGV was done by Caprioli.[2] In his series, four eyes or 17% had an elevated IOP on postoperative day 1, and one patient went on to have a second AGV placed for IOP control. Two patients experienced corneal decompensation and 33% actually experienced worsening of vision following the cataract surgery, highlighting the diseased state of many eyes that have had GDD placement.

Surgical Technique

Our preferred technique is clear cornea temporal approach in these patients. We tend to minimize the viscoelastic used in these cases, as too much viscoelastic can exit into the bleb through the tube and cause elevated IOP in the immediate postoperative period. We also tend to use a topical steroid

Table 17.1 MMC before bleb revision[5] (off-label use)

- Topical anesthetic drops
- Topical fluoroquinolone antibiotic drops
- Ophthalmic Betadine drops (Alcon, Fort Worth, TX)
- Mix 0.1 ml of preservative-free lidocaine 1% with 0.1 ml of 0.4 mg/ml MMC in a Tb syringe, drawn up with a 25-ga needle
- Switch to a 30G needle (same syringe)
- Inject temporal or nasal to the bleb
- Massage the eye with the lids closed until the lido/mito mixture is completely dissipated
- Perform needle revision

for 6–8 weeks postoperative cataract surgery to decrease any postoperative inflammation in the bleb.

The other situation that needs to be considered in this setting is the possibility of the GDD tube being too long and lying on the cataract surface. In these cases, it is best to trim the tube at the very beginning of the surgery. After the temporal entry into the anterior chamber (AC) is made with keratome, viscoelastic is re-injected to deepen the AC. A long Vaness scissors is introduced into the AC and the tube trimmed to the required length. Then the cut portion of the tube is retracted using Utratta forceps. Caution should be used not to cut the tube too short, especially if the IOP is low and the eye ball is somewhat collapsed, as the tube tends to retract more when the globe is normotensive.

Outcomes

In a small percentage of patients (20–30% in our experience), the IOP may become permanently elevated with fibrosis of the bleb from the postoperative inflammation. The majority of these patients respond to topical glaucoma medications. Some of these patients may respond to bleb revisions with mitomycin C (MMC) injection into the bleb (0.1 cc of 0.4 mg/cc concentration), especially in case of the Ahmed valve.[4–6] See Table 17.1. Some of these cases may fail to respond to all the above measures and may need a second GDD implantation in one of the other quadrants.

R. Ayyala (✉)
Department of Ophthalmology, Tulane University School of Medicine, New Orleans, LA 70112, USA
e-mail: rayyala@tulane.edu

S.M. Johnson (ed.), *Cataract Surgery in the Glaucoma Patient*, DOI 10.1007/978-0-387-09408-3_17,
© Springer Science+Business Media, LLC 2009

Summary

Cataract surgery in the presence of preexisting GDD is no different from standard cataract surgery in the majority of patients. The possibility of GDD failure, and worsening of vision from comorbidities such as reduced endothelial cell function, should be reviewed with the patients.

References

1. Sa HS, Kee C. Effect of temporal clear corneal phacoemulsification on intraocular pressure in eyes with prior Ahmed glaucoma valve insertion. *J Catract Refract Surg*. 2006;32:1011–4.

2. Gujral S, Nouri-Mahdavi K, Caprioli J. Outcomes of small-incision cataract surgery in eyes with preexisting Ahmed glaucoma valves. *Am J Ophthalmol*. 2005;140: 911–3.

3. Bhattacharyya CA, WuDunn D, Lakhani V, Hoop J, Cantor LB. Cataract surgery after tube shunts. *J Glaucoma*. 2000;9: 453–57.

4. Lam DSC, Lai JSM, Chua JKH, et al. Needling revision of glaucoma drainage device filtering blebs. *Ophthalmology*. 1998;105:1127–8

5. Shetty RK, Wartluft L, Moster M. Slit-lamp needle revision of failed filtering blebs using-high dose mitomycin C. *J Glaucoma*. 2005;14:52–6.

6. Mardelli PG, Lederer CM, Murray PL, et al. Slit lamp needle revision of failed filtering blebs using mitomycin C. *Ophthlmology*. 1996;103:1946–55.

Chapter 18

Cataract Surgery in the Primary Angle-Closure Patient

Jimmy S.M. Lai

Introduction

Primary angle-closure glaucoma (PACG) is a major cause of blindness in Asia and South Africa.[1,2] It is defined as a glaucomatous optic neuropathy secondary to ocular hypertension, caused by closure of the drainage angle. Angle closure is the result of apposition or adhesion (synechiae) of the peripheral iris to the surface of the pigmented trabeculum. The blocking of aqueous access to the trabeculum results in raised intraocular pressure. When a sufficient proportion of the trabecular meshwork is blocked, the intraocular pressure begins to rise and causes symptoms.[3] If the elevation of the intraocular pressure persists for a period of time, the optic nerve head will be damaged resulting in glaucoma. There are at least five mechanisms in the causation of angle closure listed in Table 18.1. Although pupillary block is the most common cause of angle-closure glaucoma, at least in the acute type, a thick and anteriorly positioned human lens, either combined with pupillary block or acting alone, is also an important cause of angle closure (Table 18.2).

Primary angle-closure glaucoma can be subdivided into acute and chronic subtypes. The acute form is highly symptomatic, and results from sudden appositional closure of the angle leading to a rapid rise in the intraocular pressure. The correct terminology should be acute primary angle closure, because glaucoma, that is, optic nerve damage, may not have occurred yet. A significant proportion of these eyes subsequently progress to the chronic type of primary angle-closure glaucoma. The chronic type runs a more insidious course. It is characterized by closure of at least 180° of the drainage angle by the iris tissue with the presence of manifest optic nerve tissue damage. It may be a sequel of a previous acute angle-closure attack or it may develop de novo.

Table 18.1 Mechanisms of angle closure

- Pupillary block
- Plateau Iris
- Lens induced
- Aqueous misdirection
- Mixed Mechanism

Table 18.2 Challenges of cataract surgery in angle closure

- Shallow anterior chamber
- Decreased corneal endothelial cell count
- Large lens
- Poor dilation
- Posterior synechiae
- Possible high IOP
- Possible weak zonule

The chronic type of primary angle-closure glaucoma is often referred to as chronic angle-closure glaucoma (CACG). Its prevalence increases with age, and therefore chronic angle-closure glaucoma frequently coexists with senile degenerative cataract. In patients with coexisting chronic angle-closure glaucoma and cataract requiring surgical intervention for the medically uncontrolled intraocular pressure, there are, in general, three surgical options.

- The first option is to perform a drainage operation alone, usually trabeculectomy, to control the intraocular pressure.
- The second option is to combine the trabeculectomy with removal of the cataract in one single operation.
- The third option is to perform cataract extraction alone.

Eyes with primary angle-closure glaucoma have thicker and more anteriorly positioned lenses than normal eyes.[4] The anterior chambers in these eyes are shallower and the drainage angle is narrower.[5] Many studies have shown that removal of the bulging lens significantly deepens the anterior chamber and widens the drainage angle.[6–8] It has also been shown that cataract extraction alone results in significant lowering of intraocular pressure in chronic angle-closure glaucoma eyes.[9–11] Cataract extraction alone may,

J.S.M. Lai (✉)
Queen Mary Hospital, Eye Institute and Research Center for Heart Brain and Healthy Ageing, The University of Hong Kong, Cyberport, Hong Kong, China
e-mail: laism@hku.hk

S.M. Johnson (ed.), *Cataract Surgery in the Glaucoma Patient*, DOI 10.1007/978-0-387-09408-3_18,
© Springer Science+Business Media, LLC 2009

therefore, suffice as the primary treatment for chronic angle-closure glaucoma with coexisting cataract, as it may treat both diseases with one operation.

Performing cataract extraction by phacoemulsification alone, without trabeculectomy, has the following advantages: (1) it is a fast, simple, standard and minimally invasive procedure with fast visual recovery; (2) avoidance of complications of trabeculectomy, and the need for additional surgical interventions to maintain filtration, such as laser suture lysis or needling; and (3) substantial savings in resources, including operative time and follow-up visits. In those patients whose intraocular pressure is not sufficiently controlled after phacoemulsification alone, trabeculectomy can always be performed separately at a later stage without any known compromise of the long-term outcome. The disadvantage is that there may be a postoperative pressure spike, which is undesirable in eyes with preexisting advanced glaucomatous nerve damage. Secondly, the reduction of the intraocular pressure is not immediate and it may take some time for it to be reduced to a safe and stable level.

Effect of Cataract Extraction on the Angle Structure

The width of the angle is influenced by the thickness of the human lens. When the lens is thick, the angle becomes crowded and narrow, especially if the lens is also in a more anterior position. Cataract extraction alone was shown to deepen anterior chambers and widen drainage angles in PACG eyes.[6–8] It has been reported that the angle widened by 17°, the anterior chamber deepened by 2 mm, and the intraocular pressure decreased by 6 mmHg after phacoemulsification in eyes with angle-closure glaucoma.[6]

After phacoemulsification and foldable intraocular lens implantation, ultrasound biomicroscopy revealed that the iris diaphragm shifted backward, the anterior chamber deepened by approximately 850 μm, and the angle widened by approximately 10°.[12] These findings may be of clinical significance in eyes with angle-closure glaucoma or with occludable angles. Residual angle closure is common even after laser peripheral iridotomy and cataract extraction is effective to resolve the residual angle closure in these patients.[13]

Effect of Cataract Surgery on the Intraocular Pressure

Cataract extraction alone with phacoemulsification and intraocular lens implantation in chronic angle-closure glaucoma patients with uncontrolled intraocular pressure resulted in a significant reduction in the intraocular pressure within 12 months following surgery.[9,11,14]

The deepening of the anterior chamber, the widening of the drainage angle, and the improved access of aqueous to the trabecular meshwork may all contribute to the intraocular pressure reduction, after cataract extraction by phacoemulsification. In the author's experience, in some eyes, the angle remained closed after phacoemulsification and yet the intraocular pressure still showed a significant reduction. Therefore, other factors may contribute to the intraocular pressure reduction such as flushing of the trabecular meshwork from the positive pressure during phacoemulsification, the pressure effect on the trabecular meshwork from the intraocular lens haptics, and there also may be biochemical and blood aqueous barrier alterations.

Role of Phacotrabeculectomy

In view of the advantages and beneficial effects on the angle structure and the intraocular pressure control in cataract extraction alone, the role of combined phacotrabeculectomy in the surgical treatment of chronic angle-closure glaucoma may be diminishing. It has been shown by ultrasound biomicroscopy that phacoemulsification alone resulted in greater opening of the drainage angle and greater deepening of the anterior chamber than combined phacotrabeculectomy in primary angle-closure glaucoma eyes.[15] It is uncertain whether the additional trabeculectomy procedure is needed and offers additional benefits to the outcome in these patients. It has also been shown that phacotrabeculectomy was only slightly more effective than phacoemulsification alone in controlling the intraocular pressure in chronic angle-closure glaucoma eyes with coexisting cataract. The combined surgery was, however, associated with more complications and additional drainage adjustment procedures in the postoperative period.[16]

There is one more point to consider when deciding whether phacoemulsification or phacotrabeculectomy should be done. It has been shown that a myopic shift from intraocular lens power prediction error was significantly more frequent following posterior chamber intraocular lens (IOL) implantation with phacotrabeculectomy compared with phacoemulsification.[17] Unless special precaution is taken to compensate in the IOL calculation, intraocular lens power is more accurately predicted if phacoemulsification alone is performed.

Indications for Cataract Surgery

After discussion of the effects of cataract removal on the angle structure and the intraocular pressure control, is the indication of cataract extraction different in primary angle-closure patients from that of the normal aging population? The indication for cataract surgery in patients with primary angle-closure glaucoma basically follows that of senile degenerative cataract. When the cataract is visually significant, cataract extraction is advised. Cataract removal improves vision and there may be an additional advantage of lowering the intraocular pressure after surgery. But when the cataract is minimal, the decision whether to remove the lens or not is controversial. There is now increasing evidence that lens removal is beneficial in eyes with chronic angle-closure glaucoma in terms of intraocular pressure control. On the one hand, when primary angle-closure glaucoma patients have a dense cataract, the purposes of cataract removal are to improve the vision, deepen the angle, and to lower the intraocular pressure. On the other hand, when the cataract is minimal, the purpose of lens removal is mainly to deepen the angle and lower the intraocular pressure. Ideally, removal of the bulging lens may open up the already closed angle and prevent progressive closure of unclosed angle.

Phacoemulsification with intraocular pressure implantation is thus useful when there is residual angle closure, after relief of pupillary block with laser peripheral iridotomy.

Preoperative Assessment and Medications

Cataract surgery in primary angle-closure glaucoma eyes, especially those with a previous attack of acute angle closure, is a big challenge to phaco surgeons because of shallow anterior chamber, large lens, poor mydriasis from iris atrophy, posterior synechiae or effect of long-term pilocarpine, and even zonular weakness (Figs. 18.1and 18.2).[15] See Table 8.2.

The corneal clarity may be suboptimal, and the endothelial cell count may be low. The risk of intraoperative suprachoroidal hemorrhage may increase if the preoperative intraocular pressure is high.[18]Small incision cataract surgery using phacoemulsification with foldable intraocular lens implantation is preferred because the risk of intraoperative suprachoroidal hemorrhage is less. Only in exceptional cases such as a very hard and dense nuclear cataract, or cataract with severe zonular laxity, is a larger wound with extracapsular cataract extraction performed.

A cataractous angle closure eye may have had a previous drainage operation, and the presence of a large superior bleb may interfere with wound construction in phacoemulsification (Fig. 18.3). Under those circumstances, a temporal approach has to be adopted to avoid damaging the bleb. See Chapter 16.

The preoperative assessment should include careful assessment of the stability of the lens, the degree of mydriasis

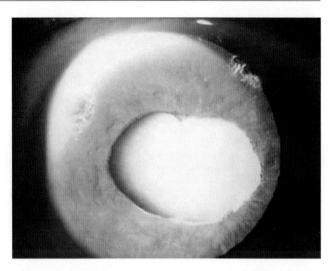

Fig. 18.1 Chronic angle-closure glaucoma eye with cataract showing a distorted pupil due to iris atrophy and posterior synechiae

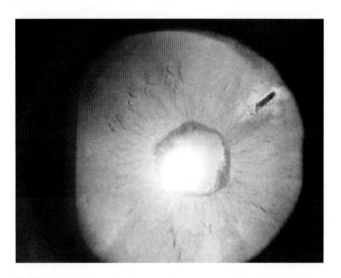

Fig. 18.2 Chronic angle-closure glaucoma eye with cataract showing extensive posterior synechiae with a small pupil

achieved with pharmacological agents, the extent and nature of the angle closure, and the cup-disc ratio. Perimetry is often unreliable in the presence of dense cataract. In eyes with extensive peripheral anterior synechiae angle closure with high intraocular pressure, it is advisable to do a combined phacotrabeculectomy because cataract extraction alone may not be able to achieve significant angle-opening and intraocular pressure lowering. In eyes that already have advanced cupping with medically uncontrolled intraocular pressure, it is also advisable to perform a combined phacotrabeculectomy because a pressure spike after phacoemulsification alone may result in a wipe-out syndrome.[19]

The endothelial cell count should be performed preoperatively. Eyes with primary angle-closure glaucoma are prone to endothelial cell damage during phacoemulsification because of shallow anterior chamber.[14] In eyes with a

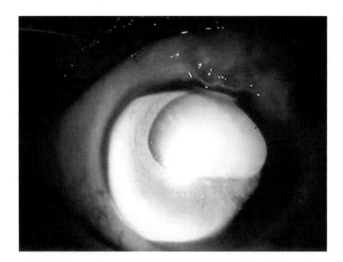

Fig. 18.3 Chronic angle-closure glaucoma eye with cataract that has undergone trabeculectomy showing the presence of a cystic bleb in the superior quadrant

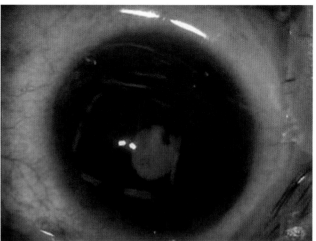

Fig. 18.4 Small pupil before the use of iris hooks

history of acute angle-closure attack, there is significant loss of endothelial cells due to the disease itself or from the laser peripheral iridotomy.[20]

All the anti-glaucoma medications, except pilocarpine and prostaglandin analogues, are continued to the date of surgery. Pilocarpine is stopped at least 2 weeks before cataract surgery to reverse the miotic effect. Since there have been reports on the possible causal relationship between prostaglandin analogue use and cystoid macular edema following cataract surgery, it is advisable to stop the medication, as well, for 1–2 weeks prior to surgery.[21,22] Since a high preoperative intraocular pressure increases the risk of intraoperative suprachoroidal hemorrhage, intravenous mannitol is sometimes used immediately prior to cataract surgery to reduce the intraocular pressure. See Table 20.4. If the preoperative intraocular pressure is above 30 mmHg on maximum medications, cataract removal alone is unlikely to lower the intraocular pressure to a safe level. In these circumstances, cataract removal needs to be combined with other intraocular pressure-lowering procedures including trabeculectomy and goniosynechialysis.

Operative Procedures

Intraoperative difficulties in eyes with primary angle-closure glaucoma stem from the presence of shallow anterior chamber, posterior synechiae, iris atrophy, large lens, and hazy cornea, as mentioned previously.

Phacoemulsification can usually be performed under topical anesthesia using Xylocaine 2% jelly.[23,24] See Chapter 2. A corneal wound is preferred because it leaves the conjunctiva uninterrupted for future filtering operation if needed.

In eyes with a small pupil, due to the presence of posterior synechiae, lysis of the synechiae is performed before performing the continuous curvilinear capsulorhexis. After breaking the synechiae, viscoelastic agent is injected into the anterior chamber to enlarge the pupil. If the pupil poorly reacts to mydriatics without the presence of posterior synechiae, 1:1000 adrenaline can be added to the infusion bottle. It is important to add the adrenaline at the start of the operation when the infusion bottle is still full to avoid it being too concentrated. Intracameral (preservative-free preferred) adrenaline (0.5 ml of 1 in 10,000) can also be used to achieve intraoperative mydriasis.[25] It is best avoided in eyes with low endothelial cell count because of the potential toxic effect on the endothelial cells by its preservatives, sodium bisulfite ($NaHSO_3$) and sodium metabisulphite ($Na_2S_2O_5$).[26,27] It is equally important to make sure that the patient has no cardiac diseases that contraindicate the use of adrenaline. Again, viscoelastic agent can be injected to force the pupil to dilate. If the above maneuvers fail, the iris can be stretched with iris pusher and iris hook. Finally, iris hooks can be used (Figs. 18.4and 18.5). Pain may be experienced by the patient during manipulation of the iris tissue. Intracameral lidocaine (0.3 ml 1% preservative-free lidocaine (50 mg/5 ml) may be added to supplement the topical anesthesia.[28] See also Chapter 3.

Because the anterior chamber is usually shallow, a copious amount of viscoelastic agent is required to maintain the anterior chamber and to flatten the anterior lens surface during introduction of instrumentation and performance of the continuous curvilinear capsulorhexis. It is important to flatten the lens surface with viscoelastic agent during continuous curvilinear capsulorhexis because a convex anterior lens surface predisposes to radial tear of the anterior capsule.

Capsule stain with either trypan blue 1% or indocyanine green 0.5% may be needed to aid with visualization of the anterior capsule in mature cataract and in dense cataract with a poor red reflex (Fig. 18.5).[29] See Table 20.5.

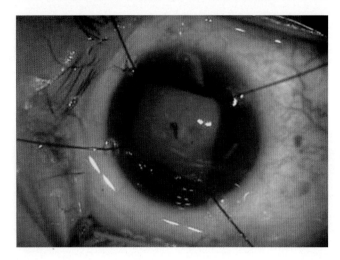

Fig. 18.5 The use of iris hooks to enlarge the pupil and capsule stain during phacoemulsification

Table 18.3 Medications to lower IOP following phacoemulsification

- Brinzolamide
- Brimonidine
- Acetazolamide
- Intracameral acetylcholine
- Timolol

The aspiration rate or the vacuum power should be reduced, in the presence of iris atrophy, to avoid aspiration of the iris tissue. Special measures should be adopted to protect the corneal endothelial cell during phacoemulsification. Use of a well-balanced irrigation solution that resembles the natural chemical properties of the aqueous is important.[30] The use of dispersive ophthalmic viscosurgical devices (OVDs) with low viscosity is preferred. The other option is to use a viscoadaptive device that possesses both cohesive and dispersive properties. These devices allow better anterior chamber depth maintenance as well as providing a longer retention time during high flow rates. They also protect the endothelial cells from the damaging effects of air bubbles.

Every step must be taken to avoid the complication of posterior capsule rupture and vitreous loss. Vitreous loss during cataract surgery in glaucoma patients adversely affects long-term intraocular pressure control.[31]

At the end of the surgery, the viscoelastic agent should be removed completely from the anterior capsule and the capsular bag to avoid a retained viscoelastic agent-induced postoperative intraocular pressure spike that can be sight-threatening in eyes with preexisting advanced optic nerve glaucomatous damage. Retained viscoelastic may cause trabecular meshwork blockage, postoperative capsular bag hyperdistension, anterior displacement of the intraocular lens optic, and capsular block from occlusion of the anterior circular opening.[32,33]

Postoperative Assessment and Medications

The operated eye is examined on the first postoperative day. The corneal clarity, the intraocular pressure, and the anterior chamber reaction are carefully assessed. Thereafter the patient is reassessed in 1–2 weeks' time and then according to clinical need. All the preoperative anti-glaucomatous medications are continued and titrated against the intraocular pressure. Pilocarpine and prostaglandin analogue should be avoided if possible. As mentioned, preoperative use of prostaglandin analogue may be associated with an increased risk for pseudophakic cystoid macular edema and prophylactic treatment with topical nonsteroidal anti-inflammatory drugs and steroids in the immediate postoperative period may be considered.[34] Routinely, topical steroid combined with antibiotic is given 6–8 times per day for a period of 2 weeks and tapered off gradually, over a period of 4–6 weeks in parallel with the subsidence of the anterior chamber reaction.

Postoperative Complications

A postoperative intraocular pressure spike is common in patients with preexisting glaucoma. In post-cataract surgery patients with raised intraocular pressure, anterior chamber paracentesis alone results in immediate control of intraocular pressure. However, the intraocular pressure reduction is transient and may rebound within an hour.[35] This intraocular pressure-lowering procedure is easy to perform under slit lamp biomicroscopy and is useful for retained viscoelastic agent-induced intraocular pressure spike. Intraocular pressure-lowering medications are also effective and will lead to a more gradual and sustained control of intraocular pressure. Multiple medications, as listed in Table 18.3, have similar effects in reducing intraocular pressures after phacoemulsification.[36]

It has been found that patients with high preoperative intraocular pressure are more likely to have intraocular pressure spikes after surgery. In a day-case setting these patients should be scheduled first on the operating list to facilitate postoperative intraocular pressure measurement and detection of intraocular pressure spike before being discharged home.[37] See Chapter 5.

Endothelial cell loss after phacoemulsification and intraocular lens implantation is around 5%.[38] A significant loss of endothelial cell may result in irreversible corneal decompensation necessitating penetrating keratoplasty. Eyes with primary angle-closure glaucoma are prone to endothelial cell damage during phacoemulsification because of

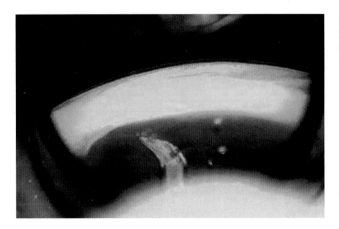

Fig. 18.6 Goniosynechialysis

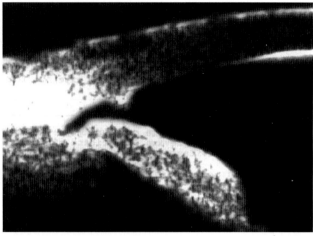

Fig. 18.8 Ultrasound biomicroscope (UBM) image of the angle after goniosynechialysis

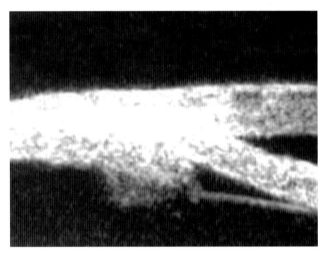

Fig. 18.7 Ultrasound biomicroscope (UBM) image of the angle before goniosynechialysis

shallow anterior chamber and large, hard cataractous lens. The cell loss can be as high as 18%.[14] The corneal endothelial cell loss after phacoemulsification in eyes with occludable angles was shown to be associated with preoperative axial length and the postoperative intraocular pressure within 24 h. To minimize corneal endothelial cell damage, it is critical to avoid an intraocular pressure spike during the early postoperative period and to exercise extreme caution intraoperatively in eyes with an axial length of less than 22.6 mm.[39] See Chapter 19.

Role of Goniosynechialysis

The objective of goniosynechialysis (GSL) is to open up the closed drainage angle by stripping the peripheral anterior synechiae from the angle wall (Figs. 18.6, 18.7, and 18.8).

The reported success rate if peripheral anterior synechiae are less than 1 year is 80%.[40,41] It is effective in phakic and

pseudophakic eyes and can be combined with phacoemulsification.[42–44] It is also effective after failed filtration surgery. There is no risk of overdrainage, suprachoroidal hemorrhage, or delayed endophthalmitis. The efficacy of goniosynechialysis for chronic peripheral anterior synechial angle closure is uncertain. Complications include optic nerve damage due to persistent high intraoperative intraocular pressure from the use of viscoelastic agent to maintain the anterior chamber throughout the procedure, postoperative intraocular pressure spike due to retained viscoelastic agent, hyphema, inflammation from manipulation of the iris tissue, and lens damage. When goniosynechialysis is combined with cataract extraction, the cataract is removed first. The anterior chamber becomes deep after cataract removal and it will facilitate the goniosynechialysis procedure. The intraocular pressure reduction may be the additive effect of the two procedures. Post-goniosynechialysis laser peripheral iridoplasty can be performed to minimize the chance of angle re-closure in future.[41,42,45] It has been reported that 180° is also effective for treating primary angle-closure glaucoma eyes with total synechial angle closure.[41,42]

Since removal of the lens has so many advantages in the surgical management of primary angle-closure glaucoma, goniosynechialysis alone is diminishing in its importance. The procedure is usually combined with cataract extraction.

Phacoemulsification in Filtered (Functioning Bleb) Primary Angle-Closure Glaucoma Eyes

Patients with primary angle-closure glaucoma may have had a prior filtering operation for the control of intraocular pressure. Cataract extraction in these eyes will have some added difficulties because of the presence of a bleb. If the bleb is large, a temporal corneal approach is adopted to avoid damaging the bleb directly. A Seidel test for bleb leakage should be performed in the preoperative assessment (Fig. 9.4). Any leak must be sealed before proceeding to phacoemulsification. The positive pressure during phacoemulsification may rupture a small cystic bleb with a very thin bleb wall. Intraoperative bleb leakage is not easily identifiable by direct observation under the operating microscope. Indocyanine green staining enables the surgeon to clearly visualize aqueous leakage from the bleb. The bleb leakage can be repaired with 10-0 nylon sutures18.1 [46] preferably on a BV or other small needle.

Previously successful bleb needling can be significantly compromised by subsequent cataract surgery.[47] Phacoemulsification significantly increased intraocular pressure even without an effect on the intrableb features as shown by ultrasound biomicroscopy imaging.[48] Eyes with higher intraocular pressure, invisible route under scleral flap, and stronger intrableb reflectivity on ultrasound biomicroscopy imaging before phacoemulsification had greater postoperative bleb failure.[48]

However, phacoemulsification in eyes with a functional filtering bleb for primary angle-closure glaucoma can be accomplished without compromising the functioning of the bleb. It has been reported that the difference between the preoperative and the postoperative intraocular pressures at all occasions during follow-up was statistically insignificant but the central anterior chamber depth was significantly deeper in the post-phacoemulsification eyes.[49] See also Chapter 16.

Summary

Primary angle-closure glaucoma often coexists with senile cataract. Increasing evidence has shown that removal of the cataract or even removal of the lens that has minimal cataract will deepen the anterior chamber, widen the drainage angle, and lower the intraocular pressure without a combined filtering operation. The outcome in terms of intraocular pressure control is as effective as cases that undergo filtering operations, at least in the short-term postoperative period. This new trend of surgical management of primary angle-closure glaucoma offers several advantages compared with traditional surgical management in the past where trabeculectomy or phacotrabeculectomy were the treatments of choice. The advantages include faster visual recovery, avoidance of complications associated with trabeculectomy, and substantial savings in medical resources. More studies are required to assess the long-term effect of cataract extraction alone on the intraocular pressure control. Cataract surgery primarily can be considered in eyes without risk of "snuff-out" or advanced visual field loss where there is time to assess the response to the cataract operation without significant risk if there is delay of lowering of IOP or need for a filtration procedure.

References

1. Congdon N, Wang F, Tielsch JM. Issues in the epidemiology and population-based screening of chronic angle-closure glaucoma. *Surv Ophthalmol.* 1992;36:411–23.
2. Salmon JF, Mermoud A, Ivey A, et al. The prevalence of primary angle-closure glaucoma and open-angle glaucoma in Mamre, Western Cape, South Africa. *Arch Ophthalmol.* 1993;111:1263–9.
3. Campbell DG. Primary angle-closure glaucoma, proportionality principle: the direct relationship between the degree of closure and the elevation of the intraocular pressure. In: Albert DM, Jakobiec FA, eds. Albert & Jakobiec principles and practice of ophthalmology clinical practice CD-ROM. Philadelphia: WM Saunders Company, 1995; Chapter 120. Records 41922–41928.
4. Lowe RF. Aetiology of the anatomical basis for primary angle-closure glaucoma. Biometrical comparisons between normal eyes and eyes with primary angle-closure glaucoma. *Br J Ophthalmol.* 1970;54:161–9.
5. Lowe RF. Causes of shallow anterior chamber in primary angle-closure glaucoma. Ultrasonic biometry of normal and angle-closure glaucoma eyes. *Am J Ophthalmol.* 1969;67:87–93.
6. Hayashi K, Hayashi H, Nakao F, Hayashi F. Changes in anterior chamber angle width and depth after intraocular lens implantation in eyes with glaucoma. *Ophthalmology.* 2000;107:698–703.
7. Kurimoto Y, Park M, Sakaue H, Kondo T. Changes in the anterior chamber configuration after small-incision cataract surgery with posterior chamber lens implantation. *Am J Ophthalmol.* 1997;124:775–80.
8. Yang CH, Hung PT. Intraocular lens position and anterior chamber angle changes after cataract extraction in eyes with primary angle-closure glaucoma. *J Cataract Refract Surg.* 1997;23:1109–13.
9. Hayashi K, Hayashi H, Nakao F, Hayashi F. Effect of cataract surgery on intraocular pressure control in glaucoma patients. *J Cataract Refract Surg.* 2001;27:1779–86.
10. Roberts TV, Francis IC, Lertusumitkul S, et al. Primary phacoemulsification for uncontrolled angle-closure glaucoma. *J Cataract Refract Surg.* 2000;26:1012–6.
11. Lai JS, Tham CC, Chan JC. The clinical outcomes of cataract extraction by phacoemulsification in eyes with primary angle-closure glaucoma (PACG) and co-existing cataract: a prospective case series. *J Glaucoma.* 2006;15:47–52.
12. Pereira FA, Cronemberger S. Ultrasound biomicroscopic study of anterior segment changes after phacoemulsification and foldable intraocular lens implantation. *Ophthalmology.* 2003;110:1799–1806.
13. Nonaka A, Kondo T, Kikuchi M, et al. Cataract surgery for residual angle closure after peripheral laser iridotomy. *Ophthalmology.* 2005;112:974–9.
14. Kubota T, Toguri I, Onizuka N, Matsuura T. Phacoemulsification and intraocular lens implantation for angle closure glaucoma after the relief of pupillary block. *Ophthalmologica.* 2003;217:325–8.
15. Tham CC, Leung DY, Kwong YY, Li FC, Lai JS. Effects of phacoemulsification versus combined phaco-trabeculectomy on drainage angle status in primary angle closure glaucoma (PACG). Unpublished data.
16. 16.Tham CC, Kwong YY, Leung DY, et al. Phacoemulsification alone versus combined phaco-trabeculectomy in medically-controlled chronic angle closure glaucoma with coexisting cataract. *Ophthalmology.* 2008 [In press].

17. Chan JC, Lai JS, Tham CC. Comparison of postoperative refractive outcome in phacotrabeculectomy and phacoemulsification with posterior chamber intraocular lens implantation. *J Glaucoma.* 2006;15:26–9.

18. Obuchowska I, Mariak Z. Risk factors of massive suprachoroidal hemorrhage during extracapsular cataract extraction surgery. *Eur J Ophthalmol.* 2005;15:712–7.

19. Costa VP, Smith M, Spaeth GL, Gandham S, Markovitz B. Loss of visual acuity after trabeculectomy. *Ophthalmology.* 1993;100:599–612.

20. Tham CC, Kwong YY, Lai JS, Lam DS. Effect of a previous acute angle closure attack on the corneal endothelial cell density in chronic angle closure glaucoma patients. *J Glaucoma.* 2006;15:482–548.

21. Altintaş O, Yüksel N, Karabaş VL, Demirci G. Cystoid macular edema associated with latanoprost after uncomplicated cataract surgery. *Eur J Ophthalmol* 2005;15:158–61.

22. Yeh PC, Ramanathan S. Latanoprost and clinically significant cystoid macular edema after uneventful phacoemulsification with intraocular lens implantation.J Cataract Refract Surg. 2002;28:1814–8.

23. Kershner RM. Topical anesthesia for small incision self-sealing cataract surgery. A prospective evaluation of the first 100 patients. *J Cataract Refract Surg.* 1993;19:290–2.

24. Duguid IG, Claoue CM, Thamby-Rajah Y, Allan BD, Dart JK, Steele AD. Topical anesthesia for phacoemulsification surgery. *Eye.* 1995;9:456–9.

25. Soong T, Soultanidis M, C.laoué C, Gallagher M, Thomson S. Safety of intracameral mydriasis in phacoemulsification cataract surgery. *J Cataract Refract Surg.* 2006;32:375–6.

26. Hull DS, Chemotti MT, Edelhauser HF, Van Horn DL, Hyndiuk RA. Effect of epinephrine on the corneal endothelium. *Am J Ophthalmol.* 1975;79:245–50.

27. Pong JC, Tang EW, Tang WW, Lai JS. Toxic anterior segment syndrome after intraocular lens repositioning with intracameral adrenaline. *J Cataract Refract Surg.* 2008 [In press].

28. Ezra DG, Nambiar A, Allan BD. Supplementary intracameral lidocaine for phacoemulsification under topical anesthesia. A meta-analysis of randomized controlled trials. *Ophthalmology.* 2008;115:455–87.

29. Chung CF, Liang CC, Lai JS, Lo ES. Safety of trypan blue 1% and indocyanine green 0.5% in assisting visualization of anterior capsule during phacoemulsification in mature cataract. *J Cataract Refract Surg.* 2005;31:938–42.

30. Nuyts RM, Edelhauser HF, Holley GP. Intraocular irrigating solution, a comparison of Hartmann's lactated Ringer's solution, BSS and BSS Plus. *Graefes Arch Clin Exp Ophthalmol* 1995;233: 655–61.

31. Sharma TK, Nessim M, Kyprianou I, Kumar V, Shah P, O'Neil E. Vitreous loss during phacoemulsification in glaucoma patients: long-term intraocular pressure control. *J Cataract Refract Surg.* 2008;34:831–4.

32. Mastropasqua L, Carpineto P, Ciancaglini M, Falconio G. Intraocular pressure changes after phacoemulsification and foldable silicone lens implantation using Healon GV. *Ophthalmologica.* 1998;212:318–21.

33. Watts P, Austin M. Retained Viscoat and intraocular pressure after phaceomulsification. *Indian J Ophthalmol.* 1999;47:237–40.

34. Henderson BA, Kim JY, Ament CS, Ferrufino-Ponce ZK, Grabowska A, Cremers SL. Clinical pseudophakic cystoid macular edema. Risk factors for development and duration after treatment. *J Cataract Refract Surg.* 2007;33:1550–8.

35. John M, Souchek J, Noblitt RL, Boleyn KL, Davis LC. Side-port incision paracentesis versus anti-glaucoma medication to control postoperative pressure rises after intraocular lens surgery. *J Cataract Refract Surg.* 1993;19:62–3.

36. Borazan M, Karalezli A, Akman A, Akova YA. Effect of antiglaucoma agents on postoperative intraocular pressure after cataract surgery with Viscoat. *J Cataract Refract Surg.* 2007;33:1941–5.

37. O'Brien PD, Ho SL, Fitzpatrick P, Power W. Risk factors for a postoperative intraocular pressure spike after phacoemulsification. *Can J Ophthalmol.* 2007 42:51–5.

38. Hayashi K, Hayashi H, Nakao F, Hayashi F. Corneal endothelial cell loss in phacoemulsification surgery with silicone intraocular lens implantation. *J Cataract Refract Surg.* 1996;22:743–7.

39. Ko YC, Liu CJ, Lau LI, Wu CW, Chou JC, Hsu WM. Factors related to corneal endothelial damage after phacoemulsification in eyes with occludable angles. *J Cataract Refract Surg.* 2008;34: 46–51.

40. Shingleton BJ, Chang MA, Bellows AR, Thomas JV. Surgical goniosynechialysis for angle-closure glaucoma. *Ophthalmology.* 1990;97:551–6.

41. Lai JS, Tham CC. Efficacy and safety of inferior 180 degrees goniosynechialysis followed by diode laser peripheral iridoplasty in the treatment of chronic angle-closure glaucoma. *J Glaucoma.* 2000;9:388–391.

42. Lai JS, Tham CC. The efficacy and safety of combined phacoemulsification, intraocular lens implantation, and limited goniosynechialysis, followed by diode laser peripheral iridoplasty, in the treatment of cataract and chronic angle-closure glaucoma. *J Glaucoma.* 2001;10:309–15.

43. Harasymowycz PJ, Papamatheakis DG, Ahmed I, et al. Phacoemulsification and goniosynechialysis in the management of unresponsive primary angle closure. *J Glaucoma.* 2005;14: 186–9.

44. Razeghinejad MR. Combined phacoemulsification and viscogonosynechialysis in patients with refractory acute angle-closure glaucoma. *J Cataract Refract Surg.* 2008;34:827–30.

45. Tanihara H, Nagata M. Argon laser gonioplasty following goniosynechialysis. *Graefes Arch Clin Exp Ophthalmol.* 1991;229:505–7.

46. Okazaki T, Kiuchi T, Kawana K, Oshika T. Indocyanine green staining facilitates detection of bleb leakage during trabeculectomy. *J Glaucoma.* 2007;16:257–9.

47. Rotchford AP, King A. Cataract surgery after needling revision of trabeculectomy blebs. *J Glaucoma.* 2007;16:562–6.

48. Wang X, Zhang H, Li S, Wang N. The effects of phacoemulsification on intraocular pressure and ultrasound biomicroscopic image of filtering bleb in eyes with cataract and functioning filtering blebs. *Eye.* 2007 Oct 12. [Epub ahead of print].

49. Khokhar S, Sindhu N, Pangtey MS. Phacoemulsification in filtered chronic angle closure glaucoma eyes. *Clin Experiment Ophthalmol.* 2002;30:256–60.

Chapter 19

Nanophthalmos

Carlos Gustavo Vasconcelos de Moraes and Remo Susanna Jr.

Introduction

Nanophthalmos (Greek: nanos = "dwarf, small"; ophthalmos = "eye") is an uncommon developmental disorder that can potentially result in sight-threatening outcomes. Most cases are bilateral and sporadic, although a pattern of autosomal recessive transmission has been described. Both sexes are equally affected.[1]

Conceptually, nanophthalmos represents a pure form of microphthalmos without any systemic abnormalities. While in microphthalmia the eye may show gross developmental defects, the nanophthalmic eye is a small but functional eye with relatively preserved anatomy.

There is still controversy regarding the possible causes of nanophthalmos. Hirsch et al.[2] suggested that a developmental arrest of the optic vesicle after the closure of the embryonic fissure results in a small eye. However, their theory does not explain some other ocular abnormalities found in this disorder to be described further. In 1982, Ryan et al.[3] proposed that a smaller-than-normal optic vesicle growing from the forebrain at the early stages of embryogenesis may be responsible for the reduced ocular size and its associated histological abnormalities.

Nanophthalmos is clinically characterized by the features listed in Table 19.1.

Singh et al.[4] described a group of nanophthalmic eyes with an average corneal diameter of 10.3 mm, an average axial length of 17.0 mm, and an average lens thickness of 5.1 mm. A linear relationship has been demonstrated between cycloplegic refraction and axial length in nanophthalmic eyes.[5] Yet, corneal and lens increased refractive power may compensate for the excessive hyperopia that would otherwise be anticipated in these eyes.[2]

C.G. Vasconcelos de Moraes (✉)
Department of Ophthalmology, Glaucoma Associates of New York, New York Eye and Ear Infirmary, New York, NY 10003, USA
e-mail: gustavousp@gmail.com

Table 19.1 Features of nanophthalmos

- Short anterior–posterior axial length
- Short corneal diameter
- Flat anterior chamber
- Abnormal and thick sclera
- Small to normal lens thickness/high lens-eye ratio
- Narrow palpebral fissure
- Eyes deeply set in the orbits

Table 19.2 Posterior segment findings in nanophthalmos

- Crowded optic discs
- Papillomacular striae and folds
- Foveal aplasia
- Yellow pigmentation

During ophthalmoscopy, uncommon findings listed in Table 19.2 may be observed. These findings could be explained by the disparity in growth between the neurosensory retina and the outer layers of the eye.[6,7] Ultrasound biomicroscopy (UBM) also shows an anteriorly placed ciliary body, reduced ciliary sulcus, and an iris aspect that resembles plateau iris configuration.[8] The sclera is thicker than in the normal eye (see Fig. 19.1) and its collagen lamellae are disorganized, with variable sizes, decreased amounts of glycosaminoglycans, and elevated fibronectin content.[9–12] Because of the abnormally thick sclera and crowded vasculature, increased amplitude of the ocular pulse may be noticed during applanation tonometry.[4]

Nanophthalmic eyes are more prone to the development of angle-closure glaucoma due to their high lens-eye volume ratio, which results in crowding of the anterior chamber. Moreover, the presence of thick and abnormal sclera predisposes nanophthalmic eyes to develop choroidal effusion and exudative retinal detachment.[1–4] The thick sclera may impede drainage of the venous blood through the vortex veins, as well as reduce the permeability to proteins, leading to uveal effusion syndrome.[13] Other complications that have been associated with nanophthalmos are listed in Table 19.3. These events may occur spontaneously or following any type

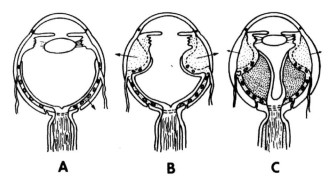

Fig. 19.1 The mechanism of uveal effusion in nanophthalmous described by Gass. (**a**) Normal eye with focal vascular leak. (**b**) Aphakic eye with transient postoperative ciliochoroidal detachment that usually resolves spontaneously within days. (**c**) Uveal effusion syndrome with increased resistance to protein outflow and uveal venous outflow caused by abnormally thick sclera

Table 19.3 Complications associated with nanophthalmos
- Choroidal effusion
- Exudative retinal detachment
- Malignant glaucoma
- Pupillary block
- Expulsive suprachoroidal hemorrhage
- Shallow anterior chamber

of intraocular intervention (e.g., peripheral laser iridotomy, cataract surgery, and filtering procedures).

Because of the increased risk of post-surgical complications, surgical treatment in nanophthalmos should be considered a last resort. The physician must carefully weigh risks and benefits before indicating surgery in this population, since these postoperative complications may cause significant visual impairment.

Key Points:

- Nanophthalmic eyes show reduced biometric measurements.
- Crowding of the anterior chamber may lead to angle-closure glaucoma.
- There is an increased risk of postoperative complications in these eyes.

Indications for Surgery

In nanophthalmic eyes, a relative pupillary block secondary to iridolenticular contact may eventually lead to development of peripheral anterior synechiae (PAS) and increased intraocular pressure (IOP) and, thus, angle-closure glaucoma (ACG). Alternatively, when nanophthalmos presents with annular ciliochoroidal effusion and ciliary body detachment, the anterior chamber angle may also be closed by physical displacement of the peripheral iris by anteriorly rotated ciliary processes.

Glaucoma treatment in nanophthalmic eyes involves peripheral laser iridotomy, gonioplasty, and use of antiglaucoma medication, when necessary. Filtering procedures may be indicated if unsatisfactory IOP control persists despite maximal tolerated therapy. The prevalence of cataract may increase with age, so that combined surgical procedures may become necessary during follow-up.

As described previously, nanophthalmic eyes present a high lens-eye volume ratio that is involved in the pathogenesis of angle-closure glaucoma. The incidence of glaucoma in these eyes is inversely correlated with the axial length and might increase with age (most cases of angle-closure glaucoma occur between 30 and 50 years of age) probably because of thickened lens diameter leading to flat anterior chamber and increased iridocorneal apposition.[14]

When the nanophthalmic patient presents with significant lens opacity and impaired visual acuity, most ophthalmologists agree that cataract surgery should be performed. However, there is continued debate about whether an eye with a transparent lens should be subjected to an intraocular procedure and thus be placed at risk for sight-threatening postoperative complications. Some authors counter that cataract surgery halts the mechanism of angle closure, as lens removal deepens the anterior chamber and decreases contact between the iris periphery and corneal endothelium, and therefore has added utility in nanophthalmos[5,14–16] (see Fig. 19.2a and b). We believe that despite this argument, there is still no consensus whether the benefits of transparent lens extraction may benefit nanophthalmic patients and prevent angle closure during long-term follow-up. Taking into account the high *rate* of complications in nanophthalmic eyes, cataract surgery should be undertaken with caution. This *decision* will depend on the biomicroscopic evaluation and the level of visual impairment *indicated* by the patient. Macular hypoplasia is one of the differential diagnoses of low vision in nanophthalmic eyes, which should be differentiated from the visual impairment caused by cataract. The use of PAM (potential acuity meter) may be helpful in these cases.

Preoperative Considerations

A complete ophthalmic evaluation is strongly recommended before any type of surgery in nanophthalmic eyes.

A careful evaluation of the eye's best corrected visual acuity (BCVA) is advisable before the procedure for both

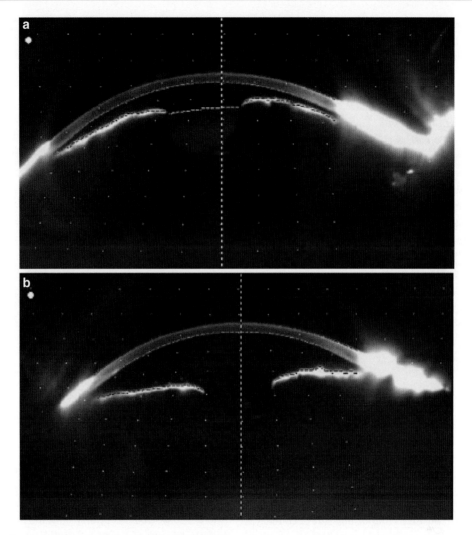

Fig. 19.2 Pentacam images of the anterior chamber of nanophthalmic eye (**a**) before and (**b**) after cataract surgery. Figures courtesy of John R. Grigg, MD, and reprinted by permission from Sharan et al.[8] Elsevier

legal purposes and to enable more detailed follow-up. Biomicroscopic evaluation should include the following: (1) presence of blepharitis or other potential sources of infection; (2) evaluation of pupil dilation, if necessary, should be monitored closely due to the increased risk of developing acute angle closure following pharmacologic mydriasis; (3) classification of the lens opacity, which can be difficult due to its poor response to miosis; (4) anterior chamber depth; (5) gonioscopy, which should be compared postoperatively; and (6) fundus evaluation, if possible. Even when appropriate fundus examination is impossible due to media opacities and/or miosis, ocular ultrasonography and biometry should be performed. Data regarding the presence of uveal effusion before surgery, axial length, and lens thickness may help in planning the procedure. The presence of glaucomatous optic neuropathy (GON) or high IOP under treatment may help decide whether combined cataract-glaucoma surgery would be beneficial.

IOL Choice

Lens power calculation remains a challenge when performing cataract surgery in nanophthalmic eyes. The maximum IOL power available may vary among different companies, most of them ranging between 30 and 40 diopters, so that placing a single intraocular lens leaving the patient with residual refractive error versus multiple intraocular lens (IOL) implantation can be considered. It has been extensively discussed in the literature whether a single high-power IOL or piggy-back lenses should be used. Cases of glaucoma have been described following piggy back IOLs, and nanophthalmic eyes may be more prone to this given their anatomy. Caution should be pursued when using this approach in these eyes.[17-19]

We recommend that the IOL power calculation be performed using the Haigis and Hoffer Q biometric formulas,[20] inserting a single piece acrylic lens in the poster chamber.[15,21] Also, the Haigis formula seems to be more accurate for open-loop lenses, whereas the Hoffer Q is more accurate for plate-haptics design. The most common complications of piggy-back implantation are interlenticular opacification, which may cause hyperopic shift and decrease in vision, and IOL anterior displacement.[22]

Using a combination of acrylic and silicone IOLs in the capsular bag may decrease the incidence of opacification postoperatively. For instance, a hydrophobic acrylic IOL may be inserted posteriorly in the capsular bag preventing capsular opacification, while a silicone IOL may be inserted more anteriorly in the ciliary sulcus. Preferably, the lens power should be calculated so that a slight hyperopia (+0.50 to +1.50) will remain postoperatively. Angle closure secondary to a piggy back IOL has been described as well as pigmentary glaucoma secondary to piggy back acrylic lenses in the sulcus.[23,24]

Prophylaxis

The use of oral steroids and intravenous acetazolamide and mannitol (see Table 20.4) preoperatively has been suggested to prevent major intraocular complications (uveal effusion, iris prolapsed, expulsive hemorrhage).[25,26]

Some drugs used during general anesthesia cause transient IOP decrease, which may be favorable during the operation. Moreover, extraconal and intraconal anesthesia may lead to intraoperative positive vitreous pressure secondary to orbital volumetric expansion. When general anesthesia is not an option, care should be taken not to infuse over 3 ml of local anesthetics intraconal. Some may prefer to use topical tetracaine or subconjunctival lidocaine with a blunt cannula. See Chapter 2.

Surgical Procedures to Prevent Uveal Effusion

The pathophysiologic mechanism of uveal effusion is not completely understood; however, it seems well accepted that the thickened sclera is part of the problem. It is thought to induce choroidal effusion by compressing the vortex veins, impeding normal venous outflow.[3,4,13]

Based on this theory, Brockhurst[27] introduced the vortex vein decompression with lamellar sclera resection, which reduced high venous pressure in the choriocapillaris, thereby reducing the leakage of fluids and proteins. He advocated that the procedure should be performed at the time of cataract surgery.

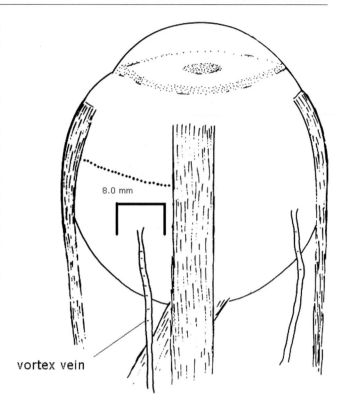

Fig. 19.3 Scleral decompression technique modified from Brockhurst

Scleral resection with vortex vein decompression is performed by excising 8 × 8 mm pieces of partial-thickness sclera between the rectus muscles in each quadrant. The sclera is dissected posteriorly until the intrascleral portion of each vortex vein is exposed and decompressed. The edges of the scleral wound are cauterized by diathermy to prevent adhesion resulting from scarring. This allows the fluid to be drained from the suprachoroidal space continuously after surgery. However, this technique was thought to be difficult and caused considerable bleeding during removal of the sclera; also, it is often difficult to identify the vortex veins, which may sometimes be hypoplastic (Fig. 19.3).

Johnson and Gass[28] reported in 1990 that uveal effusion could instead be treated by lamellar sclera resection and sclerotomy. Their technique involves the creation of rectangular 5 × 7 mm, one-half to two-thirds sclerectomies in each quadrant, centered just anterior to the equator and placed outside the meridian of each vortex vein to avoid its intrascleral course. A linear sclerostomy (approximately 2 mm) is made in the center of each sclerectomy bed and enlarged with 1- to 2-mm scleral punch. No attempt is made to drain subretinal fluid[28] (Fig. 19.4).

In the same year, Jin and Anderson[29] described a V-shaped full-thickness sclerotomy that is left unsutured to provide ongoing drainage postoperatively. They suggested making a conjunctival incision far from the limbus and

sclerectomies   sclerostomies

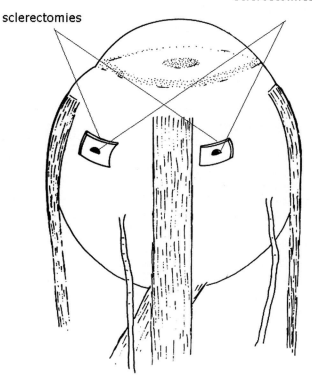

Fig. 19.4 Scleral decompression technique described by Gass

dissecting forward to make the scleral incision far forward, just behind the limbus. Next, they performed a 5 × 7 mm two-thirds thick sclerectomy and removed a 1-mm scleral piece from its bed, which allowed continuous outflow of the suprachoroidal fluid. It should be done in two quadrants, in case one sclerectomy seals over. The scleral area above the pars plana should be avoided, since there is only a thin layer of uvea separating the vitreous cavity from the orbit that can rupture and cause vitreous to prolapse through the ocular wall. Thus, sclerectomy should be performed as anteriorly as possible. After creating the scleral hole, it is left opened, and the conjunctival incision is then closed, according to personal communication from Douglas Anderson, MD (Fig. 19.5).

There are no studies comparing these three techniques in terms of efficiency in preventing uveal effusion syndrome. Yet, it is recommended that one of the scleral decompression procedures should be performed before any intraocular surgery. The authors prefer the latter one due to its simplicity.

Key Points:

• Cataract surgery should be recommended with caution in nanophthalmic eyes due to the high rate of intraoperative and postoperative complications.
• Scleral decompression is advised before surgery.

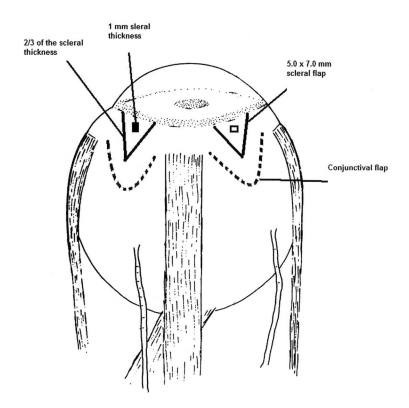

Fig. 19.5 Scleral decompression as described by Jin and Anderson

Surgical Technique

Two techniques of cataract surgery are typically performed in nanophthalmic eyes: (1) extracapsular cataract extraction (ECCE), and (2) phacoemulsification. Phacoemulsification is the recommended surgery technique, since it is performed in a closed system compared to the extracapsular technique, thereby reducing perioperative complications. In some cases, lensectomy from a posterior approach in combination with a pars plana vitrectomy may be undertaken, as in cases when the anterior chamber is extremely shallow. This procedure spares the corneal endothelium and may be technically easier to perform in terms of instrument manipulation.

Extracapsular Cataract Extraction

Detailed ECCE techniques are described in Chapter 7.

Appropriate exposure is a challenge when operating on nanophthalmic eyes, especially during ECCE. Placement of a traction suture, preferably in the superior rectus, is advisable. As described previously, nanophthalmic eyes may present with poor pupillary dilation, requiring sphincter enlargement using iris hooks, sphincterotomies, or breaking posterior synechiae with an iris spatula or Kuglen hook. See Chapter 3.

The ECCE technique allows extraction of the entire lens nucleus with minimal intraocular manipulation, using either a corneal or scleral incision. However, a sudden decrease in IOP may result in uveal effusion, secondary retinal detachment, or suprachoroidal hemorrhage. Moreover, secondary increased vitreous pressure, due to choroidal expansion, may lead to iris prolapse, posterior capsule rupture, and vitreous loss.

Care should be taken in order to avoid sudden IOP decrease after penetrating the anterior chamber and to avoid a lengthy intraoperative course.

Phacoemulsification

In 1990, Brockhurst[25] described the first case of phacoemulsification with IOL implantation in a nanophthalmic eye. However, the author documented choroidal and retinal detachments secondary to the procedure.

Faucher et al.[15] and later Wu[30] suggested that the improved control and smaller IOP fluctuation achieved with phacoemulsification and small incision cataract surgery appeared to lower the risk of uveal effusion. The improved

Table 19.4 Surgical instruments typically used during phacotrabeculectomy

- 7–0 black silk suture on a semicircular needle (traction suture)
- 10-0 nylon suture
- Westcott scissors
- Conjunctival forceps
- Colibri forceps
- #75 blade
- Scleral pocket knife
- Paracentesis slit knife
- Anterior segment infusion cannula
- Sclerectomy punch
- Sponges
- Mitomycin C
- Burato holder
- Ultrata forceps
- Vannas scissors
- Irrigation-aspiration tips
- Phaco apparatus

IOP control was attributed to the reducing of the anterior chamber crowding after lens removal.

Despite these results, it should be emphasized that this surgery is technically difficult in small eyes, which makes instrument manipulation in the anterior chamber extremely dangerous. The proximity between the ultrasound waves and the endothelium may increase the risk of corneal decompensation and postoperative edema. Similarly, the water-column tension generated by the balanced saline solution (BSS) height may lead to transitory IOP elevation and, in turn, stress the zonular bundles. Capsulorhexis should be performed carefully with appropriate size (4–6 mm diameter) under viscoelastic to avoid extension to periphery. This complication is more likely to occur in nanophthalmic eyes due to their increased vitreous pressure.

Sutureless corneal incisions may be associated with a positive Seidel test following the operations, which may result in sudden IOP lowering during blinking or minor postoperative activity. This could precipitate choroidal effusion or suprachoroidal hemorrhage. We also recommend that sclerotomies should be performed before phacoemulsification as well (see Table 19.4 for surgical instruments).

Postoperative Care

Postoperative recommendations for general cataract surgery also apply to intraocular procedures in nanophthalmic eyes. If the surgery is performed in an ambulatory surgical center, patients may return home following the procedure but should avoid Valsalva maneuver, which may predispose to choroidal effusion or suprachoroidal hemorrhages.

Antibiotic and steroid eye drops should be used postoperatively. Topical antibiotics four times a day should be tapered within the first week and topical steroids four times a day or more within the first month, depending on inflammation and the presence of complications. Careful monitoring of the anterior chamber depth is mandatory in order to detect aqueous misdirection or hemorrhagic suprachoroidal detachment, both of which usually present as flat anterior chamber in the presence of high IOP.

If fundoscopic evaluation is impaired by poor pupil dilation and the clinician suspects uveal effusion, complementary ultrasonography or ultrasound biomicroscopy (UBM) should be performed and repeated during follow-up.

Outcomes of Cataract Surgery

Most studies that have evaluated the visual outcomes following cataract surgery in nanophthalmic eyes have demonstrated improvement of the best corrected visual acuity (range 70–100%).[15,16,22,25] Yet, a significant number of eyes developed mild to serious complications that have led to visual deterioration and even phthisis bulbi. Jin and Anderson[29] reported good results following ECCE plus posterior chamber intraocular lens (PC IOL) implantation in combination with full-thickness sclerostomy. None of the nine operated eyes developed postoperative choroidal effusion, retinal detachment, or malignant glaucoma; seven eyes had improved vision. Juneman et al. reported the results of cataract surgery on 20 eyes in Germany. These patients had extracapsular cataract surgery and anterior sclerotomy was performed in one eye at the time of surgery. Initial vision improved in 16 eyes and three patients had postoperative glaucoma problems including angle closure, iris bombe, and aqueous misdirection that required intervention.[30]

Faucher et al.[15] reported a series of six nanophthalmic patients who underwent phacoemulsification with IOL implantation. Prophylactic sclerotomies were not performed in any case. All six eyes maintained or improved their visual acuity, and five of the six showed stable or improved IOP control following the procedure. The series from Wu included 12 eyes and sclerotomies were done if there was a history of choroidal effusion (2 eyes) or at the surgeon's discretion (2 eyes) and one also received mannitol. Their patients had a mean number of prior procedures of 2.5. None of the eyes lost vision with the cataract surgery but there were complications including a case of choroidal hemorrhage and two of aqueous misdirection.[31]

Cataract extraction improves the outflow facility, providing IOP control, and relieving potential glaucoma.[15,16,22]

Key Points:

- Extracapsular cataract extraction (ECCE) and phacoemulsification are often indicated in nanophthalmic eyes with significant visual impairment due to cataract. Phacoemulsification is the preferred technique.
- The surgical technique should be adapted in these eyes to avoid complications.
- Attention to postoperative complications, particularly uveal effusion and flat anterior chamber, is advised.
- Visual outcomes are usually satisfactory.

Glaucoma Treatment Versus Cataract Surgery

As described earlier, nanophthalmos is associated with the development of peripheral anterior synechiae (PAS) and angle-closure glaucoma. Peripheral laser iridotomy (PLI) is widely recommended in any case of nanophthalmos regardless of the level of glaucomatous damage.[14] If apposition persists despite PLI, peripheral iridoplasty may be indicated.

Non-penetrating glaucoma surgery is not indicated in cases of angle-closure glaucoma. Trabeculectomy may therefore be required in patients who continue presenting unsatisfactory clinical control after PLI or peripheral iridoplasty.

If significant cataract is present at the time trabeculectomy is considered, the physician may need to choose between performing a combined procedure (phacotrabeculectomy) or trabeculectomy followed by cataract extraction at a future date. The severity of the glaucoma and cataract, as well as the potential improved IOP control after lens removal as described previously should be weighed carefully against the risk of increased bleb failure and complications when performing phacotrabeculectomy.

We recommend that whenever significant cataract exists and trabeculectomy is indicated, that a combined procedure should be performed. In cases of severe glaucomatous optic neuropathy (GON), we prefer to perform the trabeculectomy first and, when the bleb is mature, to perform phacoemulsification. As a routine, we inject daily subconjunctival 5-fluorouracil (5-FU; 0.2 ml of a 50 mg/ml solution) or mitomycin-C (MMC; 0.1 ml of a 0.3 mg/ml solution) postoperatively for 4–7 days to reduce the possibility of bleb failure, which may occur in this situation, and to increase efficacy of the bleb.[32]

ECCE-Trabeculectomy

Although most surgeons prefer a combined phacoemulsification and trabeculectomy, a combined ECCE and filtration procedure can be a safe and effective alternative. A brief description of the technique follows.

After the preoperative IOP reduction has been performed, a superior rectus bridle suture should be placed. The decompression sclerostomies should be performed inferiorly to avoid overlapping with the superior scleral incisions. A superior conjunctival flap is then developed, followed by cauterization of the filtration site. The scleral sulcus is grooved and the paracentesis track made. The anterior chamber should be filled with sodium hyaluronate to avoid an intraoperative flat chamber. The further steps of a conventional ECCE should be performed. After IOL implantation, sclerectomy and a peripheral iridectomy are performed, and then the sclera is closed completely with 10-0 nylon sutures except in the area where the trabeculectomy flap is placed. Test filtration and adjust the trabeculectomy flap sutures as necessary. The conjunctiva is then closed with 10-0 nylon suture and should be water-tight. A subconjunctival injection of steroids and topical atropine are recommended.

Phacotrabeculectomy

The technique that will be discussed here is the two-site fornix-based phacotrabeculectomy, which is preferred by the authors. Before combined cataract and glaucoma surgery, some considerations should be addressed. The preoperative recommendations described herein should be remembered. Hyperosmotic agents 30 minutes before surgery followed by prophylactic sclerotomies are mandatory. These should be made inferiorly between the rectus muscles in order to spare the superior conjunctiva for the trabeculectomy. After scleral decompression, the eye may become hypotonic, which may cause difficulty for creating the surgical incisions. This problem may be overcome by injecting viscoelastic solution into the anterior chamber.

A fornix-based flap of conjunctiva and Tenon's capsule is created superiorly. After homeostasis of the episcleral blood vessels with wet-field cautery, a one-half thickness rectangular (4.0 × 2.0 mm) scleral flap (1.5 mm from the limbus) is outlined and dissected anteriorly without entry into the anterior chamber. Surgical sponges (typically three) measuring about 2.0 mm × 2.0 mm are soaked in a solution of 0.5 mg/ml MMC. The sponges are placed over the dissected bed; the superficial scleral flap and the conjunctiva-Tenon layer are then draped over the MMC-soaked sponges so that only those ocular tissues in contact with the sponge are directly exposed to MMC. After 3 minutes, the sponges are removed and MMC is irrigated away thoroughly with 20 ml balanced salt solution (BSS). A 2 × 1-mm-deep trabecular block is then removed and a peripheral iridectomy performed.

The scleral flap is closed with three interrupted 10-0 nylon sutures. The conjunctivo-Tenon's flap is closed at the limbus using two interrupted 10-0 nylon sutures with one in each side of the flap, involving the corneal limbus–Tenon–conjunctiva. After the closure, the conjunctiva should be watertight.

After the completion of the trabeculectomy, the temporal corneal incision and subsequent steps of phacoemulsification should be performed.

After IOL implantation, it is recommended to leave the viscoelastic solution in the anterior chamber. This technique aims to prevent shallowing of the anterior chamber and hyperfiltration postoperatively. The conjunctival wound can be checked with fluorescein to ensure it is watertight.

Postoperative Care and Complications

Typical postoperative care following cataract surgery also applies to any combined procedure. In addition, atropine 1% eye drops twice a day are advised during the first month of follow-up. Despite these precautions, the mere presence of a fistula may increase the risk of uveal effusion and other complications.

Intense IOP reduction in the first postoperative days should be avoided. Rather, it is recommended to maintain IOP between 15 and 20 mmHg during the first 3 days, and perform suture lysis later depending on the bleb appearance, and the ease of obtaining bleb elevation and IOP reduction with compression of the posterior lip of the wound with a cotton tip (see Fig. 9.6). Adjunctive MMC or 5-FU subconjunctival injection may be necessary within the first week since these eyes tend to show intense conjunctival scarring and fibrosis.

A diagram of a decision tree for detecting complications is described in Fig. 19.6. Most importantly, the physician should pay attention to the depth of the anterior chamber and the IOP. A brief description of the most common complications and treatment will follow and many issues related to the bleb are discussed in Chapter 9. Review of specific literature is encouraged.

Deep Anterior Chamber and Low IOP

Hyperfiltration: will be suggested by bleb appearance. Large elevated blebs are likely to present with this. Observation and tapering of the steroids are usually effective. Further intervention may be necessary, such as sutures or scleral shell.

Reduced aqueous production: this complication may be a result of subclinical ciliary body detachment or inflammation. Spontaneous remission usually occurs within days.

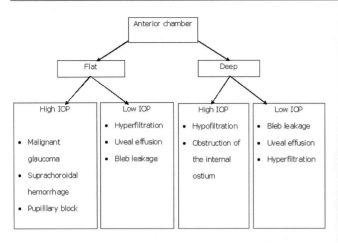

Fig. 19.6 Diagram of the differential diagnosis of complications following phacotrabeculectomy in nanophthalmos

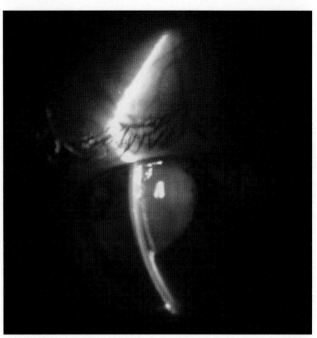

Fig. 19.7 Nanophthalmic patient presented with shallow anterior chamber (**A**) on the third postoperative day. The IOP was 43, the bleb was flat, and no choroidal detachment was noted on ocular ultrasonography. The patient was diagnosed with malignant glaucoma and was submitted to pars plana vitrectomy due to unresponsiveness to clinical treatment

Uveal effusion: fundus examination or ultrasonography may confirm the diagnosis. Topical and systemic steroids should be augmented or initiated and tapered slowly. Complete remission may take as long as 6 weeks.

Bleb leak: confirmed by positive Seidel test. Treatment may involve using bandage contact lenses or suture. A Palmberg mattress suture is very effective when the leakage occurs in the limbus.[33] Surgical re-interventions may also involve using amniotic membrane or performing conjunctiva advancement.

Flat Anterior Chamber and Low IOP

The same causative agents may be applied here. If significant flat anterior chamber (grade IV – corneal-lenticular contact) is present, prompt surgical intervention and treatment of causative agents is required.

Deep Anterior Chamber and High IOP

Hypofiltration: eye massage or suture lysis is recommended.

Obstruction of the trabeculectomy: Blood clot or iris fragments may be obstructing the aqueous humor outflow, which can be diagnosed during gonioscopy. Treatment may demand observation or applying laser to the internal ostium.

Flat Anterior Chamber and High IOP

Malignant glaucoma (aqueous misdirection): The presence of a patent iridectomy and normal fundus/echographic appearance may confirm the diagnosis. Initial treatment involves intravenous hyperosmotic agents, and topical and oral anti-glaucoma medication. YAG laser hyaloidectomy

may be successful. If the anterior chamber is significantly shallow (grade IV) for more than 5 days consider pars plana vitrectomy (see Fig. 19.7).

Suprachoroidal hemorrhage: The patient may complain of sudden severe pain and the fundus examination may reveal red/brownish choroidal detachment. If grade IV atalamia (Greek for shallow anterior chamber) is present, consider immediate drainage. If not, observe with daily ultrasonography until the blood becomes more fluid (which takes approximately 7 days), and then consider drainage (see Chapter 12).

Other Postoperative Complications

Tenon capsule's cysts: may be prevented by using subconjunctival injections of MMC and 5-FU as described previously. It may require Tenon's conjunctival needle revision (TCNR), which can also precipitate aqueous misdirection if IOP decreases by a large amount and, thus, should be performed cautiously.

Infectious complications (blebitis, endophthalmitis): urgent treatment is necessary. Large spectrum topical antibiotic (fourth-generation quinolones or fortified cephalosporins + gentamicin) should be initiated promptly. Intravitreous injections (ceftazidime and vancomycin) and pars plan vitrectomy may be considered. Consultation with a retina specialist is optimal.

Key Points:

- When significant cataract and uncontrolled glaucoma coexist, combined procedures may be indicated.
- Specific measures to avoid intraoperative complications are also warranted.
- Attention to the anterior chamber depth, bleb appearance, and IOP. This information is fundamental to detect the cause of the complication and to take appropriate actions.

Summary

Nanophthalmos is a rare eye developmental anomaly with a high risk of sight-threatening complications. Any type of surgical intervention should be undertaken with particular attention to these potential risks. Cataract extraction may result in good visual outcomes and IOP reduction if specific prophylactic procedures are employed. Nonetheless, these patients continue to have a risk for developing glaucoma after surgery, so ophthalmologists should routinely include a complete evaluation for glaucoma, especially gonioscopy, during patient follow-up. Referral to a glaucoma specialist is advised once glaucoma is diagnosed and/or the patient needs further surgical intervention.

References

1. Duke-Elder S. Anomalies in the size of the eye. In Duke-Elder S, ed. System of Ophthalmology, Vol 3, pt 2. St. Louis: CV Mosby; 1964:488.
2. Hirsch SE, Waltman SR, LaPiana FG. Bilateral nanophthalmos. Arch Ophthalmol. 1973; 89: 353.
3. Ryan EA, Zwaan J, Chylack LT. Nanophthalmos with uveal effusion: clinical and embryologic considerations. *Ophthalmology.* 1982;89: 1013–1017.
4. Singh OS, Simmons RJ, Brockhurst RJ, Temple CL. Nanophthalmos: a perspective on identification and therapy. *Ophthalmology.* 1982; 89:1006–1012.
5. Tay T, Smith JE, Berman Y, et al. Nanophthalmos in a Melanesian population. Clin Experiment Ophthalmol. 2007;35:348–354.
6. Aras C, Ozdamar A, Ustundag C, Ozkan S. Optical coherence tomographic features of papillomacular fold in posterior microphthalmos. Retina. 2005;25:665–667.
7. Kim JW, Boes DA, Kinyoun JL. Optical coherence tomography of bilateral posterior microphthalmos with papillomacular fold and novel features of retinoschisis and dialysis. Am J Ophthalmol. 2004;138:480–481.
8. Sharan S, Grigg JR, Higgins RA. Nanophthalmos: ultrasound biomicroscopy and Pentacam assessment of angle structures before and after cataract surgery. J Cataract Refract Surg. 2006;32: 1052–1055.
9. Yue BYJT, Duvall J, Goldberg MF, et al. Nanophthalmic sclera; morphologic and tissue culture studies. *Ophthalmology.* 1986;93:534–541.
10. Yue B, Kurosawa A, Duvall J, et al. Nanophthalmic sclera; fibronectin studies. *Ophthalmology.* 1988;95:56–60.
11. Stewart DH III, Streeten BW, Brockhurst RJ, et al. Abnormal scleral collagen in nanophthalmos; an ultrastructural study. Arch Ophthalmol. 1991; 109:1017–1025.
12. Yamani A, Wood I, Sugino I, et al. Abnormal collagen fibrils in nanophthalmos: a clinical and histologic study. Am J Ophthalmol. 1999;127:106–107.
13. Brockhurst RJ. Nanophthalmos with uveal effusion; a new clinical entity. Arch Ophthalmol. 1975; 93:1289–1299; correction 1976;94:583.
14. Yalvac IS, Satana B, Ozkan G, Eksioglu U, Duman S. Management of glaucoma in patients with nanophthalmos. *Eye.* 2007;9.
15. Faucher A, Hasanee K, Rootman DS. Phacoemulsification and intraocular lens implantation in nanophthalmic eyes: report of a medium-size series. J Cataract Refract Surg. 2002;28:837–842.
16. Chan FM, Lee L. Nanophthalmic cataract extraction. Clin Experiment Ophthalmol. 2004;32:535–538.
17. Chang SHL, Lim G. Secondary pigmentary glaucoma associated with piggyback intraocular lens implantation. *J Cataract Refract Surg.* 2004;30:2219–2222.
18. Iwase T, Tananka N. Elevated intraocular pressure in secondary piggyback intraocular lens implantation. *J Cataract Refract Surg.* 2005;1821–1823.
19. Garca-Feijo J, Saenz-Franes F, Martinez-de-la-Casa JM et al. Angle-closure glaucoma after piggy back intraocular lens implantation. *Eur J Ophthalmol.* 2008;18:822–826.
20. MacLaren RE, Natkunarajah M, Riaz Y, Bourne RR, Restori M, Allan BD. Biometry and formula accuracy with intraocular lenses used for cataract surgery in extreme hyperopia. Am J Ophthalmol. 2007;143:920–931.
21. Gayton JL, Apple DJ, Peng Q et al. Interlenticular opacification:clinicopathological correlation of a complication of posterior chamber piggyback intraocular lenses. J Cataract Refract Surg. 2000;26:330–336.
22. Susanna R Jr. Implantation of an intraocular lens in a case of nanophthalmos. CLAO J. 1987;13:117–118.
23. Garca-Feijo J, Saenz-Frances F, Martinez-De-La-Casa JM et al. Eur J Ophthalmol. 2008;18:822–826.
24. Iwase T, Tanaka N. Elevated intraocular pressure in secondary piggyback intraocular lens implantation. J Cataract Refract Surg. 2005;31:1821–1823.
25. Brockhurst RJ. Cataract surgery in nanophthalmic eyes. Arch Ophthalmol. 1990;108:965–967.
26. Hill WE. Consultation section: cataract surgical problem. J Cataract Refract Surg. 2000;26:1702–1704.
27. Brockhurst RJ. Vortex vein decompression for nanophthalmic uveal effusion. Arch Ophthalmol. 1980; 98:1987–1990.
28. Johnson MW, Gass DM. Surgical management of the idiopathic uveal effusion syndrome. Ophthalmology. 1990; 97: 778–785.
29. Jin JC, Anderson DR. Laser and unsutured sclerotomy in nanophthalmos. Am J Ophthalmol. 1990; 109: 575–580.
30. Junemann A, Kuchle M, Handel A, Naumann GO. Cataract surgery in nanophthalmic eyes with an axial length of less than 20.5 mm. Klin Monatsbl Augenheilkd. 1998;212:13–22.
31. Wu W, Dawson DG, Sugar A, et al. Cataract surgery in patients with nanopthalmos. J Cataract Refract Surg. 2004;30:584–590.
32. Mietz H, Jacobi PC, Krieglstein GK. Postoperative application of mitomycin for trabeculectomies. Arch Ophthalmol. 2000; 118:1341–1348.
33. Palmberg P, Zacchei A. Compression sutures-a new treatment for leaking or painful filtering blebs. Invest Ophthalmol Vis Sci. 1996;37:S444.

Chapter 20

Cataract Induced Glaucoma: Phacolytic/Phacomorphic

Sandra M. Johnson

Introduction

Lens-related glaucoma arises from a variety of pathophysiologic mechanisms. These are listed in Table 20.1 and include phacolytic glaucoma, phacomorphic glaucoma, phacoanaphylaxis, and lens particle glaucoma. Phacomorphic glaucoma and lens dislocation involve an angle-closure mechanism while the other forms are secondary open angle glaucomas. While the clinical presentations of each disorder may overlap, the choice of appropriate therapy is aided by accurate diagnosis. Both phacolytic and phacomorphic glaucoma are secondary to mature cataracts and these diseases present typically in patients in their sixth decade or older. A prospective study at an eye hospital in Nepal found that 1.5% of cataracts that presented in 1998 had phacolytic or phacomorphic glaucoma with 72% phacomorphic and 28% phacolytic glaucoma.[1]

Table 20.1 Types of lens-related glaucoma

Types of lens-related glaucoma
1. Phacolytic glaucoma
2. Phacomorphic glaucoma
3. Phacoanaphylaxis
4. Lens particle glaucoma
5. Dislocated lens

Part I: Phacolytic Glaucoma

Pathogenesis

Phacolytic glaucoma develops as lens proteins leaking from mature cataracts obstruct the trabecular meshwork and prevent aqueous humor outflow. With age and cataract

progression, the amount of high molecular weight protein in the lens increases. In immature cataracts, these proteins are found in the nucleus of the lens. With cataract maturation and protein accumulation, increasing amounts of high-molecular-weight protein are found in the liquid cortex of the lens. Eventually, additional cataract changes in the lens capsule allow release of the proteins into the aqueous humor. This damage to the lens is microscopic in nature, as the lens capsule appears grossly intact on clinical examination. The increased concentrations of high-molecular-weight protein in the aqueous humor results in obstruction of the trabecular meshwork and diminished aqueous humor outflow. In addition, the presence of lens proteins in the anterior chamber leads to inflammation and a macrophage response. It was previously believed that the accumulation of large macrophages swollen by engulfed lens proteins was the primary cause of trabecular meshwork obstruction. However, it has been experimentally determined that released lens proteins alone are sufficient to cause obstruction[2–4] (Fig. 20.1). The role of

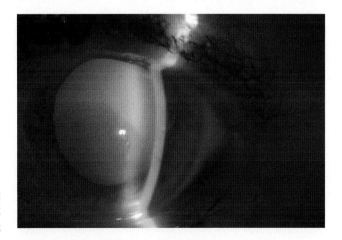

Fig. 20.1 Elderly female with a history of light perception and mature cataract in this eye presented with pain and an intraocular pressure of 69 mmHg. Slit-lamp exam revealed a morgagnian cataract. There appears to be aggregation of macrophages and/or lens proteins on the anterior surface of the lens (*arrow*). Photograph courtesy of Jared Watson, COT, University of Virginia, Department of Ophthalmology

S.M. Johnson (✉)
Department of Ophthalmology, University of Virginia School of Medicine, Charlottesville, VA 22908, USA
e-mail: catglaubk@gmail.com

heavy molecular weight proteins in pathogenesis is further confirmed as children and young patients with cataracts do not have such proteins, and subsequently do not experience phacolytic glaucoma.

Clinical Presentation

The acute intraocular pressure (IOP) elevation of phacolytic glaucoma is a medical emergency and must be quickly differentiated from other ocular conditions. The differential diagnoses of acute IOP elevation are listed in Table 20.2. The diagnostic evaluation of suspected phacolytic glaucoma is shown in Table 20.3.

Table 20.2 Differential diagnosis of acute IOP elevation

- Acute angle-closure glaucoma
- Pupillary block glaucoma
- Phacomorphic glaucoma
- Lens-particle glaucoma
- Neovascular glaucoma
- Uveitic glaucoma
- Glaucoma secondary to trauma

Table 20.3 Diagnostic evaluation of phacolytic glaucoma

Diagnostic evaluation of phacolytic glaucoma
1. History of cataract and other ocular diseases
2. Slit-lamp examination
3. Gonioscopy
4. Posterior segment evaluation
5. Diagnostic paracentesis
6. Phase-contrast microscopy and Millipore filter technique

The typical clinical presentation of phacolytic glaucoma involves an acute onset of monocular pain, redness, and decreased visual acuity in a patient with a history of gradual visual loss over months or years. The symptoms are due to an acute elevation of intraocular pressure, and thus may closely mimic acute angle-closure glaucoma. For this reason, a history of gradual vision loss secondary to progressing cataract, prior to the acute onset of symptoms, offers a vital clue to correct diagnosis. The vision is likely to be hand motions or worse.[1]

Slit-lamp examination usually reveals corneal epithelial edema. If particularly edematous, topical glycerin may aid in slit-lamp and gonioscopic examination. Oftentimes, anterior chamber flare is visible. Such flare is thought to be due to soluble lens proteins, but may also include calcium oxalate and cholesterol crystals.[5] White aggregates of particles are frequently visible in the aqueous humor and anterior lens surface. These clumps consist of scattered cells, precipitated lens proteins, and other lens materials

(Fig. 20.1). The majority of cells visible on slit-lamp examination are swollen macrophages, which appear larger and more translucent than leukocytes. Mild to modest cellular reaction is prevalent in the anterior chamber, with only very rare instances of hypopyon. There may be keratic precipitates but, unlike uveitic glaucoma, are typically not present. Finally, in nearly all cases of phacolytic glaucoma, a mature cataract will be evident. Immature cataracts rarely lead to this disease.

Gonioscopic examination of suspected phacolytic glaucoma is a necessary step in diagnosis. Examination will reveal an open iridocorneal angle. Angle recession may sometimes be seen related to a mature traumatic cataract, but oftentimes, no abnormalities are visible.

Posterior segment evaluation may also reveal abnormalities in phacolytic glaucoma. Leaking lens proteins have been reported to cause retinal perivasculitis. A mature cataract may also dislocate into the vitreous. In such cases, the other clinical signs of phacolytic glaucoma including ocular redness may be less apparent, making diagnosis more difficult. These rare occasions may produce a subacute type of phacolytic glaucoma due to the intermittent leakage of protein.[6] It may be necessary to evaluate the posterior segment with B-scan ultrasound if the mature cataract prohibits an exam.

While the clinical diagnosis of phacolytic glaucoma should not be missed, diagnostic paracentesis may help in questionable cases. Phase contrast microscopy examination of aqueous fluid typically shows engorged macrophages. Quantitative analysis of macrophages in anterior chamber fluid is not known to correlate with disease severity. Phase contrast microscopy and millipore filter technique may aid examination of aqueous fluid and identification of cells.[7] Biochemical analysis of aspirated fluid for heavy-molecular weight lens proteins has become an accepted practice, but, while diagnostic paracentesis may help to confirm the diagnosis, a diagnosis based on clinical evidence alone is made in most cases.

Management

Initial management of suspected phacolytic glaucoma involves an attempt to medically control intraocular pressure. Medical treatments to lower intraocular pressure include hyperosmotic agents, carbonic anhydrase inhibitors, topical beta-adrenergic antagonists, or alpha-adrenergic agents. In an inflamed cataractous eye with elevated intraocular pressures, a trial of topical steroids may be helpful. In phacolytic glaucoma, a temporary reduction of IOP may be achieved, but there is no long-term improvement with anti-inflammatory treatment. Thus, a diagnostic steroid trial may be useful in differentiating the elevated IOP of phacolytic glaucoma from uveitic glaucoma.

Despite the previously mentioned medical therapies, long-term IOP control is difficult to obtain without surgery. Thus, a presumed diagnosis of phacolytic glaucoma necessitates cataract extraction. In cases of dangerously elevated IOP not responding to initial medical treatment, emergent surgery may be required.

Preoperative Care

All attempts should be made to reduce IOP and inflammation prior to initiating surgery, as listed previously. Prior to surgery of the globe, it is very important to measure IOP. If a patient does not have medical contraindications, mannitol 20% can be administered intravenously preceding surgery (Table 20.4). Doctors prescribing mannitol should be educated on the use of this potent systemic medication. Digital massage, Super Pinky, or Honan balloon may be employed to help reduce IOP following a block. It has been suggested that retrobulbar or peribulbar anesthesia with epinephrine is preferred to topical or can be combined with general anesthesia in order to decrease orbital vascular congestion.[8]

Table 20.4 Mannitol

Mannitol
Dose is 1–2 g/kg infused intravenously over 30 minutes
Onset in 60 minutes, duration of effect 4–8 h
Avoid in severe renal impairment, heart failure, dehydration, intracranial bleeding, pulmonary edema, and concurrent use of diuretics or cardiac glycosides
Side effects include hypokalemia, acidosis, and hyponatremia
Further information: www.mdconsult.com

Operative Technique

For IOP that remains elevated prior to surgery, the anterior chamber should be entered by a paracentesis initially to prevent rapid decompression of the eye. Extracapsular extraction has become the primary surgical technique in phacolytic glaucoma, although severe corneal edema may make such a procedure more difficult. Microcystic edema may improve as the IOP decreases. Nevertheless, extracapsular extraction with posterior chamber intraocular lens (PC IOL) has achieved good results. McKibbin presented a series of nine eyes in which only traditional extracapsular cataract extraction was used, due to concern over phacoemulsification in eyes with a poor view due to corneal edema or inflammation.[9] The capsulotomy may prove difficult, due to a white lens, and capsular staining with trypan blue can facilitate

Table 20.5 Use of trypan blue

Use of trypan blue (Vision Blue; Dutch Ophthalmic, USA)
• Complete initial incisions
• Inject an air bubble into the anterior chamber or replace aqueous with viscoelastic
• Apply trypan blue 0.06% sterile solution over the anterior capsule
• Irrigate the dye from the eye, apply viscoelastic, and perform capsulotomy or capsulorhexis

capsulotomy or capsulorhexis (Table 20.5, Fig. 18.5).[10] If the nucleus is morgagnian (Fig. 20.1), it may be delivered through a large capsulorhexis and 6 mm wound. The use of such manual small incision cataract surgery has been reported by Venkatesh et al. in 33 patients.[11] The use of continuous curvilinear capsulorhexis for planned extracapsular cataract extraction has also been reported.[12] In the setting of liquefied cortex, hydrodissection is not necessary. If the liquefied cortex is under pressure then the capsule is prone to tears with the initial puncture for continuous curvilinear capsulorhexis (CCC), and the capsule could be fibrotic as well.[13,14] Venkatesh et al. have suggested filling the capsular bag with viscoelastic after the initial puncture of the anterior capsule and aspiration of liquid cortex, then continuing with capsulorhexis. See further discussion under phacomorphic glaucoma.[10]

Many surgeons employ phacoemulsification techniques even in mature cataracts. Chakrabarti reported on 212 white cataracts where 208 had successful phacoemulsification, although none had progressed to glaucoma.[14] Two eyes had nuclei deemed too hard for phacoemulsification. The series included 12 patients with postoperative corneal edema and this could be higher in a population with elevated IOP, since elevated IOP contributes to corneal endothelial cell loss as noted in acute angle-closure glaucoma.[15] Ermis has reported on a similar group of 82 patients with white cataracts who underwent phacoemulsification.[16] This report noted 20.7% of the eyes of the mature cataract cohort to have corneal edema versus 3.7% in the eyes that underwent phacoemulsification for a non-white cataract. No reports are known to the author on phacoemulsification employed in an eye with white cataract and phacolytic glaucoma. For phacolytic glaucoma secondary to a dislocated cataract in the vitreous cavity, referral for pars plana vitrectomy is the approach of choice.

Postoperative Care

Postoperative topical antibiotics and steroids are used as in standard cases of cataract surgery. Patients with phacolytic glaucoma may require topical glaucoma medications until the inflammatory response has subsided.[9]

Complications

Due to increased lens capsule fragility, capsule rupture is a potential complication of surgery for phacolytic or phacomorphic glaucoma.[9] In such an event, any remnant protein and lens material should be removed with sufficient irrigation of the anterior chamber and anterior vitrectomy as needed. As mentioned previously, capsulorhexis may be complicated in eyes with mature cataracts. In a series of cases reported by Prajna et al., 2 of 44 patients experienced postoperative persistent inflammation and cystoid macular edema with decreased vision.[17] Vitreous opacities, which may be related to the inflammation of this condition, may be seen postoperative and resolve.[18]

Results/Outcome

Cataract extraction for phacolytic glaucoma has shown excellent results, with IOP quickly returning to normal and significant improvements in postoperative visual acuity. One report from India on 45 eyes indicated IOP control in all patients with a follow-up ranging from 1 to 5 years. Their patients were treated with extracapsular cataract extraction (ECCE) with no IOL in 28 eyes due to contralateral aphakia.[19] Of note, only three patients demonstrated corneal clearing, after treatment with glaucoma medications. There were no differences in outcome with or without an IOL placed. A retrospective analysis of another Indian cohort of 135 eyes showed no difference at 6 months in IOP control in cataract extraction alone versus cataract extraction combined with trabeculectomy.[20] In the case series by Prajna et al., patients with delay in treatment were more likely to experience poor postoperative vision, and 4 of their 44 patients had compromised optic nerves.[17]

Part II: Phacomorphic Glaucoma

Pathogenesis, Clinical Presentation, and Management

Phacomorphic glaucoma is an angle-closure glaucoma secondary to an intumescent cataract, in an eye not predisposed to angle closure. These patients present much the same as those with phacolytic glaucoma with likely hand motion or worse vision. The IOP is very elevated; the eye is red and painful with corneal edema and a mature cataract. However, as in an eye presenting with acute angle closure, the

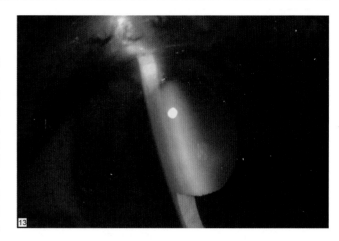

Fig. 20.2 Elderly patient with an eye with a patent iridotomy that developed angle closure. The patient presented the same day and the glaucoma was stabilized with gonioplasty and medications prior to phaco/IOL. The vision improved to 20/20 and glaucoma medications were greatly reduced. This case illustrates the overlap of classic phacomorphic glaucoma and angle closure relieved with cataract surgery. Photo courtesy of Tom Monego at Dartmouth Hitchcock Medical Center (DHMC), Lebanon, NH

pupil will be fixed and dilated and the anterior chamber shallow with the angle closed on gonioscopy. Glycerin and IOP-lowering medications may be required to decrease the corneal edema prior to gonioscopy. As in acute angle closure, this glaucoma is likely more common in females versus males due to the naturally shallower anterior chamber. There may be an element of pupillary block present in these patients and iridotomy may be beneficial, as well as iridoplasty, in aiding in IOP control[21-23] (Fig. 20.2). Medical management is much the same as for phacolytic glaucoma, with the initiation of glaucoma medications and topical steroids preoperatively. Miotics are not likely to be beneficial due to their effect on the lens iris diaphragm, and their use may cause further shallowing of the anterior chamber, although limited evidence exists regarding actual clinical results.[9] Patients are treated with topical steroids preoperatively, and surgery is scheduled promptly to avoid the development of permanent peripheral anterior synechiae.

Operative Techniques

As in phacolytic glaucoma, preoperative intravenous mannitol 20% (1 gm/kg) if tolerated may help dehydrate the vitreous, lower the intraocular pressure, and additionally allow the anterior chamber to deepen (Table 20.4). Ocular massage, Honan balloon, or Super-Pinky following the block may help decompress the eye. Gentle depression of the eye at the limbus with a 19-ga cannula, muscle hook, or other similar blunt instrument at the start of surgery may aid in pushing aqueous from the posterior into the anterior chamber to deepen it. Vitreous tap or small gauge vitrectomy may be used as an adjunct to cataract surgery to deepen the anterior chamber.[24,25] Due to the limited view in performing a pars plana vitrectomy, retinal detachment may be more likely. A rare patient may require pars plana lensectomy for cataract removal. A two-plane valved incision is helpful for avoiding iris prolapse in these eyes with a shallow anterior chamber and is an advantage of a phacoemulsification approach. Generous use of viscoelastic is recommended to protect the corneal endothelium, especially if phacoemulsification is employed. A dispersive viscoelastic is preferred.

As noted previously, capsulorhexis can be challenging in a white intumescent cataract, which is more common in phacomorphic than phacolytic glaucoma as the intumescence and intralenticular swelling contributes to the shallow anterior chamber, through the increased convexity of the lens[13] (Fig. 20.3). As mentioned above, the capsule in intumescent lenses is under pressure, which makes it prone to radial tears during initiation of capsulotomy or CCC. A needle puncture of the capsule with aspiration of liquid cortex under counter pressure of adhesive viscoelastic such as Healon V (AMO, Santa Ana, CA) or Viscoat (Alcon, Fort Worth, TX) may prevent a tear in the anterior capsule, which is under pressure.[26] Rao recommends this maneuver with entry of the needle through the limbus and not the wound to avoid loss of viscoelastic, until the lens has been decompressed. He suggests further removal of liquid cortex with a cannula. Bhattacharjee has reported a similar type of approach with the use of an endoilluminator to complete the capsulorhexis once the liquid cortex has been removed. Liquid cortex may further obstruct the view and require irrigation of the anterior chamber and replacement of the viscoelastic. He described a success rate over 96% of 84 eyes.[27] Chan described using a bent needle attached to a syringe of balanced salt solution (BSS) introduced through a partial thickness paracentesis to

perform a CCC. The BSS is used to maintain the pressure in the anterior chamber and dilute liquid cortex, as needed. He reported success in 94 cases.[28]

Results

In the case series by McKibben, five patients had phacomorphic glaucoma and had surgery within 2 days of presentation with good control of IOP postoperatively.[9] Prajna presented 49 cases of phacomorphic glaucoma from India. His cohort underwent extracapsular cataract extraction, with 44% receiving a PC IOL, and five of the patients had permanently reduced vision due to glaucomatous optic neuropathy (Fig. 20.4). The report did not address IOP control.[17]

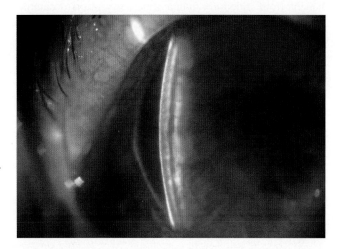

Fig. 20.4 Elderly patient with a dense cataract and a picture of angle closure who waited a week to present. There was no effect from an iridotomy and the patient underwent ECCE due to the corneal edema and very shallow anterior chamber. The glaucoma stabilized but vision remained poor. Photo courtesy of University of North Carolina ophthalmic photography, Chapel Hill, NC

Angra et al. reported on 40 cases of phacomorphic glaucoma randomized to intracapsular cataract extraction versus intracapsular cataract surgery combined with trabeculectomy in a cohort of Indian patients.[29] They achieved IOP in the normal range in 90% of patients with a combined surgical approach versus 75% with cataract surgery alone with a follow-up of 3 months. They suggested that patients with a longer duration of the glaucoma attack were more likely to develop permanent posterior anterior synechiae (PAS) and were more likely to benefit with the addition of the trabeculectomy. Chandra et al. implanted Ahmed valves (New World Medical, Rancho Cucamonga, CA) at the time of cataract surgery with PC IOL due to concern over trabeculectomy failure in inflamed eyes with phacomorphic glaucoma.[30] The report is on 15 patients with nearly 360° of preoperative PAS. The patients presented 7–15 days after

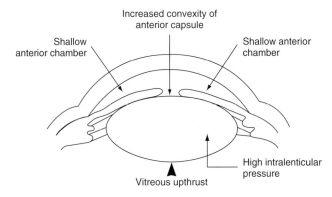

Increased convexity of
anterior capsule

Shallow
anterior chamber

Shallow anterior
chamber

High intralenticular
pressure

Vitreous upthrust

Fig. 20.3 Intralenticular pressure and shallow anterior chamber are two of the challenges in cataract extraction for phacomorphic glaucoma

the start of their glaucoma attacks, and all received systemic steroids in addition to IOP-lowering medications. Patients had normalization of IOP in the teens with follow-up of 6–46 months. Unfortunately, they did not have a control group.

Summary

Mature cataracts can result in both open and closed angle glaucoma. Due to the severity of the intraocular pressure elevation, cataract surgery should be pursued as soon as it is feasible to avoid vision loss from optic atrophy or vascular occlusions. The initiation of medical therapy including glaucoma medications and topical steroids can be helpful but not definitive treatment. Phacomorphic angle closure may benefit from iridotomy and/or iridoplasty prior to cataract surgery. The most challenging aspect of the surgery is likely the capsulorhexis. Patients with phacomorphic glaucoma may require concomitant or sequential glaucoma surgery for chronic glaucoma, especially if there is a delay in presentation and the development of synechial angle closure.

Acknowledgments The author wishes to acknowledge Devon Ghodasra for his research assistance with this chapter.

References

1. Pradhan D, Hennig A, Kumar J, Foster A. A prospective study of 413 cases of lens-induced glaucoma in Nepal. *Indian J Ophthalmol.* 2001;49:103–7.
2. Epstein DL, Jedzinak JA, Grant WM. Identification of heavy molecular weight soluble protein in aqueous humor in human phacolytic glaucoma. *Invest Ophthalmol Vis Sci.* 1978;17:398.
3. Epstein DL, Jedzinak JA, Grant WM. Obstruction of aqueous outflow by lens particles and by heavy molecular weight soluble lens proteins. *Invest Ophthalmol Vis Sci.* 1978;17:272.
4. Epstein DL. Lens-induced glaucoma. In: Epstein DL, ed. *Chandler and Grant's Glaucoma.* 3rd ed. Philadelphia, PA: Lea & Febiger; 1986:320–31.
5. Bartholomew RS, Rebello PF. Calcium oxalate crystals in the aqueous. *Am J Ophthalmol.* 1979;88:1026.
6. Pollard ZF. Phacolytic glaucoma secondary to ectopia lentis. *Ann Ophthalmol.* 1975;7:999–1001.
7. Goldberg MF: Cytological diagnosis of phacolytic glaucoma utilizing milipore filtration of the aqueous. *Br J Ophthalmol.* 1967;51:847.
8. Richter C. Lens-induced open-angle glaucoma. In: Ritch R, Shields MB, Krupin T, eds. *The Glaucomas.* 2nd ed. St. Louis: Mosby; 1996:1023–6.
9. McKibben M. Cataract extraction and intraocular lens implantation in eyes with phacomorphic or phacolytic glaucoma. *J Cataract Refract Surg.* 1996;22:633–6.
10. Jacobs DS, Cox TA, Wagoner MD, Ariyasu RG, Karp CL. Capsule staining as an adjunct to cataract surgery: a report of the American Academy of Ophthalmology. *Ophthalmology.* 2006; 113:707–13.
11. Venkatesh R, Tan CSH, Kumar TT, Ravindran RD. Safety and efficacy of manual small incision cataract surgery for phacolytic glaucoma. *Br J Ophthalmol.* 2007;91:279–81.
12. Pande M. Continuous curvilinear (cicular) capsulorhexis and planned extracapsular cataract extraction-are they compatible? *Br J Ophthalmol.* 1993;77:152–7.
13. Rao SK. Capsulorhexis in white cataracts. *J Cataract Refract Surg.* 2000;26:477–8.
14. Chakrabarti A, Singh S, Krishnadas R. Phacoemulsification in eyes with white cataract. *J Cataract Refract Surg.* 2000;26:1041–7.
15. Setala K. Corneal endothelial cell density after an attack of acute glaucoma. *Acta Ophthalmol.* 1979;57:1004–13.
16. Ermis SS, Ozturk F, Inan UU. Comparing the efficacy and safety of phacoemulsification in white mature and other types of senile cataracts. *Br J Ophthalmol.* 2003;87:1356–9.
17. Prajna NV, Ramakrishnan R, Krishnadas R, Manoharan N. Lens induced glaucomas-visual results and risk factors for final visual acuity. *Indian K Ophthalmol.* 1996;44:149–55.
18. Thomas R, Braganza A, George T, et al. Vitreous opacities in phacolytic glaucoma. *Ophthal Surg Lasers.* 1996;27:839–43.
19. Mandal AK, Gothwal VK. Intraocular pressure control and visual outcome in patients with phacolytic glaucoma managed by extracapsular cataract extraction with or without posterior chamber intraocular lens implantation. *Ophthalmic Surg Lasers.* 1998;29:880–9.
20. Braganza A, Thomas R, George T, Mermoud A. Management of phacolytic glaucoma: experience of 135 cases. *Indian J Ophthalmol.* 1998;46:139–43.
21. Tomey KF, AL-Rajhi AA. Neodymium:YAG laser iridotomy in the initial management of phacomorphic glauocoma. *Ophthalmology.* 1992;9:660–65.
22. Tham CCY, Lai JSM, Poon ASY et al. Immediate argon laser peripheral iridoplasty (ALPI) as initial treatment in angle-closure (phacomorphic glaucoma) before cataract extraction. *Eye.* 2005:19:778–83.
23. Johnson SM. Surgical intervention for phacomorphic glaucoma. *Glaucoma Today.* 2006;4:37–9.
24. Chang DF. Pars plana vitreous tap for phacoemulsification in the crowded eye. *J Cataract Refract Surg.* 2001;27:1911–14.
25. Dada T, Kumar S, Gafia R, Aggarwal A, Gupta V, Sihota R. Sutureless single-port transconjunctival para plana limited vitrectomy combined with phacoemulsification for management of phacomorphic glaucoma. *J Cataract Refract Surg.* 2007;33:951–5.
26. Rao SK, Padmanabhan P. Capsulorhexis in eyes with phacomorphic glaucoma. *J Cataract Refract Surg.* 1998;24:882–4.
27. Bhattacharjee K, Bhattacharjee H, Goswami BJ, Sarma P. Capsulorhexis in intumescent cataract. *J Cataract Refract Surg.* 1999;25:1045–7.
28. Chan DDN, Ng ACK, Leung CKS, Tse KKR. Continuous curviliner capsuolrhexis in intumescent or hypermature cataract with iquefied cortex. *J Cataract Refract Surg.* 2003;29:431–4.
29. Angra SK, Pradhan R, Garg SP. Cataract induced glaucoma-an insight into management. *Indian J Ophthalmol.* 1991;39:97–101.
30. Chandra DJ, Chaudhuri Z, Bhomaj S, Sharma P, Gupta R, Chauhan D. Combined extracapsular cataract extraction with ahmed glaucoma valve implantation in phacomorphic glaucoma. *Indian J Ophthalmol.* 2002;50:25–28.

Chapter 21

Glaucoma Related to Pseudophakia

Junping Li and Jason Much

Introduction

The term *pseudophakic glaucoma* is often used to refer to any secondary glaucoma following cataract extraction. However, elevation of intraocular pressure and glaucoma after cataract surgery may occur by a wide variety of mechanisms each with a different natural history and time course. Therefore, in describing this complex condition, it has been suggested that the general term of *glaucoma in pseudophakia* be adopted to replace *pseudophakic glaucoma*, which implies a single entity and mechanism.[1,2]

Glaucoma in pseudophakia should be distinguished from preexisting glaucoma recognized postoperatively. For example, routine postsurgical inflammation is often of little consequence in normal eyes, but may cause elevated intraocular pressure in eyes with preexisting primary open angle glaucoma with compromised aqueous outflow. Other causes of transient increased intraocular pressure in the immediate postoperative period include angle distortion or trabecular edema, early hyphema, and retained viscoelastic material. In most cases, the intraocular pressure returns to normal levels after 24 h. However, some eyes progress to a chronic glaucoma, and it is important to identify these cases early to prevent optic nerve damage.[3]

The incidence of glaucoma after cataract surgery has declined with the advent of modern extracapsular cataract surgery (ECCE). In one review of 166 cases, 71 eyes received posterior chamber intraocular lenses, 91 eyes received iris clip lenses, and 4 eyes received anterior chamber lenses.[4] See Fig. 21.1. The authors reported persistent ocular hypertension (IOP > 22 mmHg for over a month) in 15 eyes (9%), and 5 eyes (3%) required treatment. More recent studies report an incidence of secondary glaucoma after ECCE between 0

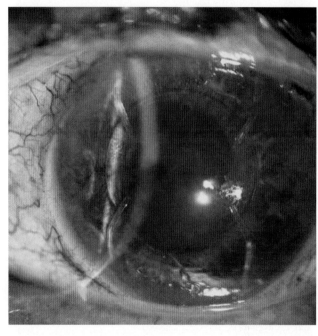

Fig. 21.1 Uveitis-glaucoma-hyphema syndrome in an 83-year-old Caucasian man 4 years after extracapsular cataract extraction with insertion of a Binkhorst iris-clip design anterior chamber intraocular lens

and 9.8%, with the rate being higher for anterior chamber lens implantation than for posterior chamber lenses.[5] Nowadays, it is generally more likely for intraocular pressure to fall by 1 or 2 mmHg or more following uncomplicated cataract surgery. See Chapter 4.

As previously mentioned, glaucoma in pseudophakia has many causes, which we have listed by time of onset in Table 21.1. These may also be classified into two broad categories based on the status of the anterior chamber angle, as shown in Table 21.2. This chapter will focus on those mechanisms of glaucoma specifically related to the intraocular lens (IOL) including the uveitis-glaucoma-hyphema (UGH) syndrome, pigment dispersion syndrome and glaucoma (PDS/PDG), and pseudophakic pupillary block.

J. Li (✉)
Clinical Ophthalmology, University of Virginia, Salem Veterans Affairs Medical Center, Salem, VA 24153, USA
e-mail: junping.li2@va.gov

S.M. Johnson (ed.), *Cataract Surgery in the Glaucoma Patient*, DOI 10.1007/978-0-387-09408-3_21,
© Springer Science+Business Media, LLC 2009

Table 21.1 Differential diagnosis of increased intraocular pressure following cataract surgery based on time of onset

Early Postoperative Period (1–7 days)
Preexisting open-angle glaucoma
Retained viscoelastic
Trabecular edema or angle distortion
Surgical hyphema
Pigment dispersion
Inflammation
Pupillary block
Aqueous misdirection
Choroidal hemorrhage or effusion
Intermediate Postoperative Period (1–7 weeks)
Preexisting open-angle glaucoma
Vitreous in the anterior chamber
Steroid-induced glaucoma
Ghost cell glaucoma
Lens particle glaucoma
Neovascular glaucoma
Late Postoperative Period (after 2 months)
Preexisting open-angle glaucoma
Ghost cell glaucoma
Uveitis-glaucoma-hyphema syndrome
Pigment dispersion
Chronic uveitis
Epithelial downgrowth or fibrous ingrowth
Pupillary block

Table 21.2 Differential diagnosis of increased intraocular pressure following cataract surgery based on status of anterior chamber angle

Open-angle glaucomas
Preexisting primary open-angle glaucoma
Retained viscoelastic
Trabecular edema or angle distortion
Surgical hyphema/Ghost cell glaucoma
Lens particle glaucoma
Steroid-induced glaucoma
Inflammation/Uveitis
Pigment dispersion
Uveitis-glaucoma-hyphema syndrome
Angle-closure glaucomas
Preexisting angle-closure glaucoma
Pupillary block
Aqueous misdirection
Choroidal hemorrhage or effusion
Neovascular glaucoma
Epithelial downgrowth or fibrous ingrowth

Uveitis-Glaucoma-Hyphema Syndrome

The uveitis-glaucoma-hyphema (UGH) syndrome was originally described by Ellingson in the late 1970s following the implantation of poorly manufactured anterior chamber intraocular lenses such as the Mark VIII designed by Peter Choyce.[6,7] The rough haptic edges, which were produced by mold injection (rather than lathe cut), caused mechanical irritation of the iris and angle structures leading to the classic triad of inflammation, hyphema, and elevated intraocular pressure. Poor fit and excessive mobility also contribute to the pathogenesis.[8–12]

Though seen much less frequently today, UGH syndrome has been reported with modern, flexible open-loop anterior chamber lenses as well as with posterior chamber lenses even when both haptics are in the capsular bag.[13–15] The mechanical etiology has been supported by several studies.[16–18] Asaria et al.[16] used electron microscopy to demonstrate melanosomes on the haptic surface, presumably derived from the iris pigment epithelium. Piette et al.[17] confirmed posterior iris chafing in nine cases of UGH syndrome using ultrasound biomicroscopy.

The clinical appearance of UGH syndrome is variable and may occur as only part of the triad.[19] See Fig. 21.1. Symptoms usually begin in the late postoperative period but may be delayed for many years after surgery. Patients often complain of blurry vision, redness, and photophobia, but pain may or may not be present. Several cases have been reported where the UGH syndrome simulated amaurosis fugax with transient white-out of vision due to recurrent hyphema.[20–23] The patients, however, described a slower onset and resolution of visual obscuration than is typical of amaurosis, and none reported no light perception. It is important to distinguish UGH syndrome from other causes of postoperative recurrent hyphema such as wound vascularization, suture trauma, and ingrowth of episcleral vessels.[24,25] Gonioscopy is key for diagnosis and may help rule out other similar causes of open angle glaucoma such as ghost cell or uveitic glaucoma.[26]

Treatment for UGH syndrome depends on its severity. Topical mydriatics or miotics are used to prevent movement of the pupil against the intraocular lens. Topical steroids control inflammation, and placement of an eye shield is beneficial to prevent eye trauma at night.[27] Temporary discontinuation of systemic anticoagulation such as warfarin may decrease the risk of persistent hyphema, provided this is safe for the patient.[28] In rare cases, medical management of the glaucoma may be adequate, and the syndrome can "burn out" when no further iris erosion occurs. More commonly, however, additional treatment is necessary, and several approaches have been described in the literature.[29,30] Nicholson[29] used fluorescein iris angiography to identify leaking vessels at the sites of haptic irritation. Argon laser photocoagulation (50-micron spots of 400 mW power and 0.2 s duration) was used to successfully ablate these vessels. John et al.[30] reported three cases of UGH syndrome successfully treated by rotation of the posterior chamber intraocular lens as an alternative to lens explantation. They made two paracenteses 180° apart perpendicular to the orientation of the lens haptics, injected viscoelastic into the anterior

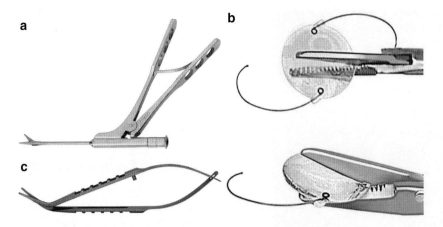

Fig. 21.2 Soft IOLs can be cut with special scissors such as (**a**) the Katena soft IOL cutter (**b**) shown cutting a lens. Figures courtesy of Katena Products, Denville, NJ. (**c**) The Storz ET-1306 Osher IOL scissors. Image courtesy of Bausch & Lomb, Rochester, NY

chamber, and rotated the intraocular lens 90°.[30] The viscoelastic was then removed from the anterior chamber with irrigation and aspiration, and acetylcholine was used to constrict the pupil.[30]

Explantation of the intraocular lens is the definitive treatment for many cases of UGH syndrome and is required for persistent cases, particularly those complicated by cystoid macular edema and/or refractory glaucoma. UGH syndrome has been a common indication for lens explantation in several reviews along with lens dislocation, pseudophakic bullous keratopathy, and incorrect lens power.[31–34] Surgical technique varies with the clinical scenario but removal of the haptics alone may be sufficient for posterior chamber lenses when the optic is fixed by the capsule.

Preoperative Preparation

It is imperative to know the style and characteristics of the IOL to be explanted, the status of the capsular support, and the original lens calculation and postoperative refraction. The type and location of placement for the new IOL should be planned in advance. Gonioscopy should be performed on every patient. If significant peripheral anterior synechiae are present, IOL explantation alone may not be enough to control the intraocular pressure. Trabeculectomy or glaucoma drainage tube may be required. In cases of UGH with non-resolving vitreous hemorrhage, concurrent vitrectomy by a retinal specialist should be coordinated. Preoperative treatment with a non-steroidal anti-inflammatory drug (NSAID) may improve patient comfort and prevent postoperative macular edema.

Instruments

Depending on the type of IOL to be explanted, different surgical instruments, equipment and supplies are needed. In general, the following should be available to the surgeon: a variety of microhooks, scissors including lens cutters, a vitrector, and ophthalmic viscosurgical devices (OVDs). See Figs. 21.2a–c and 21.3.

Operative Techniques

The lens style and location will dictate the technique of IOL removal. If the lens is in the sulcus or the capsular bag, viscodissection may be used to gently free the IOL from the anterior and/or posterior capsule. Oftentimes, space can be created at the haptic-optic junction using a dispersive OVD. When the IOL can be rotated easily in the bag or sulcus, it is prolapsed into the anterior chamber using a bimanual approach. Care must be taken to protect the corneal endothelium.

Once the lens is in the anterior chamber, there are a number of options for its removal depending on the IOL material and the desired wound size. If an anterior chamber intraocular lens (ACIOL) is to be implanted, the incision is enlarged, allowing direct removal of the posterior chamber intraocular lens (PCIOL). If a 3 mm or less incision is desired, the IOL can be cut into two or three pieces with a lens cutter or scissors[35](Figs. 21.2a, b, c and 21.3). Many acrylic PCIOLs can be refolded and removed directly through a small corneal wound. Cutting the foldable lens two-thirds across the optic usually allows its removal by subsequent gentle pulling on one haptic to lead it out of the small incision; this

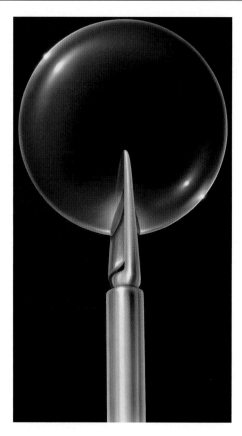

Fig. 21.3 Packer-Change 19G IOL cutter. Figure courtesy of Microsurgical Technologies, Redmond, WA

type of technique has also been described with silicone plate lenses.[36]

Most ACIOLs are easily explanted through a large corneoscleral incision. Closed-loop ACIOLs are more difficult to remove because of fibrosis around the loops in the anterior chamber angle. In such cases, the loops should be amputated from the optic, rotated back through the fibrous capsule, and then removed from the eye.[31,33]

Postoperative Care

Because of additional surgery and intraocular manipulation in an already compromised eye, it is recommended that a potent fourth-generation topical fluoroquinolone be used to prevent infection. Postoperative topical steroids and NSAIDs should be used for a longer period of time than after routine cataract surgery. Close monitoring of intraocular pressure is essential.

Outcomes

As mentioned previously, UGH is one of the most common indications for IOL explantation. In a series of 102 cases

reported by Mamalis et al., UGH was the second most frequent reason for explantation in patients with ACIOLs as well as in those with iris-fixated IOLs.[31] Of ten patients who received an ACIOL exchange, seven had an improvement in their clinical condition, two stabilized, and one worsened.

Secondary Pigmentary Glaucoma

Pigment dispersion following cataract surgery can obstruct the trabecular meshwork causing increased intraocular pressure and secondary pigmentary glaucoma.[37–40] The mechanical etiology is similar to that seen in the UGH syndrome.[41] However, secondary pigmentary glaucoma is more common with sulcus-placed posterior chamber intraocular lenses than with anterior chamber lenses. One study reported that the incidence of pigment dispersion following sulcus-based intraocular lens implantation may be as high as 16%.[42] Haptics placed in the ciliary sulcus can erode into the iris pigment epithelium, liberating pigment granules for many months after surgery. Any single-piece intraocular lens with broad, square-edged haptics such as the AcrySof (Alcon Laboratories, Inc., Fort Worth, TX) is contraindicated for sulcus placement.[43–46]

Secondary pigmentary glaucoma should be distinguished from *primary* pigmentary glaucoma, which is often diagnosed in young, myopic males with iridozonular friction, though they share many of the same clinical signs. A pigment spindle on the corneal endothelium, iris transillumination defects, and excess pigment on the iris and trabecular meshwork may be seen in both conditions. Unlike primary pigmentary glaucoma, however, secondary pigmentary glaucoma is only seen in eyes after intraocular lens implantation. In addition, iris transillumination defects appear in areas of contact between the intraocular lens and the posterior iris and not in a midperipheral radial pattern. As with the UGH syndrome, gonioscopy aids in the diagnosis. Angulated haptics and lens decentration may aggravate pigment dispersion. See Figs. 21.4 and 21.5a, b.

Most cases of secondary pigmentary glaucoma can be managed medically. If this fails, laser trabeculoplasty or trabeculectomy may be indicated. Lens explantation is rarely required[47] (Figs. 21.6 and 21.7).

Pseudophakic Pupillary Block

Pseudophakic pupillary block is another important cause of intraocular lens-related glaucoma following cataract surgery.[48–50] Most cases present in the early postoperative

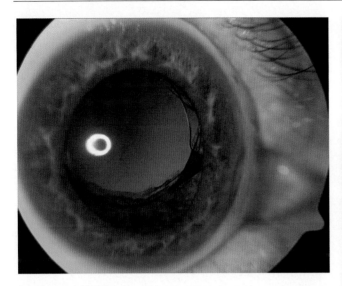

Fig. 21.4 Secondary pigmentary glaucoma in a 51-year-old Caucasian man 3 years after uncomplicated phacoemulsification and insertion of a one-piece intraocular lens in the sulcus. He had intervening pneumatic retinopexy and retinal surgery. Note the iris transillumination defect over the haptic nasally

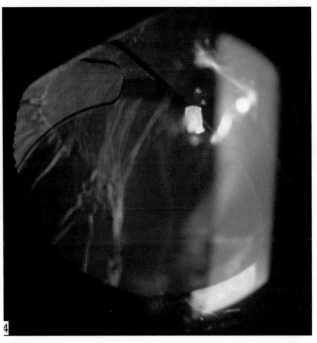

Fig. 21.6 Slit-lamp photo of an eye with PDG secondary to an Acrysof IOL in the sulcus. Note the decentration of the IOL. The glaucoma was controlled medically

period, and patients will have pain, blurry vision, and corneal edema. The pupillary space may be occluded by any surface in front of or behind the iris, including the vitreous face, capsule, or the optic of either an anterior or posterior chamber intraocular lens.[51] When an anterior chamber lens or iris-fixated lens is used, it is essential to perform a prophylactic peripheral iridectomy, otherwise the incidence of pupillary block is very high. With modern microsurgical phacoemulsification and posterior chamber intraocular lens implantation, the incidence of pupillary block is so low that a routine intraoperative peripheral iridectomy is no longer performed. However, pupillary block is still possible in this setting, especially in diabetic patients who may have increased thickness of the iris and ciliary body and possibly intense postoperative inflammation.[52,53] A prophylactic peripheral iridectomy should also be considered for cases of posterior

capsular rent or zonular dehiscence where vitreous prolapse may occlude the pupil.

Gonioscopy will confirm the closed angle with iris bombé and help distinguish pupillary block from other causes of a flat anterior chamber postoperatively, such as aqueous misdirection or choroidal hemorrhage. Ultrasound biomicroscopy and more recently optical coherence tomography (OCT; Carl Zeiss Meditec, Jena, Germany) and the Pentacam (Oculus, Lynnwood, MA) have provided valuable diagnostic imaging.[54–57]

Urgent medical and laser therapy for any form of pupillary block glaucoma will help prevent permanent peripheral anterior synechiae, which may require goniosynchialysis.[58] YAG capsulotomy is effective for capsular block as well as

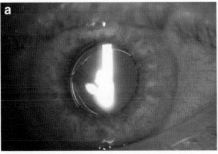
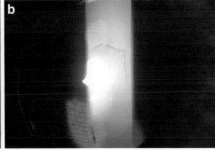

Fig. 21.5 Slit-lamp photos of a patient with PDG secondary to a piggy back IOL over an Alcon Restore IOL (Fort Worth, TX). In (**a**), note the decentration of the IOL and the TIDs at the pupillary margin. In (**b**), note the pigment deposition on the IOL at the area of the pupillary margin seen when the pupil is dilated. Photographs courtesy of Alan Lyon, Ophthalmic Photographer, University of Virginia, Charlottesville, VA

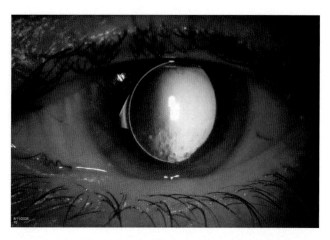

Fig. 21.7 Slit-lamp photo of patient with PDG and microhyphemas secondary to an Acrysof PC IOL (Alcon, Fort Worth, TX) in the ciliary sulcus. Note the elevation of the nasal aspect of the IOL and the iris TIDs. The patient underwent IOL exchange with resolution of hyphemas and much improved glaucoma control.[65] Photograph courtesy of Tom Monego, Ophthalmic Photographer at Dartmouth Hitchcock Medical Center, Lebanon, NH

for disruption of the anterior hyaloid face through a patent iridotomy.[59,60] If these steps fail, trabeculectomy may be indicated.

Summary

The three main mechanisms of intraocular lens-related glaucoma discussed here should be considered in all cases of glaucoma after cataract extraction and lens implantation. Reports of pigmentary glaucoma or pupillary block following insertion of posterior chamber phakic refractive lenses have already appeared in the literature.[61–64] See Fig. 21.5a, b. The consequences of persistent increased intraocular pressure postoperatively are greater for those patients with preexisting glaucoma, and early diagnosis and treatment are essential to prevent permanent vision loss.

References

1. Tomey KF, Traverso CE. The glaucomas in aphakia and pseudophakia. *Surv Ophthalmol.* 1991;36:79–112.
2. Traverso CE, Tomey KF, Gandolfo E. The glaucomas in pseudophakia. *Curr Opin Ophthalmol.* 1996;7:65–71.
3. Layden WE. Pseudophakia and glaucoma. *Ophthalmology.* 1982;89:875–9.
4. van Oye R, Gelisken O. Pseudophakic glaucoma. *Int Ophthalmol.* 1985;8:183–6.
5. Gedliczka T, Urban R. Secondary glaucoma in pseudophakia. *Klinika Oczna.* 1994;96:268–70.
6. Ellingson FT. The uveitis-glaucoma-hyphema syndrome associated with the Mark VIII anterior chamber lens implant. *J Am Intraocul Implant Soc.* 1978;4:50–3.
7. Keates RH, Ehrlich DR. "Lenses of chance" complications of anterior chamber implants. *Ophthalmology.* 1978;85:408–14.
8. Johnson SH, Kratz RP. Olson PF. Iris transillumination defect and microhyphema syndrome. *J Am Intraocul Implant Soc.* 1984;10:425–8.
9. Khan YA. Pavlin CJ, Cykiert R, Rootman DS. Uveitis-glaucoma-hyphema syndrome after handmade, anterior chamber lens implantation. *J Cataract Refract Surg.* 1997;23:1414–7.
10. Pazandak B, Johnson S, Kratz R. Faulkner GD. Recurrent intraocular hemorrhage associated with posterior chamber lens implantation. *J Am Intraocul Implant Soc.* 1983;9:327–9.
11. Apple DJ, Mamalis N, Loftfield K, et al. Complications of intraocular lenses. A historical and histopathological review. *Surv Ophthalmol.* 1984;29:1–54.
12. Maynor RC Jr. Five cases of severe anterior chamber lens implant complications. *J Am Intraocul Implant Soc.* 1984;10:223–4.
13. Aonuma H, Matsushita H, Nakajima K, Watase M, Tsushima K. Watanabe I. Uveitis-glaucoma-hyphema syndrome after posterior chamber intraocular lens implantation. *Jpn J Ophthalmol.* 1997;41:98–100.
14. Sharma A, Ibarra MS, Piltz-Seymour JR, Syed NA. An unusual case of uveitis-glaucoma-hyphema syndrome. *Am J Ophthalmol.* 2003;135:561–3.
15. Percival SBP, Das SK. UGH syndrome affecting posterior chamber lens implantation. *Am Intraocular Implant Soc J.* 1983;9:200–1.
16. Asaria RH, Salmon JF, Skinner AR, Ferguson DJ, McDonald B. Electron microscopy findings on an intraocular lens in the uveitis, glaucoma, hyphaema syndrome. *Eye.* 1997;11: 827–9.
17. Piette S, Canlas OA, Tran HV, Ishikawa H, Liebmann JM, Ritch R. Ultrasound biomicroscopy in uveitis-glaucoma-hyphema syndrome. *Am J Ophthalmol.* 2002;133:839–41.
18. Foroozan R, Tabas JG, Moster ML. Recurrent microhyphema despite intracapsular fixation of a posterior chamber intraocular lens. *J Cataract Refract Surg.* 2003;29:1632–5.
19. Berger RR, Kenyeres AM, Vlok AN. Incomplete posterior U.G.H. syndrome – different iatrogenic entity?. *Int Ophthalmol.* 1996;19:317–20.
20. Magargal LE, Goldberg RE, Uram M, Gonder JR, Brown GC. Recurrent microhyphema in the pseudophakic eye. *Ophthalmology.* 1983;90:1231–4.
21. Cates CA, Newman DK. Transient monocular visual loss due to uveitis-glaucoma-hyphaema (UGH) syndrome. *J Neurol Neurosurg Psychiatry.* 1998;65:131–2.
22. Rajak SN, Bahra A, Aburn NS, Warden NJ, Mossman SS. Recurrent anterior chamber hemorrhage from an intraocular lens simulating amaurosis fugax. *J Cataract Refract Surg.* 2007;33: 1492–3.
23. Lieppman ME. Intermittent visual "white out". A new intraocular lens complication. *Ophthalmology.* 1982;89:109–12.
24. Swan KC. Hyphema due to wound vascularization after cataract extraction. *Arch Ophthal.* 1973;89:87–90.
25. Watzke RC. Intraocular hemorrhage from vascularization of the cataract incision. *Ophthalmology.* 1980;87:19–23.
26. Summers CG, Lindstrom RL. Ghost cell glaucoma following lens implantation. *J Am Intraocul Implant Soc.* 1983;9:429–33.
27. Berger RO. Fox shield treatment of the UGH syndrome. *J Cataract Refract Surg.* 1986;12:419–21.
28. Angunawela R, Hugkulstone CE. Uveitis-glaucoma-hyphema syndrome and systemic anticoagulation. *Eye.* 2005;19:226–7.
29. Nicholson DH. Occult iris erosion. A treatable cause of recurrent hyphema in iris-supported intraocular lenses. *Ophthalmology.* 1982;89:113–20.
30. John GR, Stark WJ. Rotation of posterior chamber intraocular lenses for management of lens-associated recurring hyphemas. *Arch Ophthal.* 1992;110:963–4.

31. Mamalis N, Crandall AS, Pulsipher MW, Follett S, Monson MC. Intraocular lens explantation and exchange. A review of lens styles, clinical indications, clinical results, and visual outcome. *J Cataract Refract Surg.* 1991;17:811–8.

32. Doren GS, Stern GA, Driebe WT. Indications for and results of intraocular lens explantation. *J Cataract Refract Surg.* 1992;18:79–85.

33. Sinskey RM, Amin P, Stoppel JO. Indications for and results of a large series of intraocular lens exchanges. *J Cataract Refract Surg.* 1993;19:68–71.

34. Mamalis N. Explantation of intraocular lenses. *Curr Opin Ophthalmol.* 2000;11:289–95.

35. Por Y, Chee S. Trisection technique: a 2-snip approach to intraocular lens explantation. *J Cataract Refract Surg.* 2007;33:1151–4.

36. Osher R. Crisscross lensotomy: new explantation technique. *J Cataract Refract Surg.* 2006;32:386–8.

37. Smith JP. Pigmentary open-angle glaucoma secondary to posterior chamber intraocular lens implantation and erosion of the iris pigment epithelium. *J Am Intraocul Implant Soc.* 1985;11:174–6.

38. Masket S. Pseudophakic posterior iris chafing syndrome. *J Cataract Refract Surg.* 1986;12:252–6.

39. Watt RH. Pigment dispersion syndrome associated with silicone posterior chamber intraocular lenses. *J Cataract Refract Surg.* 1988;14:431–3.

40. Caplan MB, Brown RH, Love LL. Pseudophakic pigmentary glaucoma. *J Ophthalmol.* 1988;105:320–1.

41. Detry-Morel ML, Van Acker E, Pourjavan S, Levi N, De Potter P. Anterior segment imaging using optical coherence tomography and ultrasound biomicroscopy in secondary pigmentary glaucoma associated with in-the-bag intraocular lens. *J Cataract Refract Surg.* 2006;32:1866–9.

42. Mastropasqua L, Lobefalo L, Gallenga PE. Iris chafing in pseudophakia. *Documenta Ophthalmologica.* 1994;87(2):139–44.

43. LeBoyer RM, Werner L, Snyder ME, Mamalis N, Riemann CD, Augsberger JJ. Acute haptic-induced ciliary sulcus irritation associated with single-piece AcrySof intraocular lenses. *J Cataract Refract Surg.* 2005;31:1421–7.

44. Micheli T, Cheung LM, Sharma S, et al. Acute haptic-induced pigmentary glaucoma with an AcrySof intraocular lens. *J Cataract Refract Surg.* 2002;28:1869–72.

45. Uy HS, Chan PS. Pigment release and secondary glaucoma after implantation of single-piece acrylic intraocular lenses in the ciliary sulcus. *Am J Ophthalmol.* 2006;142:330–2.

46. Wintle R, Austin M. Pigment dispersion with elevated intraocular pressure after AcrySof intraocular lens implantation in the ciliary sulcus. *J Cataract Refract Surg.* 2001;27:642–4.

47. Samples JR, Van Buskirk EM. Pigmentary glaucoma associated with posterior chamber intraocular lenses. *Am J Ophthalmol.* 1985;100:385–8.

48. Werner D, Kaback M. Pseudophakic pupillary-block glaucoma. *Br J Ophthalmol.* 1977;61:329–33.

49. Van Buskirk EM. Pupillary block after intraocular lens implantation. *Am J Ophthalmol.* 1983;95:55–9.

50. Shrader CE, Belcher CD 3rd, Thomas JV, Simmons RJ. Murphy EB. Pupillary and iridovitreal block in pseudophakic eyes. *Ophthalmology.* 1984;91:831–7.

51. Willis DA, Stewart RH, Kimbrough RL. Pupillary block associated with posterior chamber lenses. *Ophthalmic Surg.* 1985;16:108–9.

52. Samples JR, Bellows AR, Rosenquist RC, Hutchinson BT, Fine IH, Van Buskirk EM. Pupillary block with posterior chamber intraocular lenses. *Arch Ophthal.* 1987;105:335–7.

53. Weinreb RN, Wasserstrom JP, Forman JS, Ritch R. Pseudophakic pupillary block with angle-closure glaucoma in diabetic patients. *Am J Ophthalmol.* 1986;102:325–8.

54. Aslanides IM, Libre PE, Silverman RH, et al. High frequency ultrasound imaging in pupillary block glaucoma. *Br J Ophthalmol.* 1995;79:972–6.

55. Kobayashi H, Hirose M, Kobayashi K. Ultrasound biomicroscopic analysis of pseudophakic pupillary block glaucoma induced by Soemmering's ring. *Br J Ophthalmol.* 2000;84:1142–6.

56. Sathish S, MacKinnon JR, Atta HR. Role of ultrasound biomicroscopy in managing pseudophakic pupillary block glaucoma. *J Cataract Refract Surg.* 2000;26:1836–8.

57. Mendrinos E, Dreifuss S, Dosso A, Shaarawy T. Evaluation of a pseudophakic pupillary block with an anterior segment OCT. *Br J Ophthalmol.* 2008;92:714–5.

58. Kokoris N, Macy JI. Laser iridectomy treatment of acute pseudophakic pupillary block glaucoma. *J Am Intraocul Implant Soc.* 1982;8:33–4.

59. Tomey KF, Traverso CE. Neodymium-YAG laser posterior capsulotomy for the treatment of aphakic and pseudophakic pupillary block. *Am J Ophthalmol.* 1987;104:502–7.

60. Cinotti DJ, Maltzman BA, Reiter DJ, Cinotti AA. Neodymium: YAG laser therapy for pseudophakic pupillary block. *J Cataract Refract Surg.* 1986;12:174–9.

61. Brandt JD, Mockovak ME, Chayet A. Pigmentary dispersion syndrome induced by a posterior chamber phakic refractive lens. *Am J Ophthalmol.* 2001;131:260–3.

62. Garcia-Feijoo J, Hernandez-Matamoros JL, Castillo-Gomez A. et al. Secondary glaucoma and severe endothelial damage after silicone phakic posterior chamber intraocular lens implantation. *J Cataract Refract Surg.* 2004;30:1786–9.

63. Smallman DS, Probst L, Rafuse PE. Pupillary block glaucoma secondary to posterior chamber phakic intraocular lens implantation for high myopia. *J Cataract Refract Surg.* 2004;30:905–7.

64. Chang SH, Lim G. Secondary pigmentary glaucoma associated with piggyback intraocular lens implantation. *J Cataract Refract Surg.* 2004;30:2219–22.

65. Johnson SM, Mian S, Connor C. Unusual secondary glaucoma. Glaucoma Today 2008; July/August:31–3.

Chapter 22

Cataract and Glaucoma in Retinopathy of Prematurity

Anthony J. Anfuso and M. Edward Wilson

Introduction

Effective treatment is now available for retinopathy of prematurity (ROP) using peripheral laser ablation and cryotherapy, as well as scleral buckling and/or vitrectomy for severe ROP with retinal detachment. However, with the continued improvement in survival of low birth weight and early gestational age infants, ROP remains a significant cause of childhood blindness.[1] While ROP is well known for damaging the posterior eye structures such as the retina and vitreous, ROP and its treatment can also predispose patients to develop anterior segment conditions, including cataract[2] and glaucoma[3] (Table 22.1 [4]). In fact, patients with stage V ROP have been reported to have a 30% risk of developing secondary angle-closure glaucoma[5-7] and a 50% risk of developing cataracts.[8]

Glaucoma

As traditionally described in the literature, angle-closure glaucoma associated with ROP occurs in infants and young children, corresponding with the cicatricial phase of ROP, which usually has its onset at the age of 3–6 months[9,10] (Table 22.2). Kushner suggested another possible and rare etiology when he described three cases of ciliary block glaucoma.[11] Rubeosis iridis or neovascularization of the iris commonly occurs with chronic retinal detachment due to ROP and can also lead to angle-closure glaucoma.[12] Angle-closure glaucoma has been reported after scleral buckling and after laser treatment for ROP.[13-15] Finally, angle-closure glaucoma related to pupillary block may occur later in childhood and even into adulthood in patients born with ROP.[16-19]

Table 22.1 Staging of ROP using the international classification[4]

Stage 1 – Demarcation line
  Thin structure that separates avascular retina anteriorly from the vascularized retina posteriorly
Stage 2 – Ridge
  Ridge – thickening and elevation of the retina around the demarcation line
Stage 3 – Extraretinal fibrovascular proliferation
  Extraretinal fibrovascular proliferation or neovascularization extends from the ridge into the vitreous (ridge/stage 2 ROP with extraretinal fibrovascular proliferation)
Stage 4 – Partial retinal detachment
Stage 4A – Partial extrafoveal retinal detachment
Stage 4B – Partial foveal retinal detachment
Stage 5 – Total retinal detachment
  In its most severe form, stage 5 shows a retina that is totally detached and drawn up into a fibrous mass behind the lens

Table 22.2 Cicatricial phase of ROP

Cicatricial phase of ROP
  When the acute phase ends and the regression or scarring phase begins
The fairly characteristic findings of the cicatricial phase are
  • Retinal folds
  • Dragged disk
  • Retinal pigment epithelium proliferation
  • Vitreous membranes
  • Intraretinal or subretinal exudation
  • Retinal neovascularization
  • Retinal holes
  • Retinal detachment

Hittner postulated that angle-closure glaucoma is becoming a more significant aspect of the ROP sequelae in his older ROP population. This is not only due to the increased survival of patients now reaching ages where progressive anterior segment complications may occur more frequently but also because advances in surgical technique have led to improved vision, despite initial severe retinal pathology. Thus glaucoma can be a vision-limiting factor in this population.[3]

A.J. Anfuso (✉)
University of West Virginia, Morgantown, WV, USA
e-mail: tony.anfuso@gmail.com

S.M. Johnson (ed.), *Cataract Surgery in the Glaucoma Patient*, DOI 10.1007/978-0-387-09408-3_22,
© Springer Science+Business Media, LLC 2009

Smith and Tasman reviewed 86 adult eyes with a history of ROP and found that 16% had glaucoma; 7% had narrow angle treated with iridotomy, open angle was diagnosed in nearly 6%, and the remaining 3.5% had neovascular.[20]

Smith and Shivitz presented three cases of adults with a history of ROP who presented with pupillary block glaucoma[17] and Michael presented ten eyes aged 12–45 years with a history of ROP who presented with angle-closure glaucoma.[21] In the series by Michael, two had neovascularization and the other eight had pupillary block. Ueda and Ogino reported a case of pupillary block glaucoma in a 22-year-old with a history of ROP who responded to iridotomy.[18]

Mechanism of Glaucoma

The angle-closure glaucoma in ROP patients has multiple proposed mechanisms. In infants and children with stage V ROP, the mechanism considered most likely to cause secondary angle-closure glaucoma is contraction of the retrolental membrane, during the cicatricial or scarring phase of ROP, causing anterior displacement of the lens-iris diaphragm and subsequent closure of the chamber angle[3,5,21]. Suzuki demonstrated this mechanism with high resolution ultrasonography in three cases.[19] Inflammation causing posterior synechiae formation and the subsequent development of pupillary block glaucoma can lead to angle closure in ROP eyes.[7,11] A thickened lens and shallow anterior chamber are malformations commonly noted in ROP and could also lead to pupillary block as well as account for the high degree of

Table 22.3 Non-retinal sequelae to ROP

- Rubeosis
- Thick lens
- Shallow anterior chamber
- Myopia
- Cataract
- Glaucoma

myopia often seen in children with ROP.[7,22–24] (Table 22.3). In a small cohort of children, McLoone used biometry with the IOL Master (Zeiss Meditec, Dublin, CA) to verify that eyes with a history of prior ROP had myopia associated with steeper corneas and shallower anterior chambers compared to control eyes with no history of ROP.[25]

Whatever the exact mechanism, there often is a reduced passage of aqueous humor from the posterior chamber to the anterior chamber, as iridectomy/iridotomy has frequently been successful in curing the glaucoma episode[16,17,19–21,26] (Fig.22.1a, b).

Initial Management

As mentioned previously, pupillary block is commonly the cause of glaucoma in ROP patients, and therefore iridectomy/iridotomy should be considered an initial treatment. In the three cases of babies, who had had prior treatment for ROP as infants, reported by Suzuki, the ultrasound was able to show opening of the angle following the iridectomy.[19] Additionally, Walton recommended prophylactic iridectomy when signs of cicatrization and shallowing of the

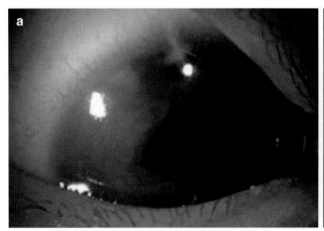
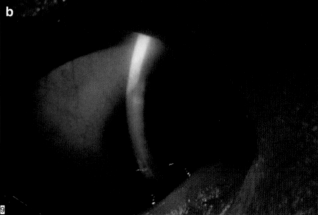

Fig. 22.1 (a) Eye of an 8-year-old adopted child followed for suspected ROP with retinopathy with macular dragging, high myopia in this eye, and angle-closure glaucoma following a dilated exam. A peripheral iridectomy was done, due to her age and nystagmus with good control of the IOP. Cataract surgery will be done when her angle further narrows, PAS develops, or elevated IOP ensues. (b) Note her shallow anterior chamber, despite iridectomy thought secondary to a large lens secondary to ROP. Photographs courtesy of Tom Monego, ophthalmic photographer, Dartmouth Hitchcock Medical Center, Lebanon, NH

Table 22.4 Cycloplegia in treating ciliary block glaucoma

Cycloplegia in treating ciliary block glaucoma

- Relax the ciliary muscle, which increases zonular tension and pulls the lens-iris diaphragm posteriorly
- May be required indefinitely, due to the anterior rotation of the ciliary body
- Miotics are contraindicated in ciliary block glaucoma as they have the opposite effect of cycloplegia

anterior chamber are seen and are progressing, even when no signs of glaucoma are present.[1,12] Walton found that in some patients, following peripheral iridectomy, continued shallowing of the anterior chamber produced apposition of the coloboma in the iris against the peripheral cornea leading to ineffectiveness of the iridectomy. To avoid this complication, he therefore recommended a sector iridectomy.

However, iridotomy/iridectomy has not been universally beneficial, suggesting that pupillary block is not the sole form of glaucoma in ROP.[16,27]

Corticosteroids and cycloplegics have had some degree of success in treating glaucoma in ROP eyes[11,27] (Table 22.4). Corticosteroids were shown often to be successful at controlling IOP and eliminating ocular discomfort. However, patients often experienced a rebound effect when attempting to discontinue corticosteroids, leading Pollard to conclude that they cannot be considered a definitive treatment[16] and cycloplegics are sometimes unsuccessful in treating pupillary block, due to posterior synechiae formation, during the cicatricial phase of ROP, which inhibits pupil dilation.[16]

After reporting ciliary block glaucoma in ROP eyes, Kushner made two recommendations: (1) If after dilation of ROP eyes there is noticeable deepening of the anterior chamber, suspect ciliary block glaucoma, and (2) if ROP eyes in acute angle glaucoma are unresponsive to miotic therapy, consider treating with a cycloplegic.[27] So while medical treatments such as steroids and cycloplegics may not always provide the definitive treatment, they should be explored prior to surgery. Kushner argues that medical treatment as opposed to surgery may be less costly, and provide less risk to the patient, as well as less emotional trauma to the parents, especially where there may be very limited visual potential.

Surgical Management

When iridectomy and medical management fail, surgical management including lensectomy, tube shunt implantation, cyclo-destructive procedures, or trabeculectomy is the next step in management[8] (Fig.22.2a, b). In cases of rubeotic glaucoma, management is often difficult, but includes shunt implantation in eyes with vision and cyclodestructive procedures in blind eyes.[8]

Indications for Surgery

Lensectomy, which can effectively treat both pupillary and ciliary block glaucoma by lessening the anterior displacement of the iris and reducing angle closure, remains an effective means of controlling acute angle glaucoma in ROP.[8] Pollard reported that lensectomy was universally successful in controlling pain and lowering IOP in eyes with a history of ROP, although visual outcome was poor, due to retinal detachment and cicatricial changes[1,16,24,28] Because lensectomy can keep the eye in a pain-free state, it is a preferred alternative to enucleation in a young infant, as early enucleation can lead to decreased growth of the bony orbit and facial asymmetry.[29] This disfiguring asymmetry, as well as the possible problems and fitting of a prosthesis are thus avoided According to Hittner, the most successful treatment in stage V ROP is lens aspiration.[2] Intraocular surgery on a blind eye was deemed indicated in these cases to avoid enucleation. However, efforts to reattach the retina are resulting in improved vision in some cases.[1,9,30–32] Rarely, only one eye develops severe cicatricial changes with angle closure, while the other eye is relatively free of ROP malformations. In this situation, Pollard recommends considering the alternatives to lensectomy – including enucleation, retrobulbar alcohol, or cyclocryotherapy – in order to avoid the rare development of sympathetic ophthalmia in the good eye.[16]

Cataract

Cataracts occur more commonly in ROP patients as compared to general population. Low birth weight and prematurity are risk factors for both ROP and cataracts.[33,34]Like glaucoma, cataracts also occur at a greater frequency over time, now that treatment modalities have preserved vision in eyes that would have otherwise been lost. Transpupillary laser photocoagulation is now the standard treatment for threshold ROP. Compared to cryotherapy, laser photocoagulation results in better structural and functional outcomes. However, laser-treated eyes have a higher incidence of secondary cataracts than cryo-treated eyes.[35–37] In 1997, Gold reported 68 cataracts in association with ROP treatment.[38] Sixty-two percent were associated with argon laser, 31% with diode laser, and 7% with cryotherapy.

Lens opacities associated with ROP comes in three types. First, focal punctuate or vacuolated opacities may occur at the subcapsular level. These are usually transient and visually insignificant.[39,40] Second, progressive lens opacities may occur in patients without retinal detachment. Most of

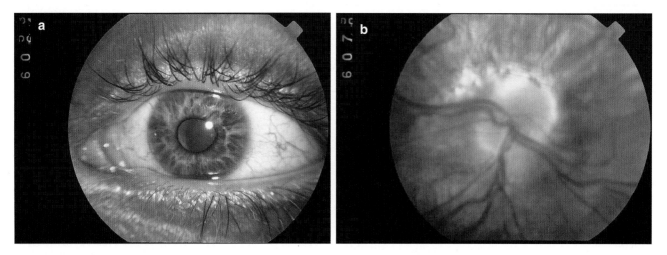

Fig. 22.2 (**a**) Slit and (**b**) fundus photo of a 23-year-old patient with a history of prematurity, high myopia, shallow anterior chamber, and angle closure. Cataract surgery was pursued. Photographs courtesy of Dr. Elizabeth Sharpe, Charleston, SC

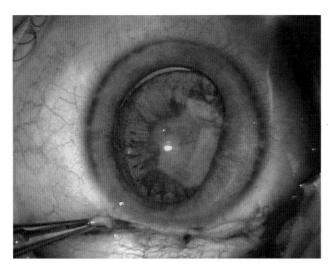

Fig. 22.3 Preoperative appearance of an infant eye status post treatment for ROP to undergo cataract removal. Photo courtesy of Dr. M. Edward Wilson, Storm Eye Institute, Charleston, SC

these eyes have had transpupillary laser treatment or "lens-sparing" vitrectomy. These cataracts may progress rapidly or much more slowly, but they almost always eventually obstruct the entire visual axis and require surgery (Fig.22.3). One study reported a median interval of 3 weeks for diagnosis of cataract after laser photocoagulation.[41] These patients may also develop glaucoma. The third type of cataract is one that develops as a result of cicatricial ROP with retinal detachment, which is also associated with glaucoma as discussed previously. In one series,[8] 54.6% (17/31) of eyes treated for advanced ROP had cataracts. In the series reported by Smith and Tasman, 83.7% of the 86 adult eyes aged 45–56 years with a history of ROP had cataract or cataract surgery.[20]

Operative Techniques

The two approaches to lensectomy in grade V ROP are pars plana lensectomy versus lensectomy via the limbal approach. A pars plana lensectomy can be combined with an attempt at retinal repair. Pars plan lensectomy with anterior vitrectomy was used successfully by Pollard for five eyes reported with angle closure, after the age of 2.[28] The limbal approach is easier and more consistent, as the pars plana entry may be difficult in these immature eyes with retinal detachment. Even when the anterior chamber is extremely shallow, an anterior corneal entry can usually be made with the assistance of a viscous ophthalmic viscosurgical device (OVD).

A visually significant cataract after laser treatment or vitrectomy for ROP is approached much like childhood cataracts in children without ROP.[2] At times the anterior capsule can be fibrotic, but a vitrectorhexis can still be easily performed.[2] IOL (intraocular lens) calculations can be performed using an immersion A-scan ultrasound unit and a portable keratometer in the operating room, after the child is under general anesthesia for cataract surgery. IOLs are implanted routinely, unless the child is in the early months of life and has microphthalmia. Most commonly, a single-piece hydrophobic acrylic IOL is implanted in children. In anticipation of myopic shift of refraction, the IOL power for a child undergoing cataract surgery should be customized based on many characteristics – especially age, laterality (one eye or both), amblyopia status (dense or mild), likely compliance with glasses, and family history of myopia. For a child with ROP and cataract, slightly higher hypermetropia may be considered in anticipation of developing more myopia, especially if treated with cryotherapy.[42]

A primary posterior capsulectomy and anterior vitrectomy is performed for children who are younger than 6 years of age. If previous vitrectomy has been performed as part of the ROP treatment, the surgeon must be aware that the posterior capsule may have been violated during the previous surgery. Lens surgery and glaucoma surgery can be done together when necessary in eyes with previous treatment for ROP. The vitrector handpiece is often used to create a peripheral iridectomy, since in young children it is also used to perform the capsulotomy, lens aspiration, posterior capsulotomy, and anterior vitrectomy.

Outcomes

In all 15 patients in a report by Pollard,[16] lensectomy cured the glaucoma. Eight patients presented with acute angle-closure glaucoma and the other seven had a chronic glaucoma. All vision remained extremely poor in the range of light perception to hand motion due to the prior ROP, but all eyes remained pain-free and had resolution of their glaucoma. This was a similar outcome to his cohort of five patients with a history of ROP who presented with glaucoma and were treated with pars plana lensectomy with anterior vitrectomy.[28] Thus, Pollard suggested lensectomy via the limbal/corneal approach be considered in infants with grade V ROP and secondary angle-closure glaucoma. Blodi warned of potentially disastrous complications in opening an eye in such patients.[5] At times, the lensectomy is merely a precursor to the inevitable enucleation. Lambert and coauthors[41] reported a high rate of progression to total retinal detachment and phthisis after cataract surgery in patients with a history of transpupillary laser photocoagulation, even when the retina is attached at the time of cataract surgery.

Other reports show a more encouraging surgical outcome for cataract surgery with posterior chamber IOL implantation in children and adults with a past history of ROP.[43–45] Yu reported on eight eyes with a history of ROP with cataract treated with lensectomy, posterior capsulectomy, and anterior vitrectomy with posterior chamber IOL.[43] All the patients were under the age of 2. Two eyes of the same patient required cryotherapy and scleral buckle at the time of the lensectomy. Two eyes were able to have vision measured at 20/60 at the last follow-up and the others were central steady maintained fixation at the last recorded follow-up. These eyes did not have glaucoma. Krolicki reported on cataract surgery in ten adults with a history of ROP.[44] Eight eyes had improved vision. Six of the eyes had coexisting glaucoma and the control improved following cataract surgery. One eye developed a retinal detachment. Farr reported on 21 adult eyes with a history of ROP who underwent cataract surgery.[45] Eight eyes had narrow angle glaucoma and five with open angle. Two eyes had angle closure treated with iridectomy and one eye had phacomorphic glaucoma that

resolved with the cataract extraction, otherwise in their series, the glaucoma control did not improve. No patient lost vision with the surgery and 18 had improved vision.

Summary

In summary, ROP remains a leading cause of vision impairment in children. Glaucoma and cataract can result from the ROP or from the treatment needed to control the ROP. Stage V ROP has a very high association with glaucoma and cataract. However, glaucoma and cataract can also occur in infants, children, and young adults after successful treatment for ROP with preservation of vision. General principles of pediatric anterior segment surgery should be followed for cataract surgery in children. A history of prematurity should be sought in patients with angle closure and other findings of ROP, such as high myopia and evidence of prior retinopathy. Cataract surgery should be considered in the treatment of the angle-closure glaucoma in these eyes. Based on the report by Farr, open angle glaucoma associated with a history or ROP and concurrent cataract are unlikely to experience improved glaucoma control with cataract surgery.[45] The risk of retinal detachment needs to be discussed with the patients and the posterior segments monitored.

References

1. Ritch R, Shields MB, Krupin T, eds. *The Glaucomas.* 2nd ed., St. Louis: Mosby; 1996:941–3.
2. Wilson ME, Trivedi RH, Pandey SK, eds. *Pediatric Cataract Surgery: Techniques, Complications, and Management.* Philadelphia, PA: Lippincott Williams and Wilkins 2005:179–83.
3. Hittner HM, Rhodes LM, McPherson AR. Anterior segment abnormalities in cicatricial retinopathy of prematurity. *Ophthalmology.* 1979;86(5):803–16.
4. International Committee for the Classification of Retinopathy of Prematurity. The international classification of retinopathy of prematurity revisited. *Arch Ophthalmol.* 2005;123:991–9.
5. Blodi FC. Symposium: retrolental fibroplasia (retinopathy of prematurity). Management. *Trans Am Acad Ophthalmol Otolaryngol.* 1955;59:35–8.
6. Kwitko M. Secondary glaucoma in infancy and childhood. In Kwitko M, ed. *Glaucoma in Infants and Children,* New York: Appleton-Century-Crofts; 1973
7. Hartnett ME, Gilbert MM, Richardson TM, Krug JH, Jr, Hirose T, Anterior segment evaluation of infants with retinopathy of prematurity. *Ophthalmology.* 1990;97(1):122–30.
8. Knight-Nanan DM, Algawi K, Bowell R, O'Keefe M. Advanced cicatricial retinopathy of prematurity – outcome and complications. *Br J Ophthalmol.* 1996;80:343–45.
9. Shields MB. *Textbook of Glaucoma.* 2nd ed. Baltimore: Williams and Wilkins, 1987:272.
10. McCormick AQ, Pratt-Johnson JA. Angle closure glaucoma in infancy. *Ophthalmic Surg.* 1971:2:91–3.

11. Kushner BJ, Sondheimer S. Medical treatment of glaucoma associated with retinopathy of prematurity. *Am J Ophthalmol.* 1982;94:313–7.

12. Walton DS. Retrolental ibroplasia with glaucoma. In Chandler DA, Grant WM, eds. *Glaocoma.* 2nd ed. Philadelphia: Lea and Febiger; 1979:361–2.

13. Lee GA, Lee LR, Gole GA. Angle-closure glaucoma after laser treatment for retinopathy of prematurity. *J AAPOS.* 1998;2:383–4.

14. Halperin LS, Schoch LH. Angle closure glaucoma after scleral buckling for retinopathy of prematurity. Case report. *Arch Ophthalmol.* 1988;106:453

15. Trigler L, Weaver G, O'Neil JW, Barondes MJ, Freedman SF. Case series of angle-closure glaucoma after laser treatment for retinopathy of prematurity. *J AASPO.* 2005;9:17–21.

16. Pollard ZF. Lensectomy for secondary angle-closure glaucoma in advanced cicatricial retrolental fibroplasia. *Ophthalmology.* 1984; 91(4):395–8.

17. Smith J, Shivitz I. Angle-closure glaucoma in adults with cicatricial retinopathy of prematurity. *Arch Ophthalmol.* 1984;102: 371–2.

18. Ueda N, Ogino N. Angle-closure glaucoma with papillary block mechanism in cicatricial retinopathy of prematurity. *Ophthalmologica.* 1988;196:15–8.

19. Suzuki A, Kondo N, Terasaki H. High resolution ultrasonography in eyes with angle closure glaucoma associated with the cicatricial stage of retinopathy of prematurity. *Jpn J Ophthalmol.* 2005;49:312–4.

20. Smith BT, Tasman WS. Retinopathy of prematurity: late complications in the baby boomer generation (1946–64). *Trans Am Ophthalmol Soc.* 2005;103:225–36.

21. Michael AJ, Pesin SR, Katz LJ, Tasman WS. Management of late-onset angle-closure glaucoma associated with retinopathy of prematurity. *Ophthalmology.* 1991;98(7):1093–8.

22. Gordon RA, Donzis PB. Myopia associated with retinopathy of prematurity. *Ophthalmology.* 1986;93:1593–8.

23. Ritch R, Chang BM, Liebmann JM. Angle closure in younger patients. *Ophthalmology.* 2003;110(10):1880–9.

24. Choi MY, Park IK, Yu YS. Long term refractive outcome in eyes of preterm infants with and without retinopathy of prematurity: comparison of keratometric value, axial length, anterior chamber depth, and lens thickness. *Br J Ophthalmol.* 2000;84:138–43.

25. McLoone EM, O'Keefe M, McLoone SF, Lanigan BM. Long-term refractive and biometric outcomes following diode laser therapy for retinopathy or prematurity. *J AAPOS,* 2006;5:454–9.

26. Johnson DR, Swan KC. Retrolental fibroplasia – a continuing problem. *Trans Pac Coast Otoophthalmol Soc Annu Meet.* 1966;47:129–33.

27. Kushner BJ. Ciliary block glaucoma in retinopathy of prematurity. *Arch Ophthalmol.* 1982 July;100(7):1078–9.

28. Pollard ZF. Secondary angle-closure glaucoma in cicatricial retrolental fibroplasia. *Am J Ophthalmol.* 1980;89(5):651–3.

29. Kennedy RE. The effect of early enucleation on the orbit in animals and humans. *Adv Ophthalmic Plast Reconstr Surg.* 1992;9: 1–39.

30. Machemer R. Closed vitrectomy for severe retrolental fibroplasia in the infant. *Ophthalmology.* 1983;90:436.

31. Trese MT. Surgical results of Stage V retrolental fibroplasia and timing of surgical repair. *Ophthalmology.* 1984;91:461.

32. Ferrone PJ, Trese MT, Williams GA, Cox MS. Good visual acuity in an adult population with marked posterior segment changes secondary to retinopathy of prematurity. *Retina.* 1998;18: 335–8.

33. SanGiovanni JP, Chew EY, Reed GF, Remaley NA, Bateman JB, Sugimoto TA, et al. Infantile cataract in the collaborative perinatal project:prevalence and risk factors. *Arch Ophthalmol.* 2002;120:1559–65.

34. Repka MX, Summers CG, Palmer EA, Dobson V, Tung B, Davis B. The incidence of ophthalmic interventions in children with birth weights less than 1251 grams. Results through 5 $\frac{1}{2}$ years. Cryotherapy for Retinopathy of Prematurity Cooperative Group. *Ophthalmology.* 1998;105:1621–7.

35. Christiansen SP, Bradford JD. Cataract in infants treated with argon laser photocoagulation for threshold retinopathy of prematurity. *Am J Ophthalmol.* 1995;119:175–80.

36. Christiansen SP, Bradford JD. Cataracts following diode laser photoablation for retinopathy of prematurity. *Arch Ophthamol.* 1997;115:275–6.

37. Kaiser RS, Trese MT. Iris atrophy, cataracts, and hypotony following peripheral ablation for threshold retinopathy of prematurity. *Arch Ophthalmol.* 1995;119:615–7.

38. Gold RS. Cataracts associated with treatment for retinopathy of prematurity. *J Pediatr Ophthalmol Strabismus.* 1997;34:123–4.

39. Alden ER, Kalina RE, Hodson WA. Transient cataracts in low-birthweight infants. *J Pediatr.* 1973;82:314–8.

40. Drack AV, Burke JP, Pulido JS, Keech RV. Transient punctuate lenticular opacities as a complication of argon laser photoablation in an infant with retinopathy of prematurity. *Am J Ophthalmol.* 1992;113:583–4.

41. Lambert SR, Capone A, Jr, Cingle KA, Drack AV. Cataract and phthisis bulbi after laser photoablation for threshold retinopathy of prematurity. *Am J Ophthalmol.* 2000;129:585–91.

42. Trivedi RH, Wilson ME. IOL power calculation for children. In: Garg A, Lin, eds. *Mastering Intraocular Lenses.* New Delhi: Jaypee Brothers Medical Publishers; Chapter 9, 2007:84–91.

43. Yu YS, Kim SJ, Chang BL. Cataract surgery in children with and without retinopathy of prematurity. *J Cataract Refract Surg.* 2004;30:96–101.

44. Krolicki TJ, Tasman W. Cataract extraction in adults with retinopathy of prematurity. *Arch Ophthalmol.* 1995;113:173–7.

45. Farr AK, Stark WJ, Haller JA. Cataract surgery by phacoemulsification in adults with retinopathy of prematurity. *Am J Ophthalmol.* 2001;132:306–10.

Chapter 23

Cataract Surgery in the Hypotonous Eye

Devon Ghodasra and Sandra M. Johnson

Introduction

Hypotony refers to low intraocular pressure (IOP) and is statistically defined in many sources as IOP less than 6.5 mmHg.[1] Because visual sequelae are variable and often absent below such a statistical definition for hypotony, this chapter primarily refers to hypotony as low IOP causing clinically significant complications.

Pathophysiology

In general, hypotony can be the result of two processes: increased outflow of aqueous humor and/or decreased aqueous humor production or inflow from the ciliary body. Table 23.1 lists the causes of hypotony.

Table 23.1 Causes of hypotony

- Ocular surgery or trauma
- Ciliochoroidal detachment
- Ciliary effusion
- Rhegmatogenous retinal detachment
- Cyclodialysis cleft
- Iridocyclitis
- Ocular ischemia
- Traction ciliary body detachment
- Pharmacologic aqueous suppressants
- Chemical from antimetabolites
- Laser or cryo cyclodestruction
- Systemic hypertonicity or acidosis

D. Ghodasra (✉)
School of Medicine, Medical College of Georgia, Augusta, GA 30912, USA
e-mail: devonghodasra@gmail.com

Hypotony Due to Inadequate Inflow of Aqueous

One general etiology of hypotony involves inadequate aqueous humor production by the ciliary body. Inadequate aqueous humor production is usually considered after structural processes have been ruled out. Such cases include iridocyclitis, ocular ischemia, traction ciliary body detachment, aqueous suppressants; chemical toxicity from antimetabolites, laser or cryo-cyclodestruction; systemic hypertonicity, or acidosis.[2–4] Iridocyclitis is a known etiology of hypotony. Inflammation increases the permeability of the blood-aqueous barrier, which decreases aqueous humor production and disrupts the transport processes of the ciliary body epithelium.[5,6] This in turn leads to ciliary edema. A self-perpetuating cycle may develop as low IOP is known to increase choroidal effusions and contribute to the development of ciliochoroidal detachment associated with low IOP.[7] In advanced cases of ocular inflammation, ciliary body vasculitis may result in diminished blood flow and further decrease ciliary body production of aqueous humor.

Hypotony Due to Increased Outflow

Because each of the causes of hypotony may be managed differently, a thorough investigation of the cause should be undertaken in order to initiate appropriate treatment. Evaluation usually begins with a history of any procedures, trauma and other ocular history, and an ocular examination to seek structural causes that may lead to the increased outflow of aqueous humor. These include wound leak secondary to ocular surgery or trauma, ciliochoroidal detachment, rhegmatogenous retinal detachment, and cyclodialysis cleft.

Among the causes of postoperative hypotony, overfiltration related to trabeculectomy is likely the most common cause of chronic hypotony and is the focus of this chapter. Although post-trabeculectomy hypotony is usually self-limited, the likelihood of visual complications increases with

S.M. Johnson (ed.), *Cataract Surgery in the Glaucoma Patient*, DOI 10.1007/978-0-387-09408-3_23,
© Springer Science+Business Media, LLC 2009

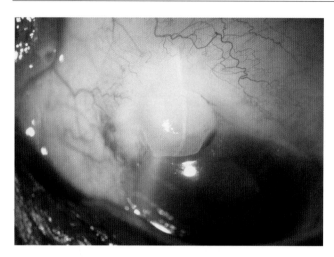

Fig. 23.1 Thin avascular bleb after a trabeculectomy with MMC in a patient with chronic hypotony with IOP maximum of 6 mmHg and 6–9 mmHg following cataract surgery. Photo courtesy of Michael Stanley, ophthalmic photographer, Medical College of Georgia, Augusta

the use of antimetabolites such as mitomycin-C (MMC) and 5-fluorouracil (5-FU) at the time of surgery and longer duration of hypotony.[8,9] Blebs that are very thin and avascular are more commonly associated with increased filtration leading to clinically significant hypotony (Fig. 23.1). Other risk factors for hypotony following filtration surgery include myopia and young age as well as male gender.[10]

Suspected sites of wound leakage can be evaluated with a Seidel test, in which fluorescein stain is painted on a bleb or wound and observed with a cobalt blue light, watching for confirmatory dilution by leaking aqueous (Fig. 9.4). Ciliochoroidal detachment and the resulting choroidal effusion lead to increased uveoscleral outflow. These processes may also be associated with reduced aqueous humor production. Rhegmatogenous retinal detachment may also lead to hypotony as posterior chamber aqueous fluid is shunted from the posterior segment through the retinal break.[11,12] In addition, iridocyclitis associated with retinal detachment may decrease aqueous humor production as discussed above. Finally, cyclodialysis clefts seen after ocular trauma or surgery are associated with hypotony. The separation of the ciliary body from the scleral spur increases uveoscleral outflow as aqueous humor flows into the supracilliary space.[13] The search for the cause of hypotony is as important as the diagnosis of hypotony, and the diagnostic evaluation of hypotony is summarized in Table 23.2[14] (Fig. 23.2). A treatment plan can be formulated once the etiology is elucidated.[15]

Clinical Manifestations

Chronic hypotony may result in several structural changes that can subsequently lead to a variety of visual symptoms.

Table 23.2 Diagnostic evaluation of hypotony

1. History of visual complaints
2. History of past eye disease, surgery, or trauma
3. History of systemic and ocular medications
4. Central corneal thickness
5. Gonioscopy for cyclodialysis cleft
6. Seidel's test
7. Ultrasonic biomicroscopy for cyclodialysis cleft
8. Ophthalmoscopy for retinal or choroidal detachment
9. Ultrasonography for posterior segment evaluation
10. Optical coherence tomography
11. Exploratory surgery

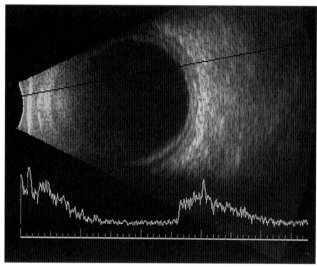

Fig. 23.2 Image of a B-scan ultrasound demonstrating a low-lying choroidal effusion that can be associated with hypotony

The IOP level at which structural and visual complications arise are variable between individuals. Individuals with reduced central corneal thickness may be less likely to develop hypotony maculopathy.[16] Increased cataract progression is often seen in chronic hypotony.[17–19] A shallow anterior chamber is associated with hypotony and may increase the rate of cataract formation through posterior synechiae. Also, abnormal lens metabolism during hypotony, with reduced aqueous, is also thought to contribute to transient lenticular opacification[20] and may contribute to a more gradual development of cataract. Several other factors may increase the likelihood of cataract progression, including preexisting cataract and administration of topical and systemic corticosteroids to treat the hypotony. In general, cataract maturation has been noted following glaucoma filtration surgeries and reported in several major clinical trials, which included trabeculectomy treatment.[21,22] The reported incidence of cataract formation varies. In older studies, it has been suggested that as many as half of patients have significant visual complications secondary to cataract 6–12 years after trabeculectomy.[23,24] Additionally, there may be rapid development of cataracts in lenses that are injured during a glaucoma procedure, such as by a forceps during iridectomy or a cannula during anterior chamber reformation.[25] Additional structural changes secondary to chronic hypotony are listed in Table 23.3.

Table 23.3 Ocular complications of hypotony

- Cataract progression
- Corneal edema and folds
- Corneal astigmatism
- Posterior synechiae
- Anterior synechiae
- Macular edema
- Chorioretinal folds
- Maculopathy

A variety of visual sequelae may arise from the structural changes associated with hypotony.[7] Reduction in visual acuity may be due to several of the structural changes. Changing corneal astigmatism and its effect on refraction is a common reason for worsening visual acuity. Corneal and macular edema in addition to chorioretinal folds may lead to a hyperopic shift. A myopic shift may result from shallowing of the anterior chamber. Cataract progression and hypotonous maculopathy can also contribute to deteriorating visual acuity[26] (Fig. 23.3). Ocular pain and discomfort are additional complaints in hypotonous patients, and these symptoms may arise from iridocyclitis that is associated with the alterations of the blood-aqueous barrier.[7] As noted previously, the appearance of symptoms does not exactly correlate with particular IOP levels, and the presence or absence of symptoms is variable between patients.

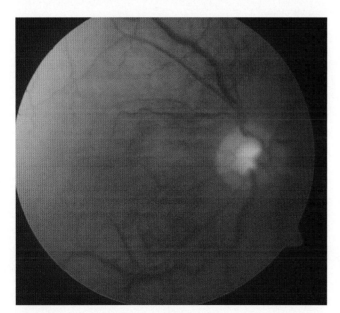

Fig. 23.3 Macular striae in a patient with IOP below 7 mmHg and blurred vision following a trabeculectomy with MMC. Photo courtesy of Michael Stanley, ophthalmic photographer, Medical College of Georgia, Augusta

Management

Because IOP levels do not always parallel clinically significant symptoms, there is no simple pressure value at which therapy is suggested. Instead, the primary reason for initiating therapy for hypotony is deterioration in vision that significantly affects the patient's lifestyle. Other considerations include a persistent wound or bleb leak that increases the chance for infection, especially if there is a history of prior ocular infections or poor patient hygiene. There is a range of medical and surgical techniques in the management of hypotony that are beyond the scope of this chapter; these are listed in Table 23.4.[27-34]

Table 23.4 Treatment options for hypotony[27,28]

Wound leak
    Cyanoacrylate glue
    Aqueous suppressant
    Therapeutic/bandage contact lens
    Collagen shield
    Surgical revision
    Torpedo patch
Overfiltration
    Bandage contact lens
    Simmons shell tamponade
    Symblepharon ring
    Trichloracetic acid to bleb
    Autologous blood injection
    External conjunctival cryopexy
    Laser grid technique to bleb
    Compression sutures
    Surgical revision
    Cataract extraction
Chronic choroidal effusion
    Drainage of choroidal fluid (Chapter 12)
Cyclodialysis cleft [27]
    Topical atropine drops
    Argon laser
    Surgical repair

Cataract Surgery

While not primarily intended as a therapy to increase intraocular pressure in hypotony related to overfiltration, cataract extraction in the setting of preexisting hypotony has shown some therapeutic potential in alleviating hypotony. The theory is that the inflammation secondary to the cataract procedure will impair some of the bleb function.[35-38] The initial study on two patients with post-filtration post trabeculectomy showed that hypotony resolved following large-incision extracapsular or intracapsular cataract extraction.[39] In 1980, Mackool reported three patients with three etiologies of hypotony and three methods of cataract extraction where all three patients had reversal of the low IOP and improved vision for 16 months or more postoperatively.[40] Sibayan et al. reported on two patients in 1997 who underwent clear cornea phacoemulsification with posterior chamber IOL who showed improvement in vision and hypotony but with persistent IOP control and filtration through their prior trabeculectomy.[41] The authors suggested that the postoperative rise in IOP was most likely the result of inflammatory compromise of the filtering bleb. Chen et al. reported improved vision in 18 of 19 patients with hypotony who underwent cataract surgery. Thirteen had phacoemulsification and the others had traditional extracapsular cataract extraction (ECCE). Three required further intervention for hypotony and two eyes underwent bleb needling.[42] Doyle and Smith have further suggested that maximizing viscoelastic use and minimizing anti-inflammatory medication may lead to even better outcomes in hypotony patients post-phacoemulsification.[43] They propose that leaving viscoelastic in eyes at the end of surgery leads to decreased aqueous flow through overfiltering blebs, while the increased inflammation secondary to limiting anti-inflammatory medications leads to decreased bleb size and function. In all of the preceding trials, cataract extraction in hypotony patients also led to marked improvements in visual acuity. Thus, it can be concluded from the limited current data that phacoemulsification and extracapsular extraction are effective techniques in improving vision and simultaneously elevating IOP in post-filtration eyes with hypotony.

Preoperative Care

Due to the additional concern of low IOP in patients with hypotony, a thorough preoperative examination is vital prior to cataract extraction. As discussed previously, the etiology of the hypotony needs to be confirmed. An extensive history including comorbid medical problems, medications, allergies, and previous eye disease or surgeries should be elicited. Physical exam begins with evaluation of refraction and visual acuity in addition to potential acuity testing. Anterior segment evaluation should include both slit lamp and gonioscopic examination. Dilated examination of the fundus is required, and B-scan ultrasonography may be needed in the presence of mature opaque cataracts. Optical coherence tomography (OCT, Zeiss Meditec, Dublin, CA) may be helpful in diagnosing hypotony maculopathy and macular folds.[44] Preoperative measurement of IOP is crucial and baseline central corneal thickness may be helpful. A history of vision loss coincident with hypotony can assist in confirming the etiology of the vision loss. Counseling about unknown visual recovery should be done as chronic hypotony maculopathy can cause permanent visual changes.

The patient also needs to be counseled about the difficulty in accurately predicting refractive outcome. The axial length has been shown to be reduced following trabeculectomy.[45,46] If a surgeon expects to correct the hypotony, then it would be reasonable to use pre-trabeculectomy measurements for IOL calculation[47] (Table 23.5).

Table 23.5 Preoperative measurements for IOL calculation for an eye with hypotony undergoing cataract surgery. Note the unpredictable nature of the predictions

Study of IOL calculations in a hypotonous right eye (OD)
1. Preoperative refraction +1.00 + 0.75 × 80 OD
   $$-1.00 \text{ left eye (OS)}$$
2. History of cataract surgery OS with a 19.5D IOL placed with a goal of −2.7D
   OD was myopic at that time, OS was not hypotonous but post trabeculectomy:
   A hyperopic shift was obtained of +1.7
   IOL calculations suggested a 15.5D lens for plano OD
   IOL Master Used (Carl Zeiss, Dublin, CA)
3. Repeated measurements pre-op surgery OD with IOL master:
   Axial length: OD 23.84 mm OS 25.18 mm
   Keratometry: K1 42.35   K1 43.38
                K2 43.83   K2 43.89
IOL calculations suggest 20.5D lens for plano OD and now 15.5D lens for plano OS
   17D predicts −0.92 OS
4. 17.5D IOL chosen in attempt to avoid anisometropia
   • Approximately minus 1D outcome if the axial length normalized and an effective hyperopic shift occurred as suspected OS
                          OR
   • Approximately plus 2D if the axial length did not change
5. Outcome +1.25 + 1.25 × 90, which reflected minimal myopic shift and increase in the axial length despite the improved IOP and no anisometropia

Operative Technique

As with all ocular surgeries, there are additional potential challenges to consider in patients who have previously undergone surgery. The operative technique of phacoemulsification used by Doyle and Smith involved a clear corneal incision, although a temporal scleral tunnel technique could aid in inducing scarring of a bleb extending temporally. Meticulous wound closure would be necessary to avoid postoperative bleb or wound leak. Post-trabeculectomy patients undergoing cataract extract may have more conjunctival scarring than a patient naïve to ocular surgery. Such scarring may make dissection more difficult and increases the risk of conjunctival tears. The bleb should be assessed for leaks at the end of the surgery and any injury repaired.

Doyle and Smith used Viscoat (Alcon, Fort Worth, TX) and implanted foldable silicone intraocular lenses, which may be more reactive than acrylic ones.[43,48] Their operative procedure was reported as unchanged from accepted clinical practices except for three modifications: (1) preoperative anti-inflammatory eye drops were withheld, (2) viscoelastic was not removed at the end of the case, and (3) postoperative anti-inflammatory eye drop use was minimized.

However, wound construction is not as easy in an eye with low IOP, and an initial paracentesis with injection of viscoelastic, to deepen the anterior chamber, helps to create a normotensive eye for a controlled cataract incision. Posterior synechiae, which may be responsible for the cataract progression and associated with hypotony, often makes visualization for capsulotomy or capsulorhexis more difficult and if present need to be lysed. In hypotonous eyes, the anterior chamber may be shallower than normal; during the procedure the bottle of irrigation solution may need to be raised to ensure an adequate working space to avoid injuring the corneal endothelium and viscoelastics used generously to cover the corneal endothelium. There may be an excess of fluid exiting through a preexisting bleb, resulting in pooling of fluid on the cornea and obscuration of the surgeon's view. A small conjunctival incision can be made in an inferior quadrant, away from the bleb, to allow escape of the excess subconjunctival fluid. Anterior synechiae, which should be noted on preoperative gonioscopic examination, may hinder implantation of an anterior chamber lens.

Cantor and coauthors combined cataract extraction with drainage of choroidal fluid in 5 of 63 reported cases who had drainage of choroidal effusions. In all five, the effusions resolved by 7 weeks postoperative. An additional five patients in their report underwent cataract surgery at the time of a second drainage procedure and effusions resolved by 8 weeks postoperative.[30] It is likely that the hypotony contributed to the cataracts and that the cataract extraction contributed to improvement of the hypotony.

Complications

Complications were not highly prevalent in previous studies of hypotony patients undergoing cataract extraction. In their technique of phacoemulsification, Doyle and Smith observed a serious postoperative IOP spike in one of nine patients that was treated with needling.[43] They propose this was most likely secondary to leaving viscoelastic in the eye at the conclusion of the case and minimizing use of anti-inflammatory medications, which were intended to elevate the IOP but not as high. Inadequate titration could be a problem in patients with advanced glaucoma at risk for "snuff out" where a high IOP, even for a short time, could be deleterious. The authors did not note any additional complications in their other eight patients. Chen et al. note the need for glaucoma medications in two of their patients postoperatively and need for bleb

needling in two others.[42] A higher risk of phthisis with additional ocular surgery is likely in eyes where hypotony is primarily due to a decreased aqueous production, which could coexist with a filtering bleb in uveitic or ischemic eyes, for example.

Postoperative Care

As suggested by Doyle and Smith, minimal use of anti-inflammatory eye drops after surgery may aid in raising and maintaining pressures.[43] In their study, dexamethasone was limited to twice daily for 1–2 weeks. In patients with hypotony undergoing cataract extraction, follow-up should also be pursued more frequently than traditionally recommended. It is important to vigilantly monitor IOP, inflammation, and bleb height during follow-up. The ophthalmologist must also watch for under filtration and injurious rise of IOP, especially if the post-trabeculectomy patient had undergone successful treatment of hypotony by some other method (Table 23.4) prior to cataract extraction. Other complications related to decreased anti-inflammatory drops may occur, such as macular edema, and should be monitored for. If hypotony persists, other methods to reverse it can be employed as in the Chen series.[42]

Summary

In general, cataract extraction for hypotony has a good overall prognosis and low risk of complication when overfiltration or increased aqueous outflow is the mechanism of hypotony. It would not prohibit further intervention for the bleb postoperatively if the desired outcome was not achieved. The major complication is elevated IOP, and the IOP should be closely monitored to avoid further glaucomatous damage. The intraocular lens calculation and choice can be a challenge in eyes with hypotony. These eyes usually measure a shorter axial length, which may increase if their IOP elevates. Pre-trabeculectomy measurements should be reviewed if available and measurements of the other eye, as well as the refractive status of the contralateral eye.

References

1. Pedeson JE, Hypotony. In Tasman W, Jaeget EA, eds. *Duanes's Clinical Ophthalmology*. Baltimore: Lippincott Williams & Wilkins 2001:3. Chapter 58.
2. Nuyts RM, Felten PC, Pels E, et al. Histoplathologic effects of mitomycin C after trabeculectomy in human glaucomatous eyes with persistent hypotony. *Am J Ophthalmol*. 1994;118:225–37.

3. Vela MA, Campbell DG. Hypotony and ciliochoroidal detachment following pharmocolgic aqueous suppressant therapy in previously filtered patients. *Ophthalmology*. 1985;92:50–7.

4. Pathanapitoon K, Kunavisarut P. Choroidal detachment after topical prostaglandin analogs: case review. *J Med Assoc Thai*. 2005;88:1134–6.

5. Toris C. Pederson J. Aqueous humaor dynamics in experimental iridocyclitis. *Invest Ophthalmol Vis Sci*. 1987;28:477–81.

6. Bito LZ, Camras C, Gunn GC, Resul B. The ocular hypotensive effects and side effects of prostaglandins on the eyes of experimental animals. In: Bito LZ, Sijernschantz J, eds. *The Ocular Effects of Prostaglandins and Other Eiccosanoids*. New York: Alan R. Liss. 1989;349–68.

7. Leen MM, Mills RP. Prevention and management of hypotony after glaucoma surgery. *Int Ophthalmol Clin*. 1999;39:87–101.

8. Suner IJ, Greenfield DS, Miller MP, Nicolela MT, Palmberg PF. Hypotony maculopathy after filtering surgery with mitomycin C. Incidence and treatments. *Ophthalmology*. 1997;104:207–14.

9. Stamper RL, McMenemy MG, Lieberman MF. Hypotonous maculopathy after trabeculectomy with subconjunctival 5-fluorouracil. *Am J Ophthalmol*. 1992;114:544–53.

10. Fanin LA, Schiffman JC, Budenz DL. Rick factors for hypotony maculopathy. *Ophthalmology*. 2003;110:1185–91.

11. Solberg T, Ytrehus T, Ringvold A. Hypotony and retinal detachment. *Acta Ophthalmol*. 1986;64:26–32.

12. Ringvold A. Evidence that hypotony in retinal detachment is due to subretinal juxtapapillary fluid drainage. *Acta Ophthalmol*. 1980;58:652–8.

13. Joo SH, Ko MK, Choe JK. Outflow of aqueous humor following cyclodialysis or ciliochoroidal detachment in rabbit. *Korean J Ophthalmol*. 1989;3:65–9.

14. Pederson JE. Ocular hypotony. In: Ritch R, Shields MB, Krupin T. eds. *The Glaucomas*. Vol 3. St. Louis: Mosby 1996:385–95.

15. Fine HF, Biscette O, Chang S, Schiff WM. Ocular hypotony: a review. *Compr Ophthalmol Update*. January-February 2007;8:29–37.

16. Nicolela MT, Carrillo MM, Yan DB, Rafuse PE. Relationship between central corneal thickness and hypotony maculopathy after trabeculectomy. *Ophthalmology*. 2007;114:1266–71.

17. D'Ermo F, Bonomi L, Doro D. A critical analysis of the long term results of trabeculectomy. *Am J Ophthalmol*. 1968;66:1034–41.

18. Akato SK, Goulstine DB, Rosenthal AR. Long-term post trabeculectomy intraocular pressures. *Acta Ophthalmol*. 1992;70:312–6.

19. Tournquest G, Drolsum LK. Trabeculectomies. A long-term study. Acta Ophthalmol. 1991;69:450–4.

20. Pillai S, Mahmood MA, Limaye SR. Transient lenticular opacification following trabeculectomy. *Ophthalmic Surg*. 1988;19:508–9.

21. Lichter PR, Musch DC, Gillespie BW et al. Interim clinical outcomes in the collaborative initial glaucoma treatment study comparing initial treatment randomized to medications or surgery. *Ophthamology*. 2001;108:1943–53.

22. CNTGSG. The effectiveness of intraocular pressure reduction in the treatment of normal tension glaucoma. *Am J Ophthamol*. 1998;126:498–505.

23. Popovic V, Sjostrand J. Long-term outcome following trabeculectomy. I. Retrospective analysis of intraocular pressure regulation and cataract formation. *Acta Ophthalmol*. 1991;69:299–304.

24. Vesti E. Development of cataract after trabeculectomy. *Acta Ophthalmol*. 1993;71:777–81.

25. Sugar HS. Postoperative cataract in successfully filtering glaucomatous eyes. *Am J Ophthalmol*. 1970;69:740–6.

26. Dellaporta A. Fundus changes in postoperative hypotony. *AJO*. 1995;40:781–5.

27. Aminlari A, Callahan CE. Medical, laser and surgical management of inadvertent cyclodialysis cleft with hypotony. *Arch Ophthalmol*. 2004;122:399–404.

28. Liebman JM, Ritch R. Complications of glaucoma filtering surgery. In: Ritch R, Shields MB, Krupin T, eds. *The Glaucomas, Vol III. Glaucoma Therapy*. 2nd ed. St Louis, Missouri: Mosby; 1996:1722–3.

29. Liebmann JM, Sokol J, Ritch R. Management of chronic Hypotony after glaucoma filtration surgery. *J Glaucoma*. 1996;5(3):210–20.

30. WuDunn D, Ryser D, Cantor LB. Surgical drainage of choroidal effusions following glaucoma surgery. *J Glaucoma*. 2005;14:103–8.

31. Schwartz GF, Robin AL, Wilson RP, et al. Resuturing the scleral flap leaks to resolution of hypotony maculopathy. *J Glaucoma*. 1996;5:246–51.

32. Mayuyama K, Shirato S. Efficacy and safety of transconjunctival scleral flap resuturing for hypotony after glaucoma filtering sutgery. *Graefe's Arch Clin Exp Ophthalmol*. 2008;246:1751–6.

33. Nuyts RM, Greve EL, Geijssen HC, Langerhorst CT. Treatment of hypotonous maculopathy after trabeculectomy with mitomycin C. *Am J Ophthalmol*. 1994;118:322–31.

34. O'Connell SR, Majji AB, Humayun MS, de Juan E, Jr. The surgical management of hypotony. *Ophthalmology*. February 2000;107(2):318–23.

35. Oyakawa RT, Maumenee AE. Clear-cornea cataract extraction in eyes with functioning filtering blebs. *Am J Ophthalmol*. 1982;93:294–8.

36. Antonios SR, Traverso CE, Tomey KF. Extracapsular cataract extraction using a temporal limbal approach after filtering operations. *Arch Ophthalmol*. 1988;106:608–10.

37. Chen PP, Weaver YK, Budenz DL, Parrish RK II. Trabeculectomy function after cataract extraction. *Ophthalmology*. 1998;105:1928–35.

38. Park HJ, Kwon YH, Weitzman M, Caprioli J. Temporal corneal phacoemulsification in patients with filtered glaucoma. *Arch Ophthalmol*. 1997;115:1375–80.

39. Avasthi P, Sood AK, Prakash O. Ocular hypotony prior to cataract surgery. Int Surg. 1973;58:693–5.

40. Mackool RJ. Mature secondary cataracts and reversible ocular hypotension. *Ophthalmic Surg*. 1980;11(4):256–8.

41. Sibayan SA, Igarashi S, Kasahara N, et al. Cataract extraction as a means of treating postfiltration hypotony maculopathy. *Ophthalmic Surg Lasers*. 1997;28(3):241–3.

42. Chen PP, Budenz DL, Parrish RK, 2nd. Cataract extraction and hypotony after trabeculectomy. *Arch Ophthalmol*. 2001;119:783.

43. Doyle JW, Smith MF. Effect of phacoemulsification surgery on hypotony following trabeculectomy surgery. *Arch Ophthalmol*. 2000;118(6):763–5.

44. Budenz D, Schwartz K, Gedde SJ. Occult hypotony maculopathy diagnosed with optical coherence tomography. *Arch Ophthalmol*. 2005;123:113–4.

45. Cashwell LF, Martin CA. Axial length decrease accompanying successful glaucoma filtration surgery. *Ophthalmology*. 1999;106:302–8.

46. Brown SVL. Discussion of the article by Cashwell and Martin: axial length decrease accompanying successful glaucoma filtration surgery. *Ophthalmology*. 1999;106:2311.

47. Tan, H, Wu S. Refractive error with optimum intraocular lens power calculation after glaucoma filtering surgery. *J Catract Refract Surg*. 2004;30:2595–7.

48. Serpa JE, Wishart PK. Comparison of PMMA, foldable silicone and foldable acrylic hydrophobic intraocular lenses in combined phacoemulsification and trabeculectomy. *Arq Bras Oftalmol*. 2005;68:29–35.

Appendix: Index of Major Figures and Tables

Clinical Figures and Tables

Fig. 1.1 Bullous keratopathy showing irregular ocular surface and stromal edema

Fig. 1.2 Iridocorneal (ICE) Syndrome showing polycoria, corectopia, ectropian uveae, iris nodules, and iris stromal atrophy

Fig. 1.3 Keratic precipitates in uveitic glaucoma

Fig. 1.4 (a) Gonioscopic view of superior angle pre-cataract extraction in angle closure glaucoma. **(b)** Gonioscopic view of superior angle post-cataract extraction in angle closure glaucoma

Fig. 1.5 Gonioscopic view showing peripheral anterior synechiae following cataract extraction

Fig. 1.6 (a) Retroillumination of the iris demonstrating transillumination defects in pigment dispersion syndrome. **(b)** Gonioscopic view of increased pigmentation of the posterior trabecular meshwork in pigment dispersion syndrome

Fig. 1.7 Pseudoexfoliation (PXF) syndrome with material deposited on anterior lens capsule and pupil margin

Fig. 1.8 Shunt vessels at the disc following branch retinal vein occlusion

Fig. 1.9 Disc hemorrhage at 7 o'clock at the disc rim

Fig. 1.10 Ultrasound of eye filled with silicone oil. The silicone oil artifactually "elongates" the axial length of the globe

Fig. 1.11 Silicone oil droplets in anterior chamber of aphakic eye

Fig. 1.12 (a) Humphrey Field Analysis (Central 24.2) demonstrating glaucomatous field loss in the presence of dense nuclear sclerosis. **(b)** Humphrey Field Analysis (Central 24.2) demonstrating improvement in MD and to a lesser extent the PSD following cataract surgery

Fig. 1.13 (a) Narrowing of the anterior chamber pre-cataract surgery. **(b)** Widening of the anterior chamber post-cataract surgery

Fig. 1.14 (a) Anomalous cupping at the disc in a healthy patient. **(b)** OCT scan confirming normal nerve fiber layer

Fig. 1.15 (a) Visante anterior segment image of angle-closure glaucoma demonstrating closing of angle and shallow anterior chamber. **(b)** Visante anterior segment image of angle-closure glaucoma demonstrating angle opening following cataract removal

Fig. 2.1 A drop of topical anesthetic (proparacaine) is instilled in the eye

Fig. 2.2 Xylocaine (lidocaine) 2% Jelly (Astra Zeneca) is placed in the eye in the preoperative area and allowed to remain in place for about 5 minutes before the patient is prepped and draped in the operating room

Fig. 2.3 (a) 1% non-preserved lidocaine (Xylocaine) is **(b)** introduced into the anterior chamber via a paracentesis with a 27-gauge cannula

Fig. 3.1 Eye with small pupil, chronic angle closure, and posterior synechiae

Fig. 3.2 (b) bimanual iris stretching technique, using Kuglen hooks

Fig. 3.4 (a) Iris retractors in place

Fig. 4.1 Aqueous vein (70 long) with various degrees of compression against Schlemm's canal (SC) external wall (EW) by trabecular meshwork (TM) at IOP of 25 mmHg. *White arrows* designate areas of compression. Minimal compression **(a,b)**. Marked compression with lumen closure **(c,d)**

Fig. 4.2 In vivo composite image showing a 49-year-old (*left*) and a 25-year-old (*right*); lens growth displaces the uveal tract anteriorly with age

Fig. 4.3 In vivo composite image showing both eyes of a 74-year-old patient with a monocular implantation of the

S.M. Johnson (ed.), *Cataract Surgery in the Glaucoma Patient*, DOI 10.1007/978-0-387-09408-3,
© Springer Science+Business Media, LLC 2009

Alcon Acrysof; the uveal tract returns to an anterioposterior position of relative youth with IOL implantation

Fig. 4.4 These slit lamp photos are from the same patient. (**a**) Shows the anterior chamber preoperatively; (**b**) shows the deeper anterior chamber post-cataract surgery. The patient also reduced topical glaucoma medications

Fig. 6.1 Fundus photo demonstrating a disc with advanced glaucomatous damage

Fig. 6.2 (**a**) Visual field grayscale image of a left eye with a dense inferior nasal step and field loss superior near fixation. (**b**) A 10 degree visual field demonstrating advanced visual field loss

Fig. 6.3 Retinal nerve fiber (RNFL) assessment by ocular coherence tomorgraphy (Zeiss Meditec, Dublin, CA). Note the decreased RNFL in one eye versus the other consistent with a more advanced glaucoma status

Fig. 6.14 (**a**) Slit lamp photograph of a diffuse bleb following a combined procedure. At 1 year of follow-up, IOP remained 10–12 mmHg without medications. (**b**) Close-up of the low lying bleb. (**c**) Fundus photo of the disc of the patient

Fig. 8.4 A diffuse bleb that is neither avascular nor focal

Fig. 9.1 Slit-lamp photo of a failing bleb with increased vascularity

Fig. 9.2 Slit-lamp photo of a normal healthy bleb

Fig. 9.3 Slit-lamp photo of an encysted bleb. Note the tense surface

Fig. 11.1 A slit lamp photograph of an eye 1 day following a combined AGV and a cataract surgery with PC IOL. Note the well-formed anterior chamber with no bleeding due to retained viscoelastic. The AGV tube is behind the iris and over the PC IOL

Fig. 11.2 Slit lamp photo of a patient with uveitis who underwent implantation of an AGV, lysis of posterior synechiae, superior scleral tunnel cataract extraction by phacoemulsification with implantation of PC IOL, and peripheral iridectomy due to the granulomatous nature of her disease. A capsulotomy was done several months postoperatively

Fig. 11.8 The final appearance of the eye after cataract surgery and before implantation of a GDD

Fig. 11.10 A 7-0 Vicryl suture is placed through the 12 o'clock limbus to help position the eye inferiorly and obtain adequate exposure of the superior conjunctiva

Fig. 12.1 B-scan ultrasound image that illustrates suprachoroidal hemorrhage with clot contraction and liquefaction

Fig. 12.3 (**a, b**) These fundus photographs illustrate the near resolution of a low-lying serous choroidal effusion

Fig. 12.4 This fundus photograph shows resolving hemorrhagic choroidal detachment. Note the wrinkling of the retina on the domed surface

Fig. 12.5 Illustration of a choroidal tap. The conjunctiva has been opened 5 mm from the limbus in the quadrant. A blade is being used to scratch down through the sclera to the level of the suprachoroidal space to allow exit of the fluid

Fig. 13.4 Treated ciliary processes

Fig. 14.3 The conjunctival peritomy. Note the anterior tag of conjunctiva at the limbus left behind to facilitate closure at the conclusion of the case

Fig. 14.5 Under the scleral flap, the white hue of the scleral spur is visible in between corneal tissue anteriorly and the sclera posteriorly

Fig. 14.9 The sutures placed into the scleral flap and surgical sponges evaluating flow out of the site. Note that the Ex-PRESS shunt footplate can be seen through the scleral flap as well as in the anterior chamber

Fig. 14.10 The conjunctiva is closed with 10-0 Vicryl in a running horizontal mattress suture and a slipknot at the end to ensure watertight closure

Fig. 14.13 An anterior segment OCT image of the canal, which is distended and expanded by the presence of the intra-canalicular suture

Fig. 14.17 The trabeculodescemet window is fashioned. A slow percolation of aqueous humor through Descemet's membrane is commonly seen. In this figure, pigmentation is visible centrally where the inner wall of Schlemm's canal and trabecular meshwork remain

Fig. 14.24 In this case, a perforation of the fine trabeculodescemet window occurred during the dissection of the deep scleral flap. A separate entry is made into the anterior chamber through the deep flap (which is not excised) and an Ex-PRESS shunt inserted. Here the footplate can be seen through the deep scleral flap as well as in the anterior chamber

Fig. 14.28 A gonioscopic view of the iStent approaching the angle mounted on the injector shaft

Fig. 14.29 The iStent seen engaging the trabecular meshwork during insertion

Fig. 14.30 The iStent is released from the injector once it is seated in the canal

Fig. 14.31 High magnification viewing under the microscope with a gonioprism confirms that the stent is satisfactorily seated in the canal

Fig. 14.33 The Trabectome tip incising the trabecular meshwork

Fig. 14.34 After incision into the canal, reflux of heme is commonly seen

Fig. 14.35 The trabectome actively ablating trabecular tissue and inner wall of Schlemm's canal

Fig. 15.1 A slit lamp photo of a dilated pupil revealing the lens with the zones associated with pseudoexfoliation syndrome

Table 15.1 Clinical manifestations of Pseudoexfoliation

Table 15.2 Signs of weak zonules

Fig. 16.1 A low, moderately vascular bleb in the presence of a nuclear sclerotic cataract and pseudoexfoliation syndrome

Fig. 16.2 The blue haptic of a three-piece IOL prolapsing through a surgical peripheral iridectomy

Fig. 18.1 Chronic angle-closure glaucoma eye with cataract showing a distorted pupil due to iris atrophy, posterior synechiae

Fig. 18.2 Chronic angle-closure glaucoma eye with cataract showing extensive posterior synechiae with a small pupil

Fig. 18.3 Chronic angle-closure glaucoma eye with cataract that has undergone trabeculectomy showing the presence of a cystic bleb in the superior quadrant

Fig. 18.4 Small pupil before the use of iris hooks

Fig. 18.5 The use of iris hooks to enlarge the pupil and capsule stain during phacoemulsification

Fig. 18.7 Ultrasound biomicroscope (UBM) image of the angle before goniosynechialysis

Fig. 18.8 Ultrasound biomicroscope (UBM) image of the angle after goniosynechialysis

Fig. 19.2 Pentacam images of the anterior chamber of nanophthalmic eye (**a**) before and (**b**) after cataract surgery

Fig. 19.7 Nanophthalmic patient presented with shallow anterior chamber (**a**) on the third postoperative day. The IOP was 43, the bleb was flat, and no choroidal detachment was noted on ocular ultrasonography. The patient was diagnosed with malignant glaucoma and was submitted to pars plana vitrectomy due to unresponsiveness to clinical treatment

Fig. 20.1 Elderly female with a history of light perception and mature cataract in this eye presented with pain and an intraocular pressure of 69 mmHg. Slit lamp exam revealed a morgagnian cataract. There appears to be aggregation of macrophages and/or lens proteins on the anterior surface of the lens (*arrow*)

Fig. 20.3 Intralenticular pressure and shallow anterior chamber are two of the challenges in cataract extraction for phacomorphic glaucoma

Fig. 20.4 Elderly patient with a dense cataract and a picture of angle closure who waited a week to present. There was no effect from an iridotomy and the patient underwent ECCE, due to the corneal edema and very shallow anterior chamber. The glaucoma stabilized but vision remained poor

Fig. 21.1 Uveitis-glaucoma-hyphema syndrome in an 83-year-old Caucasian man 4 years after extracapsular cataract extraction with insertion of a Binkhorst iris-clip design anterior chamber intraocular lens

Fig. 21.4 Secondary pigmentary glaucoma in a 51-year-old Caucasian man 3 years after uncomplicated phacoemulsification and insertion of a one-piece intraocular lens in the sulcus. He had intervening pneumatic retinopexy and retinal surgery. Note the iris transillumination defect over the haptic nasally

Fig. 21.5 Slit lamp photos of a patient with PDG secondary to a piggy back IOL over an Alcon Restore IOL (Fort Worth, TX). (**a**) Note the decentration of the IOL and the TIDs at the pupillary margin. (**b**) Note the pigment deposition on the IOL at the area of the pupillary margin seen when the pupil is dilated

Fig. 21.6 Slit lamp photo of an eye with PDG secondary to an Acrysof IOL in the sulcus. Note the decentration of the IOL. The glaucoma was controlled medically

Fig. 22.1 (**a**) Eye of an 8-year-old adopted child followed for suspected ROP with retinopathy with macular dragging, high myopia in this eye, and angle closure glaucoma following a dilated exam. A peripheral iridectomy was done, due to her age and nystagmus with good control of the IOP. Cataract surgery will be done when her angle further narrows, PAS develops, or elevated IOP ensues. (**b**) Note her shallow anterior chamber, despite iridectomy thought secondary to a large lens secondary to ROP

Fig. 22.2 (**a**) Slit and (**b**) fundus photo of a 23-year old patient with a history of prematurity, high myopia, shallow anterior chamber, and angle closure. Cataract surgery was pursued

Fig. 22.3 Preoperative appearance of an infant eye status post treatment for ROP to undergo cataract removal

Fig. 23.1 Thin avascular bleb after a trabeculectomy with MMC in a patient with chronic hypotony with IOP maximum of 6 mmHg and 6–9 mmHg following cataract surgery

Fig. 23.2 Image of a B-scan ultrasound demonstrating a low-lying choroidal effusion that can be associated with hypotony

Fig. 23.3 Macular striae in a patient with IOP below 7 mmHg and blurred vision following a trabeculectomy with MMC

Instructional Tables and Figures

Fig. 3.1 Eye with small pupil, chronic angle closure, and posterior synechiae

Fig. 3.2 (**a**) Kuglen iris manipulator tip. (**b**) bimanual iris stretching technique, using Kuglen hooks

Table 4.5 Mean IOP changes with iridectomies, iridotomies, or trabeculectomies

Table 4.6 Eyes with trabeculectomies before Phaco/IOL

Fig. 4.8 Pre-surgical and Final Mean IOP from other studies and the authors' P/L/S study

Fig. 4.11 IOP changes for the same glaucoma eyes at one year, and 6 through 10 years following surgery

Fig. 4.12 One year and final IOP changes for glaucoma eyes for patients (**a**) 80 years and older, (**b**) 70–79 years, (**c**) younger than 70 years

Fig. 4.13 Comparison of the benefits of phaco/IOL alone versus glaucoma drops for eyes with OHT or glaucoma

Fig. 4.14 Comparison of the benefits of phaco/IOL versus trabeculectomy for glaucoma eyes

Table 5.1 Medications to lower postoperative IOP

Table 5.2 Anterior chamber decompression

Fig. 5.1 The bevel up needle is used to depress the posterior lip of the paracentesis

Table 6.1 Disadvantages of combined surgery versus cataract surgery alone

Table 6.2 Preoperative ocular assessment

Table 6.3 Complications associated with glaucoma triple procedure with MMC

Table 6.4 Common minor procedures post trabeculectomy

Table 7.1 Methods of nucleus extraction in MSICS

Fig. 7.5 *Trypan blue* assisted continuous curvilinear capsulorhexis in a mature white cataract

Table 8.1 Moorfields eye hospital (more flow) regimen

Fig. 8.1 Graph showing anterior chamber flare following trabeculectomy alone (*black line*) and phacoemulsification (*dotted line*). Although there is a higher peak with trabeculectomy, the flare following cataract surgery persists for a much longer period despite the eye being clinically quiet

Fig. 8.3 Strategies in antimetabolite delivery and associated surgical techniques that increase safety and improve bleb appearance dramatically

Table 9.1 Risk factors for bleb failure

Table 9.2 Secondary glaucomas

Table 9.3 The most common complications for trabeculectomy in the TVT

Table 9.4 Clinical signs suggesting a high likelihood of bleb failure

Table 9.5 Causes of sclerostomy obstruction

Table 9.6 Bleb evaluation in the immediate postoperative period

Table 9.7 Bleb needling

Fig. 9.4 Slit lamp photo of a bleb painted with fluorescein (Siedel test), which demonstrates an area of aqueous dilution corresponding with a bleb leak

Fig. 9.5 Digital massage throughout the lower lid to push aqueous up through a scarring scleral flap

Fig. 9.6 Carlos traverso maneuver. The cotton tip applicator soaked in topical anesthetic is used to depress the edge of the scleral flap to encourage flow. This is done with topical anesthetic drops administered beforehand

Fig. 9.7 Bleb needling. In (**a**) the needle enters the conjunctiva away from the bleb. (**b**) The needle is used to lyse adhesions restricting bleb formation

Table 10.1 Lenses for laser suture lysis

Table 11.1 Indications for glaucoma tube implant

Table 12.1 Clinical settings in which choroidal detachment may occur

Table 12.2 Risk factors for SCH

Table 12.3 Prophylactic measures to avoid choroidal effusions

Table 12.4 Consequences of prolonged absence of the anterior chamber

Table 13.1 Tips for ECP success

Table 14.1 Short- and long-term risks of traditional filtration surgery

Table 14.2 Possible complications unique to tube shunts

Fig. 14.12 A graph indicating the increase in trans-inner wall flow of aqueous humor when a suture in Schlemm's canal is placed on tension

Fig. 14.44 The current treatment landscape in glaucoma with IOP lowering plotted versus risk to the patient

Table 16.1 Intracameral tissue plasminogen activator (TPA) for anterior chamber fibrinolysis (off-label use)

Table 16.2 Visualizing anterior chamber vitreous

Table 16.3 Steroids for post-surgical inflammation control

Table 16.4 Summary of reports on the effect of cataract removal on IOP

Fig. 16.3 *Ab interno* bleb revision. (**a**) A goniolens can be used intraoperatively to view the sclerostomy. (**b**) A cyclo-dialysis spatula or iris sweep can be used to probe the sclerectomy and raise the scleral flap from an internal approach

Fig. 16.4 *Ab externo* bleb revision. A 25- or 27-gauge needle enters under the conjunctiva about 5 mm from the avascular bleb and lyses subconjunctival adhesions with small sweeping motions

Table 17.1 MMC before bleb revision (off-label use)

Table 19.1 Features of nanophthalmos

Table 19.2 Posterior segment findings in nanophthalmos

Table 19.3 Complications associated with nanophthalmos

Fig. 19.1 The mechanism of uveal effusion in nanophthalmous described by Gass. (**a**) Normal eye with focal vascular leak. (**b**) Aphakic eye with transient postoperative ciliochoroidal detachment that usually resolves spontaneously within days. (**c**) Uveal effusion syndrome with increased resistance to protein outflow and uveal venous outflow caused by abnormally thick sclera

Fig. 19.3 Scleral decompression technique modified from Brockhurst

Fig. 19.4 Scleral decompression technique described by Gass

Fig. 19.5 Scleral decompression as described by Jin and Anderson

Fig. 19.6 Diagram of the differential diagnosis of complications following phacotrabeculectomy in nanophthalmos

Table 20.1 Types of lens-related glaucoma

Table 20.2 Differential diagnosis of acute IOP elevation

Table 20.3 Diagnostic evaluation of phacolytic glaucoma

Table 20.4 Mannitol

Table 20.5 Use of trypan blue

Fig. 20.2 Elderly patient with an eye with a patent iridotomy that developed angle closure. The patient presented the same day and the glaucoma was stabilized with gonioplasty and medications prior to phaco/IOL. The vision improved to 20/20 and glaucoma medications were greatly reduced. This case illustrates the overlap of classic phacomorphic glaucoma and angle closure relieved with cataract surgery

Table 21.1 Differential diagnosis of increased intraocular pressure following cataract surgery based on time of onset

Table 21.2 Differential diagnosis of increased intraocular pressure following cataract surgery based on status of anterior chamber angle

Table 22.1 Staging of ROP using the international classification

Table 22.2 Cicatricial phase of ROP

Table 22.3 Non-retinal sequelae to ROP

Fig. 22.1 Stage V ROP

Table 23.1 Causes of hypotony

Table 23.2 Diagnostic evaluation of hypotony

Table 23.3 Ocular complications of hypotony

Table 23.4 Treatment options for hypotony

Instruments

Fig. 2.4 (**a**) Steven's sub-Tenon cannula. (**b**) A close-up of the tip

Fig. 2.5 E4999 Connor Anesthesia Cannula

Fig. 3.2 (**a**) Kuglen iris manipulator tip

Fig. 3.3 Beehler pupil dilator device

Fig. 3.4 (**b**) The appearance of iris retractors

Fig. 3.5 (**a**) Morcher 5S pupil dilator (**b**) Geuder pupil dilator injector

Fig. 3.6 (**a**) Graether 2000 pupil expander and (**b**) injector

Fig. 3.7 (**a**) Perfect pupil device and (**b**) injector

Fig. 3.8 (**a**) Malyugin ring and (**b**) inserted ring

Fig. 6.4 Conjunctival forceps designed not to tear the delicate conjunctival tissue. (**a**) Duckworth and Kent DK 2-100 forceps. (**b**) Fechtner K5-1820 conjunctival forceps (**c**) close-up of Fechtner forceps

Fig. 6.10 (**a**) Kelly Descemet's Punch. (**b**) The punch is used to create the sclerostomy

Fig. 6.13 Storz EO390 Tooke knife

Fig. 8.2 (**a**) T Clamp made by Duckworth-and-Kent. (**b**) T-clamp No 2-686

Fig. 8.5 Sutures being adjusted through the conjunctiva with specialized forceps to ensure gradual lowering of intraocular pressure after antimetabolite use

Fig. 10.1 Hoskins lens

Fig. 10.2 Ritch lens

Fig. 10.3 The view of a 10-0 nylon suture after placement of a Hoskins lens

Fig. 11.3 Collar button manipulator, which is useful for lysis of posterior synechiae and pupil stretching

Fig. 11.12 Ahmed glaucoma valve is primed with balanced salt solution (BSS) with a 27-gauge cannula

Fig. 11.15 Baerveldt glaucoma implants (BGI). (**a**) Baerveldt 250 (**b**) Baerveldt 350

Fig. 13.1 ECP probe

Fig. 13.2 ECP console

Fig. 13.3 ECP surgical set-up

Fig. 14.1 Schematic diagram of the Ex-PRESS shunt models and their specifications

Fig. 14.8 The handle of the Ex-PRESS shunt injector revealing the central metal wire that will be displaced upon compression of the surgeon's index finger on the plastic bridge

Fig. 14.11 A schematic diagram of the microcatheter used to cannulate Schlemm's canal. The catheter consists of a bulbous atraumatic tip, a true lumen, a central support wire to add rigidity to the catheter, and an optical fiber to transmit light to the tip

Fig. 14.26 Photograph of the Glaukos iStent

Fig. 14.27 A blunt 27-gauge cannula is used to stroke the iris gently with the injection of a very small amount of acetylcholine to induce miosis in the area of angle surgery

Fig. 14.32 A schematic diagram of the Trabectome handpiece and tip

Fig. 14.36 A photograph of the SOLX gold microshunt

Fig. 14.37 A schematic diagram of the interior of the shunt with the two plates separated

Fig. 14.40 The gold microshunt is handled with care at the wings posteriorly with a non-toothed forceps

Fig. 15.2 Hooks designed to stabilize the capsule. (**a, b**) Mackool Cataract Support System MH-105

Fig. 15.3 Photo of a Morscher MR 1400 capsular tension ring

Fig. 15.4 Modified capsular tension rings: Cionni rings (**a**) MRiL (**b**) M2L

Fig. 18.5 The use of iris hooks to enlarge the pupil and capsule stain during phacoemulsification

Table 19.4 Surgical instruments typically used during phacotrabeculectomy

Fig. 21.2 Soft IOLs can be cut with special scissors such as (**a**) the Katena soft IOL cutter (**b**) shown cutting a lens. (**c**) and the Storz ET-1306 Osher IOL scissors

Fig. 21.3 Packer-Change 19G IOL cutter

Index

A

ACA, *see* Anterior chamber angle
AccuMap severity index, 6
ACD, *see* Anterior chamber depth
Acetazolamide, for IOP treatment, 52
ACG, *see* Angle-closure glaucoma
ACIOL, *see* Anterior chamber intraocular lens
ACP, *see* Anterior capsular phimosis
Advanced Glaucoma Intervention Study, 67, 91
Advanced glaucomatous optic nerve atrophy, therapy, 10
AGIS, *see* Advanced Glaucoma Intervention Study
AGV, *see* Ahmed glaucoma valve
Ahmed glaucoma valve, 109, 112–113
American Society of Cataract and Refractive Surgery, 21
Anesthesia, in glaucoma patients
    current status, 21
    general anesthesia, 20–21
    monitoring, 20
    preoperative assessment and preparation, 17
    retrobulbar and peribulbar techniques, 20
    sub-Tenon's anesthesia, 18–19
    topical ocular anesthesia, 17–18
    See also Glaucoma patients, cataract surgery
Angle closure
    cataract surgery challenges, 189
    mechanisms, 189
        See also Primary angle-closure glaucoma
Angle-closure glaucoma, 8, 41, 198
    and ROP, 221
        See also Retinopathy of prematurity
Anterior capsular phimosis, 172
Anterior chamber angle, 8
Anterior chamber depth, 8
Anterior chamber intraocular lens, 179, 215
Anterior segment, imaging technologies, 8
Anterior segment optical coherence tomography, 143
Antimetabolite trabeculectomy and cataract extraction
    complications, 88–89
    instrumentation, 85
    operative techniques, 85–87
    postoperative care, 87
    for surgery, 83–85
    surgical outcomes, 87–88
    See also Cataract extraction, glaucoma devices
Anti-vascular endothelial growth factor (Anti-VEGF), 181
Aqueous misdirection glaucoma, surgical approach, 14
Ascorbic acid, role, 162
ASCRS, *see* American Society of Cataract and Refractive Surgery
ASI, *see* AccuMap severity index
AS-OCT, *see* Anterior segment optical coherence tomography
Atropine drug, application, 204

B

Baerveldt glaucoma implant, 109, 113–114
Balanced saline solution, 64, 77, 137, 170, 179
BCVA, *see* Best corrected visual acuity
Beehler pupil dilator device, usage, 28
Best corrected visual acuity, 198
BGI, *see* Baerveldt glaucoma implant
Bimanual technique, for pupil expansion, 28–29
Bleb failure
    identification, 94–96
    management, 96–99
    prevention
        antimetabolites in, 93
        postoperative regimen, 94
        surgical techniques, 93–94
    risk factors, 91–93
    See also Glaucoma patients, cataract surgery
Brinzolamide, for IOP treatment, 53
BSS, *see* Balanced saline solution

C

CACG, *see* Chronic angle-closure glaucoma
Canaloplasty, role, 142
Capsular tension ring, 166
Capsule contraction syndrome, 171

Capsulorhexis, in white intumescent cataract, 211
    See also Cataract induced glaucoma
Capsulorrhexis (CCC), 165
Capsulotomy, in cataract and glaucoma management, 76
Cataract and glaucoma management, MSICS-Trab in
    cataract surgery
        capsulotomy, 76
        conjunctival flap and scleral dissection, 74–76
        epinucleus removal, cortex aspiration, and IOL
            implantation, 80
        hydrodissection, 76–77
        nucleus extraction, 78–80
        nucleus prolapse into anterior chamber, 77–78
        surgical outcomes, 82
        trabeculectomy, 80–82
    methodology for, 74
Cataract extraction and GDD implantation
    outcomes, 187
    surgical technique in, 187
Cataract extraction, glaucoma devices, 135–136
    Ex-PRESS shunt
        data related to combined surgery, 140–141
        indications for surgery, 136–137
        instrumentation and operative technique, 137–139
        postoperative concern and complications, 139–140
    non-penetrating schlemm's canaloplasty
        indications for surgery, 141–142
        instrumentation and operative technique, 142–146
        outcomes, 147–148
        postoperative concern and complications, 146–147
    suprachoroidal goldmicro-shunt
        indications for surgery, 153–154
        instrumentation and operative technique, 154–156
        postoperative concerns and complications, 156
    trabecular micro-bypass stent
        indications for surgery, 148–149
        instrumentation and operative technique, 149–150
        postoperative care and complications, 151
    trabecular micro-electrocautery
        indications for surgery, 151–152
        instrumentation and operative surgery, 152
        postoperative concerns and complications, 152–153
Cataract induced glaucoma
    phacolytic glaucoma
        clinical presentation, 208
        complications, 210
        management, 208–209
        operative technique, 209
        outcomes, 210
        pathogenesis, 207–208
        postoperative care, 209
        preoperative care, 209
    phacomorphic glaucoma

        clinical features, 210
        operative techniques, 210–211
        outcomes, 211–212
Cataract-induced visual loss, 3
Cataract, in ROP, 223–224
    operative techniques, 224–225
    outcomes, 225
    See also Retinopathy of prematurity
Cataract surgery
    in hypotonous eye, 229–230
        clinical manifestations, 228–229
        complications, 231
        management, 229
        operative technique, 230–231
        pathophysiology, 227–228
        postoperative care, 231
        preoperative care, 230
    IOP diagnosis in, 214
    in nanophthalmos, 203
        See also Nanophthalmos
    trabeculectomy bleb in
        complications, 182
        indications for surgery, 177–178
        instrumentation and operative techniques, 178–181
        outcomes, 181–182
        postoperative care, 181
Cataract surgery, in glaucoma patients
    antimetabolite trabeculectomy and cataract extraction
        complications, 88–89
        instrumentation, 85
        operative techniques, 85–87
        postoperative care, 87
        for surgery, 83–85
        surgical outcomes, 87–88
    clinical history, 3
    consent process for, 8–10
    in developing countries, MSICS-Trab in, 73–74
    effect on IOP and anatomy, 37
    examination
        anterior segment imaging, 8
        field analysis, 5–6
        nerve fiber layer imaging, 8
        specular microscopy, 7–8
        ultrasonic biometry, 6–7
    glaucoma drainage devices
        indications for surgery, 109
        operative techniques, 109–114
        postoperative care, 114–116
        surgical outcomes, 116–117
    intraocular pressure elevation after, 51
        clinical presentation, 52
        etiology, 51
        in glaucoma, 52

guidelines, 54
medical treatment, 52–54
OVDs role in, 51–52
local anesthesia
general anesthesia, 20–21
monitoring, 20
preoperative assessment and preparation, 17
present status, 21
retrobulbar and peribulbar techniques, 20
sub-Tenon's anesthesia, 18–19
topical ocular anesthesia, 17–18
preoperative assessment, 10–11
cornea, 3–4
gonioscopic assessment, 4
optic nerve rim thinning, 4–5
silicone oil retinal tamponade, 5
surgical approach
for cataract, 11–12
combined surgery, 13–14
drainage surgery, 12–13
for glaucoma and cataract, 12
and trabeculectomy surgery, 59–61
approach, 63–64
disadvantages, 62
presurgical assessment, 59–61
surgical outcomes, 67–70
techniques, 64–67
Cataract surgery and XFS
clinical implications of, 161–163
complications in eyes with
ACP, 172
CCS, 171
combined cataract and glaucoma surgery in, 172
corneal changes in, 170
ECCE, 168
intraoperative complications in, 168–170
IOL, 171
PCO, 172
postoperative care and complications, 173
postoperative complications, 170–171
preoperative evaluation, 168
surgical techniques in, 172–173
intraocular pressure changes, 163–164
operative techniques in eyes
management of zonular weakness in, 166–167
preoperative examination, 164
small pupil management, 164–165
zonular weakness in, 165–166
Cataract, surgical procedures, 11–12
Cataract treatment
complications, 133
indications for surgery, 129–130
instrumentation, 130–131

operative technique, 131–132
outcomes, 132–133
postoperative care, 132
CCC, see Continuous curvilinear capsulorhexis
CCS, see Capsule contraction syndrome
Central retinal apposition, 125–126
Choroidal detachment
definition, 119
medical management, 122–123
outcomes, 126
serous, 119–120
SCH, 120–121
ultrasound in SCH, 121–122
surgical management of, 124–126
Choroidal tap, procedure, 124
Chronic angle-closure glaucoma, 41, 189
CIGITS, see Collaborative Initial Glaucoma Treatment
Study
Clot lysis time, for suprachoroidal hemorrhage, 126
CME, see Cystoid macular edema
Collaborative Initial Glaucoma Treatment Study, 67, 94
Collaborative Initial Glaucoma Treatment Trial, 6
Conjunctival flap and scleral dissection, in cataract surgery,
74–76
Continuous curvilinear capsulorhexis, 76, 209
Corneal changes, in XFS, 170
See also Exfoliation syndrome
Cortical cataract and glaucoma, difference, 3
Corticosteroids, role, 223
See also Retinopathy of prematurity
Corticosteroids, usage, 181
CTR, see Capsular tension ring
Cyclophotocoagulation and phacoemulsification, in
glaucoma and cataract surgery, 13
Cycloplegia, in ciliary block glaucoma treatment, 223
Cystoid macular edema, 33

D
Decision tree for phaco/IOL, for OHT treatment, 45–46
Dexamethasone drug, application, 122–123
Dispersive viscoelastics, for cataract surgery, 28
Dorzolamide, for IOP treatment, 53

E
ECCE, see Extracapsular cataract extraction
ECCE-trabeculectomy, 203–204
Echothiophate, application, 21
ECP, see Endoscopic cyclophotocoagulation
Endoscopic cyclophotocoagulation, 129
advantages, 132
cataract extraction, 130
ciliary processes and, 131
outcomes, 132–133

Endoscopic cyclophotocoagulation (*cont.*)
    phacoemulsification and intraocular lens implantation
            with, 133
    postoperative management, 132
    tips for, 132
Exfoliation syndrome, 161
    cataract surgery for eyes with
        ACP, 172
        CCS, 171
        combined cataract and glaucoma surgery, 172
        corneal changes, 170
        ECCE, 168
        intraoperative complications, 168–170
        IOL, 171
        PCO, 172
        postoperative care and complications, 173
        postoperative complications, 170–171
        preoperative evaluation, 168
        surgical techniques, 172–173
    clinical implications, 161–163
    intraocular pressure changes, 163–164
    operative techniques
        management of zonular weakness in, 166–167
        preoperative examination, 164
        small pupil management in, 164–165
        zonular weakness in, 165–166
    pathophysiology, 161
Exfoliative glaucoma, 161, 172
Ex-PRESS mini glaucoma shunt, in cataract extraction
    data related to combined surgery, 140–141
    indications for surgery, 136–137
    instrumentation and operative technique, 137–139
    postoperative concern and complications, 139–140
    See also Cataract extraction, glaucoma devices
Extracapsular cataract extraction, 59, 74, 168, 181, 202, 210
Extracapsular extraction technique, in phacolytic glaucoma,
        209

F
FFSS, *see* Fluorouracil Filtering Surgery Study
Fish hook technique, for cataract surgery, 80
5-Fluorouracil, 12, 86
Fluorouracil Filtering Surgery Study, 91
Fornix-based flaps, advantage, 94
5-FU, *see* 5-fluorouracil

G
Gauge vitrectomy, in cataract surgery, 211
    See also Cataract induced glaucoma
GDD, *see* Glaucoma drainage device
Glaucoma and cataract patients, surgical approach for, 12
Glaucoma devices, in cataract extraction, 135–136
    Ex-PRESS shunt

        data related to combined surgery, 140–141
        indications for surgery, 136–137
        instrumentation and operative technique, 137–139
        postoperative complications, 139–140
    non-penetrating schlemm's canaloplasty
        indications for surgery, 141–142
        instrumentation and operative technique, 142–146
        outcomes, 147–148
        postoperative complications, 146–147
    suprachoroidal goldmicro-shunt
        indications for surgery, 153–154
        instrumentation and operative technique, 154–156
        postoperative complications, 156
    trabecular micro-bypass stent
        indications for surgery, 148–149
        instrumentation and operative technique, 149–150
        postoperative care and complications, 151
    trabecular micro-electrocautery
        indications for surgery, 151–152
        instrumentation and operative surgery, 152
        postoperative complications, 152–153
Glaucoma drainage device, 187
    implantation and cataract extraction
        outcomes, 187
        surgical technique, 187
    indications for surgery, 109
    operative techniques, 109–114
    postoperative care, 114–116
    surgical outcomes, 116–117
Glaucoma, in ROP, 221–222
    cause, 222
    corticosteroids, 223
    initial management, 222–223
    mechanism, 222
    See also Retinopathy of prematurity
Glaucoma medications, after cataract surgery, 37
Glaucoma patients, cataract surgery
    antimetabolite trabeculectomy and cataract extraction
        complications, 88–89
        instrumentation, 85
        operative techniques, 85–87
        postoperative care, 87
        for surgery, 83–85
        surgical outcomes, 87–88
    clinical history, 3
    consent process, 8–10
    in developing countries, MSICS-Trab in, 73–74
    effect on IOP and anatomy, 37
    examination
        anterior segment imaging, 8
        field analysis, 5–6
        nerve fiber layer imaging, 8
        specular microscopy, 7–8

ultrasonic biometry, 6–7
glaucoma drainage devices
indications for surgery, 109
operative techniques, 109–114
postoperative care, 114–116
surgical outcomes, 116–117
intraocular pressure elevation after, 51
clinical presentation, 52
etiology, 51
in glaucoma, 52
guidelines, 54
medical treatment, 52–54
OVDs role in, 51–52
local anesthesia
general anesthesia, 20–21
monitoring, 20
preoperative assessment and preparation, 17
present status, 21
retrobulbar and peribulbar techniques, 20
sub-Tenon's anesthesia, 18–19
topical ocular anesthesia, 17–18
preoperative assessment
cornea, 3–4
gonioscopic assessment, 4
optic nerve rim thinning, 4–5
silicone oil retinal tamponade, 5
preoperative preparation, 10–11
surgical approach
for cataract, 11–12
combined surgery, 13–14
drainage surgery, 12–13
for glaucoma and cataract, 12
and trabeculectomy surgery, 59–61
approach, 62–64
disadvantages, 62
presurgical assessment, 59–61
surgical outcomes, 67–70
techniques, 64–67
Glaucomatous optic neuropathy, 199, 203
Glaucoma treatment
and cataract surgery, 203
ECCE-trabeculectomy, 203–204
phacotrabeculectomy, 204
postoperative care and complications, 204–206
complications, 133
indications for surgery, 129–130
instrumentation in, 130–131
in nanophthalmic eyes, 198
See also Nanophthalmos
operative technique, 131–132
outcomes in, 132–133
postoperative care, 132
See also Cataract induced glaucoma

GON, see Glaucomatous optic neuropathy
Gonioscopic assessment, for glaucoma patients, 4
Goniosynechialysis (GSL), 194

H
Haigis formula, usage, 200
See also Nanophthalmos
Healon 5 OVDs, 52
Healon5, role, 131
Hoffer Q formula, usage, 200
See also Nanophthalmos
HPMC, see Hydroxyl propyl methyl cellulose
Human lens, developmental stages, 35
Hydrodissection, in cataract and glaucoma management, 76–77
Hydroxyl propyl methyl cellulose, 75
Hypotonous eye
cataract surgery in, 229–230
complications, 231
operative technique, 230–231
postoperative care, 231
preoperative care, 230
causes, 227
clinical manifestations, 228–229
diagnostic evaluation, 228
management, 229
ocular complications, 229
pathophysiology, 227–228
treatment options, 229
Hypotony
definition, 227
and suprachoroidal hemorrhage, 120
See also Suprachoroidal hemorrhage

I
ICC, see Intraclass correlation coefficient
ICE syndrome, see Iridocorneal endothelial syndrome
IFIS, see Intraoperative floppy iris syndrome
Indiana Bleb Appearance Grading Scale, for bleb, 95
Intracameral carbachol intraocular solution, for IOP treatment, 53
Intracameral injection of local anesthetics, role, 18
Intracameral trypan blue, role, 181
Intraclass correlation coefficient, 95
Intraocular lens, 5, 137, 171
Intraocular lens-related glaucoma, cause, 216
See also Pseudophakia and glaucoma
Intraocular pressure, 3, 19, 119, 129, 135
age effect on controling, 45
cataract removal on, 182
cataract surgery effect on, 190
corneal phacoemulsification on, 187
diagnosis of, 208, 214

Intraocular pressure (*cont.*)
   effect of cataract surgery on, 37, 43–45
   elevation after cataract surgery, 51
      clinical presentation, 52
      etiology, 51
      in glaucoma, 52
      guidelines, 54
      medical treatment, 52–54
      OVDs role, 51–52
   and microcystic edema, 209
   and phacolytic glaucoma, 208
   in phacomorphic glaucoma, 210
   reduction, 209
      laser suture lysis, 105–106
      non-glaucoma and glaucoma eyes, 37–43
      releasable suture technique, 106–107
   spikes, role, 130
   XFS, 163–164
   See also Glaucoma patients, cataract surgery;
      Trabeculectomy
Intraocular surgery and suprachoroidal hemorrhage
      development, 120
   See also Suprachoroidal hemorrhage
Intraoperative floppy iris syndrome, 24, 178
Intraoperative gonioscopy
   role, 180
   usage, 155
IOL, *see* Intraocular lens
IOP, *see* Intraocular pressure
Iridocorneal endothelial syndrome, 3, 27
Iris expansion retractors, for small pupil, 29–30
Iris prolapse, 31–33
   See also Pupil, small
Irrigating vectis technique, for cataract surgery, 78
iScience device, usage, 141
iScience microcatheter, role, 145

K

Kaplan–Meier survival curve analysis, advantage, 133
   See also Cataract treatment
Kelly's Descemet's membrane punch, usage, 80
Kissing choroidals, *see* Central retinal apposition
Kissing suprachoroidal hemorrhage, characteristics, 120

L

Laser endoscope, usage, 130
Laser suture lysis
   complications and outcomes, 106
   techniques, 105–106
   See also Trabeculectomy
Latanoprost, for IOP treatment, 53
Lensectomy, application, 223
   See also Retinopathy of prematurity

Lens-related glaucoma, types, 207
Limbus-based flaps, advantage, 94
LOXL1, *see* Lysyl oxidase-like protein 1
LSL, *see* Laser suture lysis
Lysyl oxidase-like protein 1, 161

M

Magnetic resonance imaging, 36
Mannitol, application, 209
Manual Small Incision Cataract Surgery, 74
Manual Small Incision Cataract Surgery Combined with
      Trabeculectomy
   in cataract and glaucoma management
      capsulotomy, 76
      conjunctival flap and scleral dissection, 74–76
      epinucleus removal, cortex aspiration, and IOL
         implantation, 80
      hydrodissection, 76–77
      methodology, 74
      nucleus extraction, 78–80
      surgical outcomes, 82
      trabeculectomy, 80–82
Manual technique, for pupil expansion, 28
Marfan's patients, cataract, 21
Medical management, of choroidal detachment, 122–123
   See also Choroidal detachment
Merocel, role, 144
Microincision bimanual phacotrabeculectomy, 13
Miochol®-E, role, 149
   See also Trabecular micro-bypass stent
Mitomycin-C, 83, 106, 138, 187
Mitomycin C augmented trabeculectomy, 63
MMC, *see* Mitomycin-C
Modified blumenthal technique, for cataract surgery, 79–80
Moorfields Bleb Grading System, for bleb, 95
Moorfields Florida "More Flow" regime, usage, 84
Moorfield's safe surgery technique, 65–66
MRI, *see* Magnetic resonance imaging
MSICS, *see* Manual Small Incision Cataract Surgery
MSICS-Trab, *see* Manual Small Incision Cataract Surgery
      Combined with Trabeculectomy
Myotonic dystrophy patients, cataract, 21

N

NAG, *see* Narrow angle glaucoma
Nanophthalmos
   characteristics, 197
   complications, 198
   definition, 197
   glaucoma treatment *versus* cataract surgery, 203
      ECCE-trabeculectomy, 203–204
      phacotrabeculectomy, 204
      postoperative care and complications, 204–206

indications for surgery, 198–199
IOL choice, 199–200
outcomes of cataract surgery, 203
posterior segment findings, 197
surgical technique, 202
    ECCE techniques, 202
    phacoemulsification, 202
    postoperative care, 202–203
uveal effusion, 198
uveal effusion prevention, 200–201
Narrow angle glaucoma, 40
Neodymium:YAG laser, usage, 151
    See also Trabecular micro-bypass stent
Nerve fiber layer, imaging, 8
    See also Glaucoma patients, cataract surgery
Non-penetrating schlemm's canaloplasty
    indications for surgery, 141–142
    instrumentation and operative technique, 142–146
    outcomes, 147–148
    postoperative concern and complications, 146–147
    See also Cataract extraction, glaucoma devices
Non-steroidal anti-inflammatory drops, 24
Non-steroidal anti-inflammatory drug, 168, 215
NSAIDs, *see* Non-steroidal anti-inflammatory drops;
        Non-steroidal anti-inflammatory drug

O
OAG, *see* Open angle glaucoma
OCT, *see* Optical coherence tomography
Ocular hypertensive, 38
OHT, *see* Ocular hypertensive
Open angle glaucoma, 14, 40
Ophthalmic viscosurgical devices, 51–52, 140, 193, 215,
        224
Optical coherence tomography, 8, 230
Optic nerve rim thinning, in glaucoma patients, 4–5
OVDs, *see* Ophthalmic viscosurgical devices

P
PACG, *see* Primary angle-closure glaucoma
Pachymetry, *see* Specular microscopy, for cataract
        measurement
PAM, *see* Potential acuity meters
Parasympathomimetics, effects, 23
Pars plana lensectomy, role, 211
    See also Cataract induced glaucoma
PAS, *see* Peripheral anterior synechiae; Posterior anterior
        synechiae
Pattern standard deviation, 5
PCIOL, *see* Posterior chamber intraocular lens
PCO, *see* Posterior capsular opacification
PDS/PDG, *see* Pigment dispersion syndrome and glaucoma
Peribulbar anesthesia, glaucoma patients, 20

Peripheral anterior synechiae, 147, 198, 203
Peripheral iridotomy, for glaucoma patients, 11
Peripheral laser iridotomy, 203
Phacoemulsification
    and Ahmed valve implantation, 13
    and cataract extraction, 190
    in nanophthalmos, 202
        See also Nanophthalmos
    in PACG eyes, 194–195
        See also Primary angle-closure glaucoma (PACG)
            patient, cataract surgery
    techniques, in cataracts, 209
        See also Cataract induced glaucoma
    usage, 74
Phaco/IOL *versus* glaucoma drops, advantages, 47
Phacolytic glaucoma
    clinical presentation, 208
    complications, 210
    diagnostic evaluation, 208
    management, 208–209
    operative technique, 209
    outcomes, 210
    pathogenesis in, 207–208
    post/pre-operative care, 209
Phacomorphic glaucoma, 37
    challenges in cataract extraction, 211
    clinical features, 210
    operative techniques, 210–211
    outcomes, 211–212
Phacosandwich technique, for cataract surgery, 78–79
Phacotrabeculectomy, role, 190
    See also Primary angle-closure glaucoma (PACG)
            patient, cataract surgery
Phacotrabeculectomy technique, 204
    See also Glaucoma treatment
Phacotrabeculectomy with mitomycin-C (phacotrabMMC),
        13
Pigment dispersion syndrome and glaucoma, 213
Pilocarpine drug, application, 192
Pilocarpine, effects, 23
PLI, *see* Peripheral laser iridotomy
PMMA, *see* Polymethyl methacrylate
POAG, *see* Primary open angle glaucoma
Polymethyl methacrylate, 123, 164, 179
Polyvinyl alcohol sponges, 85
Posterior anterior synechiae, 67, 211
Posterior capsular opacification, 172
Posterior chamber intraocular lens, 62–63, 203, 209, 215
Postoperative intraocular pressure spike, 193–194
    See also Primary angle-closure glaucoma (PACG)
            patient, cataract surgery
Postoperative suprachoroidal hemorrhage, definition, 120
Potential acuity meters, 177, 198

Prednisone drug, application, 123
Primary angle-closure glaucoma (PACG) patient, cataract
          surgery, 189–190
     angle structure, 190
     definition, 189
     indications for surgery, 190–191
          operative procedures, 192–193
          postoperative assessment and medications, 193
          preoperative assessment and medications,
               191–192
     IOP, 190
     phacotrabeculectomy in, 190
     postoperative complications, 193–194
          GSL role, 194
          phacoemulsification, 194–195
Primary open angle glaucoma, 8
Prophylactic measures and choroidal effusions avoidance,
          121
Protein accumulation, in lens nucleus, 207
     See also Cataract induced glaucoma
PSD, see Pattern standard deviation
Pseudoexfoliation syndrome, 26, 37
Pseudoexfoliative material, 4
Pseudophakia and glaucoma, 213–214
     pseudophakic pupillary block, 216–218
     secondary pigmentary glaucoma, 216
     UGH syndrome, 214–215
          instruments, 215
          operative techniques, 215–216
          outcomes, 216
          postoperative care, 216
          preoperative preparation, 215
Pseudophakic glaucoma, definition, 213
Pseudophakic patients and ECP, 131
Pseudophakic pupillary block, 216–218
     See also Pseudophakia and glaucoma
Pupil, small
     altered pupil, 27
     bimanual technique, 28–29
     and chronic uveitis, 26–27
     definition, 23
     etiology, 23
     expansion rings, 30–31
     intraoperative challenges in eyes with, 31–33
     intraoperative iris expansion, 28
     iris expansion retractors for, 29–30
     medication causing
          parasympathomimetics, 23
          surgical techniques, 24–25
          systemic alpha-1 blockers, 24
     with narrow angle glaucomas, 25
     with prior intraocular glaucoma surgery,
          25–26

and pseudoexfoliation syndrome, 26
     pupil expansion rings for, 30–31
     surgical planning for, 27
     surgical techniques, 27–28
     See also Glaucoma patients, cataract surgery
Pupillary block and angle closure glaucoma, 189
     See also Primary angle-closure glaucoma (PACG)
          patient, cataract surgery
PVA sponges, see Polyvinyl alcohol sponges
PXF material, see Pseudoexfoliative material
PXF syndrome, see Pseudoexfoliation syndrome

R
Randomized control trials (RCT), 88
Releasable suture technique, 106–107
     See also Trabeculectomy
Retinal nerve fiber layer, 8
Retinal perivasculitis, cause, 208
     See also Cataract induced glaucoma
Retinopathy of prematurity, 221
     cataract in, 223–224
          operative techniques, 224–225
          outcomes, 225
     cicatricial phase, 221
     glaucoma, 221–222
          initial management, 222–223
          mechanism, 222
     non-retinal sequelae, 222
     staging, 221
     surgical management, 223
Retrobulbar anesthesia
     for glaucoma patients, 20
     usage, 110
Rhegmatogenous retinal detachments, 125
RNFL, see Retinal nerve fiber layer
ROP, see Retinopathy of prematurity

S
SCH, see Suprachoroidal hemorrhage
Schlemm's canal, in glaucoma patients,
          141–142
Scleral decompression technique, 200–201
     See also Nanophthalmos
Scleral flap dissection, for Ex-PRESS shunt, 138
Scleral lake, role, 146
     See also Cataract extraction, glaucoma devices
Scleral tunnel incisions, in cataract surgery, 131
Scleratome blade, usage, 64
Secondary cataract (SC), 172
Secondary pigmentary glaucoma, 216
     See also Pseudophakia and glaucoma
Sedation, in cataract surgery, 20
Serous choroidal detachment, 119–120

Short wavelength automated perimetry, 179

Sinskey hook, usage, 77

Small incision cataract surgery and glaucoma
  pathogenesis, 35–37
  surgical technique, 37

Snuff syndrome, *see* Wipe-out, in glaucoma patients

Sodium hyaluronate, role, 131

Specular microscopy, for cataract measurement, 7–8
  See also Glaucoma patients, cataract surgery

Steroids, for post-surgical inflammation control, 181
  See also Trabeculectomy

Sub-Tenon's anesthesia, for glaucoma patients, 18–19

Suprachoroidal goldmicro-shunt, in cataract extraction
  indications for surgery, 153–154
  instrumentation and operative technique, 154–156
  postoperative concerns and complications, 156
  See also Cataract extraction, glaucoma devices

Suprachoroidal hemorrhage, 120–122

Surgical goniosynechialysis, usage, 181

Surgical management, of choroidal detachment,
  124–126
  See also Choroidal detachment

Surgical technique
  ECCE techniques, 202
  in GDD implantation and cataract extraction, 187
  in nanophthalmos, 202
  phacoemulsification, 202
  postoperative care, 202–203
  See also Cataract extraction and GDD implantation;
    Nanophthalmos

SWAP, *see* Short wavelength automated perimetry

T

TCC, *see* Temporal clear corneal

TCNR, *see* Tenon's conjunctival needle revision

TCPD, *see* Trabecular-ciliary process distance

TDW, *see* TrabeculoDescemet window

Temporal clear corneal, 178

Tenon's conjunctival needle revision, 205

Tetracaine, effects, 18

Timolol, for IOP treatment, 53

Tissue plasminogen activator, 97, 116, 178

Topical epinephrine, usage, 21

Topical ocular anesthesia, for glaucoma patients,
  17–18

TPA, *see* Tissue plasminogen activator

Trabecular aspiration (TA), 163

Trabecular-ciliary process distance, 12

Trabecular meshwork (TM) stiffening, 35

Trabecular micro-bypass stent
  indications for surgery, 148–149
  instrumentation and operative technique, 149–150
  postoperative care and complications, 151

See also Cataract extraction, glaucoma devices

Trabecular micro-electrocautery
  indications for surgery, 151–152
  instrumentation and operative surgery, 152
  postoperative concerns and complications, 152–153
  See also Cataract extraction, glaucoma devices

Trabeculectomy
  bleb, in cataract surgery
    complications, 182
    indications for surgery, 177–178
    instrumentation and operative techniques, 178–181
    outcomes, 181–182
    postoperative care, 181
  and cataract surgery
    approach, 63–64
    disadvantages, 62
    presurgical assessment, 59–61
    surgical outcomes, 67–70
    techniques for, 64–67
  in glaucoma and cataract management, 80–82
  See also Antimetabolite trabeculectomy and cataract
    extraction

Trabeculectomy with mitomycin-C, 13

TrabeculoDescemet window, 142

Trabeculoplasty, usage, 46

trabMMC, *see* Trabeculectomy with mitomycin-C

Traction retinal detachments, 125

Travoprost, for IOP treatment, 53

Trypan blue, usage, 209

Tube shunts, complications, 135

Tube *vs.* Trab study, 94

TVT study, *see* Tube *vs.* Trab study

U

UBM, *see* Ultrasound biomicroscopy

UGH syndrome, *see* Uveitis-glaucoma-hyphema

Ultrasonic biometry, for cataract measurement, 6–7
  See also Glaucoma patients, cataract surgery

Ultrasound biomicroscopy, 12, 197, 203, 217

Ultrasound, in SCH, 121–122
  See also Suprachoroidal hemorrhage

Utrata's capsule-holding forceps, usage, 80

Uveal effusion prevention, surgical procedures in,
  200–201
  See also Nanophthalmos

Uveal effusion syndrome, characteristics, 120

Uveitis and small pupil, 26–27

Uveitis-glaucoma-hyphema syndrome, 213–215
  instruments, 215
  operative techniques, 215–216
  outcomes, 216
  postoperative care, 216
  preoperative preparation, 215

V

Visante anterior segment imaging, 8, 10
Viscocanalostomy, procedure, 141
    See also Cataract extraction, glaucoma devices
Vitrectomy techniques, in choroidal detachment, 125
    See also Choroidal detachment
Vitreoretinal surgery, in suprachoroidal
        hemorrhages, 126

W

Wipe-out, in glaucoma patients, 21
Wound-healing modulators, usage, 74

X

XFG, *see* Exfoliative glaucoma
XFS, *see* Exfoliation syndrome

Y

YAG capsulotomy, usage, 217–218
    See also Pseudophakia and glaucoma
YAG laser, role, 148

Z

Zonular weakness management, in XFS, 166–167
    See also Cataract surgery and XFS